74

Psychiatry and
General Practice Today

Edited by
IAN PULLEN
GREG WILKINSON
ALASTAIR WRIGHT
DENIS PEREIRA GRAY

Psychiatry and General Practice Today

THE ROYAL COLLEGE OF PSYCHIATRISTS &
THE ROYAL COLLEGE OF GENERAL PRACTITIONERS

British Library Cataloguing-in-Publication Data
Psychiatry and General Practice Today
I. Pullen, Ian M.
616.89

ISBN 0-902241-50-8

Distributed in North America
by American Psychiatric Press, Inc.
ISBN 0-880486-15-5

Phototypeset by Dobbie Typesetting Limited, Tavistock, Devon
Printed in Great Britain by Bell and Bain Ltd, Glasgow

Contents

List of contributors   vii
Foreword   ix
Editors' preface   xi
The legislative framework today   xiii

Part I. The context

1 General practice and psychiatry – a general practice perspective
   Denis Pereira Gray   3
2 Psychiatry and general practice – a psychiatric perspective
   Geraldine Strathdee   22
3 Epidemiology of mental disorder in general practice
   David Goldberg   36
4 Law and ethics   *Derek Chiswick*   45

Part II. Clinical problems

5 Loss, grief and psychosocial transitions
   Colin Murray Parkes   63
6 Family and marital relationships   *Denis Pereira Gray*   77
7 Depression   *Alastair Wright*   93
8 Anxiety   *Lynne M. Drummond*   112
9 Alcohol problems   *James Dunbar*   135
10 Older people   *Idris Williams*   153
11 Emergencies, crises and violence   *Richard Westcott*   170
12 Personality problems   *Peter Tyrer*   180
13 Schizophrenia   *Tom Burns and Tony Kendrick*   194
14 Drug abuse   *Judy Greenwood*   209

v

15 Sleep problems   *Ian Pullen and Greg Wilkinson*   221
16 Benzodiazepines in general practice
   Kieran Sweeney and Margaret Cormack   235

Part III. Psychosocial management

17 Communication between general practitioners and
   psychiatrists   *Michael King and Ian Pullen*   251
18 Teamwork in the community
   Tony Kendrick, André Tylee and Tom Burns   265
19 Counselling and psychotherapy   *Michael Sheldon*   280
20 Cognitive behaviour therapy   *Janine Scott*   294
21 The prevention of mental illness in primary care
   Denis Pereira Gray, Alastair Wright, Greg Wilkinson,
   Rachel Jenkins and Keith Lloyd   311

Part IV. Training and research

22 Training for general practitioners in psychiatry
   Linda Gask   337
23 Training for psychiatrists in general practice
   Tom Burns   350
24 Research potential in general practice
   Greg Wilkinson and Alastair Wright   360

Index   *Compiled by John Gibson*   371

Contributors

Tom Burns, MD, FRCPsych, Professor of Community Psychiatry, St George's Hospital Medical School, Cranmer Terrace, London SW17 0RE

Derek Chiswick, MPhil, FRCPsych, Consultant Forensic Psychiatrist, Royal Edinburgh Hospital, Morningside Park, Edinburgh EH10 5HF

Margaret Cormack, MA, MPsychol, PhD, Director, Wessex Regional Training Course in Clinical Psychology, Knowle Hospital, Fareham, Hants PO17 5NA

Lynne M. Drummond, MRCP, MRCPsych, Senior Lecturer, Department of Mental Health Sciences, St George's Hospital Medical School, Cranmer Terrace, London SW17 0RE

James Dunbar, TD, MD, FRCGP, Clinical Tutor, Department of General Practice, University of Dundee, Dundee

Linda Gask, MSc, PhD, MRCPsych, Senior Lecturer/Honorary Consultant Psychiatrist, University of Manchester/Department of Community Psychiatry Academic Unit, Royal Preston Hospital, Sharoe Green Lane, Preston PR2 4HT

David Goldberg, MA, MSc, DM, FRCP, FRCP(Ed), FRCPsych, Director, Research and Development, Institute of Psychiatry, Denmark Hill, London SE5 8AF

Judy Greenwood, MRCPsych, Consultant Psychiatrist, Community Drug Problem Service, Royal Edinburgh Hospital, The Andrew Duncan Clinic, Morningside Park, Edinburgh EH10 5HF

Rachel Jenkins, MA, MD, FRCPsych, Consultant Psychiatrist, Section of Epidemiology and General Practice, Institute of Psychiatry, London SE5 8AF

Tony Kendrick, BSc, MRCGP, Mental Health Foundation Research Fellow, Division of General Practice and Primary Care, St George's Hospital Medical School, Hunter Wing, Level 6, Cranmer Terrace, London SW17 0RE

Michael King, MD, PhD, MRCP, FRCGP, MRCPsych, Senior Lecturer of Academic Psychiatry, Royal Free Hospital School of Medicine, Rowland Hill Street, London NW3 2QG

Colin Murray Parkes, MD, FRCPsych, Consultant Psychiatrist, St Christopher's Hospice, Lawrie Park Road, London SE26 6DZ

Keith Lloyd, MSc, MRCPsych, Senior Registrar, Section of Epidemiology and General Practice, Institute of Psychiatry, London SE5 8AF

Denis Pereira Gray, OBE, MA, FRCGP, Director, Postgraduate Medical School, University of Exeter EX2 5DW

Ian Pullen, FRCPsych, Consultant Psychiatrist, Department of Psychiatry, Royal Edinburgh Hospital, Morningside Park, Edinburgh EH10 5HF

Janine Scott, MD, MRCPsych, Senior Lecturer, University Department of Psychiatry, Royal Victoria Infirmary, Newcastle upon Tyne NE1 4LP

Michael Sheldon, MB, FRCGP, Senior Lecturer, Department of General Practice, St Bartholomew's Hospital Medical College, London EC1M 6BQ

Geraldine Strathdee, MRCPsych, Consultant Psychiatrist in Rehabilitation and Community Care, The Maudsley Hospital, Denmark Hill, London SE5 8AZ

Kieran Sweeney, MA, MRCGP, Research Fellow, Institute of General Practice, University of Exeter, 34 Denmark Road, Exeter EX1 1SF

André Tylee, FRCGP, Department of Medicine, Division of General Practice and Primary Care, St George's Hospital Medical School, Jenner Wing – Level 0, Cranmer Terrace, London SW17 0RE

Peter Tyrer, BA, MD, FRCP, FRCPsych, Professor of Community Psychiatry, St Charles Hospital, London W10 6DZ

Richard Westcott, MA, MRCGP, General Practitioner, 4 Paradise Lawn, South Molton, Devon EX36 3DJ

Greg Wilkinson, MPhil, FRCP, FRCPsych, Professor of Psychiatry, Department of Psychiatry, The London Hospital Medical College, 3rd Floor – Alexandra Wing, Turner Street, London E1 2AD

Idris Williams, MD, FRCGP, Professor of General Practice, University of Nottingham, Queen's Medical School, Clifton Boulevard, Nottingham NG7 2UH

Alastair Wright, MD, FRCGP, General Practitioner, 5 Alburne Crescent, Glenrothes, Fife KY7 5RE

Foreword

General practice has always stood for personal medicine and its application to health and disease for people in their families and homes. Psychiatry has always stood for scientific study of mental health and its application to mental and emotional problems of all kinds. Recognition of these disciplines has been relatively slow to emerge, and in both the research base took some time to build up; university departments and chairs in our subjects were established later than in many other fields. Although the Royal Medico-Psychological Association and its predecessors had a long and distinguished history (Berrios & Freeman, 1991) it was not until 1952 that the Royal College of General Practitioners was founded (Fry *et al*, 1983) and in 1971 the Royal College of Psychiatrists.

Our two Colleges are both committed to fostering and developing the highest standard of research in both general practice and psychiatry, and in seeking to translate research findings into the highest possible standard of clinical practice.

We believe that general practitioners and psychiatrists have much to learn from each other and that there are many reasons why they should collaborate for the benefit of their patients. Both subjects have been misunderstood in the past, and indeed of both it has been said that they are "the other half of medicine".

We are both encouraged by the publication of this book, produced by two Royal Colleges working in partnership. It has equal numbers of editors and authors from both disciplines. It is our joint view that disturbances of the emotions have never been the subject of as much research or education as they deserve, and both our Colleges are committed to enhancing these for all concerned in the Health Service.

Within psychiatry there is a large body of knowledge and research about mental and emotional illness and we wish to share it more widely. General practice has the greatest experience of dealing with these problems day to day and over many years, and it is similarly our wish to share that experience more widely. Our aim is that the standards of care that patients receive should be as high as possible.

We thank the editors and authors who have contributed to this book, which will form a useful contribution to the development of our two disciplines.

Fiona Caldicott
President, Royal College of Psychiatrists

Bill Styles
Chairman of Council, Royal College of General Practitioners

References

BERRIOS, G. E. & FREEMAN, H. (eds) (1991) *150 Years of British Psychiatry, 1841–1991.* London: Gaskell.

FRY, J., LORD HUNT OF FAWLEY & PINSENT, R. J. F. H. (1983) *A History of the Royal College of General Practitioners. The First 25 Years.* Lancaster: MTP.

Editors' preface

This book is about the assessment and treatment of people with psychiatric disorders in general practice and how general practitioners and psychiatrists can collaborate effectively.

The editors and authors are psychiatrists and general practitioners with an interest in developing closer working relationships between primary and secondary care. It is the first joint venture of this kind between the Royal College of Psychiatrists and the Royal College of General Practitioners and draws on the expertise of Members and Fellows of both Colleges.

The book is aimed at general practitioners, psychiatrists, and trainees in both disciplines. A growing number of clinical attachments between psychiatrists and general practitioners have developed over the last decade and this trend appears to be increasing.

The reasons for this trend are not hard to find: practitioners enjoy working together in this way for patients' benefit; general practitioners and psychiatrists have become aware of the true extent of psychiatric morbidity in general practice and of the benefits of early recognition and treatment; and, there is a historical and political movement to care for many more people with long-term mental disorders within the community.

Psychiatry and General Practice Today is a practical, clinical source book. The book covers historical aspects, clinical syndromes, modern treatment approaches, and research and prevention. It attempts to give a comprehensive and up-to-date view of the subject which is relevant to clinical practice.

The theme that pervades the book is partnership. Partnership extends beyond general practitioners and psychiatrists and encompasses the involvement of patients and their relatives and other members of the primary care and community psychiatric teams. The approach is pragmatic and draws upon the full range of psychopharmacological, psychological and social interventions.

Special attention has been given to research and prevention in psychiatry in general practice. These topics have been included to promote interest and action. They will require intensive development and evaluation as the subject advances.

The field is in rapid development and expansion. Watts & Watts published the first survey of psychiatric disorders in a general practice in 1952, and showed that a large proportion of consultations were due to psychiatric problems. In 1956 McCrae began the first specialist psychiatric clinical service at the Sighthill Health Centre in Edinburgh (Dean, 1972). Shepherd and colleagues published the first large-scale epidemiologically-based survey of psychiatric disorder in general practice in 1966.

From these beginnings the subject has become established in clinical practice throughout the world where similar health care systems exist. Current reforms in the Health Service in the United Kingdom indicate that this style of practice will be encouraged and endorsed and is likely to be emulated by other disciplines.

References

DEAN, R. M. (1972) Sighthill – the evolution of a health centre. *Journal of the Royal College of General Practitioners*, **22**, 161–168.

SHEPHERD, M., COOPER, B., BROWN, A. C., *et al* (1966)   *Psychiatric Illness in General Practice*. Oxford: Oxford University Press.

WATTS, C. A. H. & WATTS, B. (1952) *Psychiatry in General Practice*. London: J. & A. Churchill.

The legislative framework today

The implementation of the NHS and community care changes throughout the United Kingdom marks the culmination of a series of major health and social care reforms. The extent to which the aims of value for money and improved consumer choice through the introduction of competitive internal markets have been achieved has yet to be evaluated. The advent of fund-holding practices which can purchase psychiatric care for their patients, and care management whereby care managers purchase community care for their clients, presents an opportunity for improved services for mentally ill people in the community, as well as the risk of the fragmentation of services.

Background chronology

The 1962 *Hospital Plan* launched a programme of mental hospital closure in England and Wales and a programme for community care. The 1975 White Paper *Better Services for the Mentally Ill* set targets for bed closures and proposed a network of health and social services in the community. A critical Audit Commission report in 1986 entitled *Making a Reality Out of Community Care* led to a government report *Community Care – Agenda for Action* (Griffiths, 1988). Known as the *Griffith's report*, this formed the basis of the *National Health Service and Community Care Act* 1990, which came into force on 1 April 1993. This Act laid down the organisational structure for community care. The structure defines the GP as a key identifier of need and as a link between the local authority and the health authority. Social security monies previously allocated to residential and nursing home care have been transferred to local authorities, who will become the purchasers of community care for individuals. The emphasis will shift to purchasing services from the voluntary and private sectors rather than services run by local authorities. A distinction will be made between health care (the responsibility of health authorities) and social care (to be purchased by the local authorities).

Case/care management

Case management involves: continuity of care, accessible services, titrating support to need, facilitating independence, patient advocacy, and advocacy for services (Thornicroft, 1993). The 1990 Act made it the responsibility of local authorities to:

(a) to carry out an assessment of an individual's need for any service
(b) to decide whether the need calls for the provision of any services.

By 1991 the term 'care manager' appeared on the grounds that the term 'case' was demeaning. Care managers are clearly identified as the purchaser and not the provider of services.

The GP is a key identifier of need and can request a 'needs assessment' by the local authority, as can relatives, carers or anyone else concerned.

Discharge planning

Although discharge planning has always appeared desirable, it is now mandatory. No discharge from hospital should occur without a clearly agreed discharge plan. The discharge or community care plan should set out clearly which named professional has agreed to provide what service and must be agreed with the patient. The GP will be a crucial provider of services for most discharged patients and should be involved in pre-discharge discussions.

Countdown to community care

By April 1992 local authorities were to draw up community care plans and care programmes were introduced for severely mentally ill people. In December 1992 health authorities (health boards in Scotland) were to draw up plans on good practice in discharging patients from hospital. On 1 April 1993, local authorities took over the lead responsibility; care management started; users and carers were to have more say in planning, assessment, and choice of services; GPs were to get regular information about local care services, make referrals for care providing basic clinical information to care managers (with the patient's permission); and the processes were to be monitored (Groves, 1993). The implementation of the Act raised the spectre of greater choice for patients and carers with ready access to needs assessment and the purchasing, on their behalf, of the care of their choice.

Potential shortcomings

Sir Roy Griffiths (1993) drew attention to two key recommendations in his report that were not accepted by the government: the ring fencing of government money for community care and the establishment of a minister for community care to give a higher profile to the subject. He acknowledged that

> "there is a feeling by general practitioners that they have been involved only at a comparative late stage in the initial preparations [for community care]. The changes for general practitioners are not great, what is needed is . . . that when they do become involved in referring people to the social services it is done in an effective, disciplined way (as in the case of referrals to consultants) with written referral and follow up." (Griffiths, 1993)

A GP (Morris, 1993) spelled out the background to the working relationship between GPs and social workers.

> "The two professions tend to be suspicious of each other, have little understanding of each other's roles, and have very different cultures. Social workers operate in teams, take measured approaches to problems, and rarely take decisions on their own. GPs work mainly as individuals . . . and have to take decisions quickly."

The process of needs assessment in this form is new, and it appears that some social services teams have become overwhelmed by requests for assessments, with an increasing length of time before assessments can be made. This causes delay in discharge of patients from psychiatric units and may lead to potentially avoidable hospital admissions.

The distinction between social and health care is not entirely clear but, since who pays for what is subsequently provided hinges on this decision, it is an area which is likely to provoke disputes between the purchasers of care, especially if they have to manage with very tight budgets.

Fund-holding general practitioners and the psychiatric team

Fund-holding GPs are already using contracts to spell out what they expect from hospital services and some aspects of community health services, and this may in time be extended to social aspects of community care. The advent of fund-holding has given some GPs the opportunity to negotiate quality standards for their patients which may be different from those negotiated by health authorities for most patients. This period of change has caused some anxiety to psychiatrists as leaders of the psychiatric team. Will referral patterns become distorted by financial pressures? As emergency cases are treated at no cost to the fund-holding GP, will there be a temptation to delay referral until it becomes an emergency? Where differential charges have been negotiated for referral to different professions within the team, will there be a tendency to refer to nurses rather than psychiatrists? Finally, what will happen where the psychiatrist recommends intensive out-patient treatment (at considerable cost to the GP's fund) which the GP is not prepared to fund?

To balance these psychiatrists' fears there are a number of important principles which favour the fundholding initiative. Firstly, it enables psychiatrists to deal with fellow doctors on a doctor-to-doctor basis. Secondly, decision-taking in primary care is devolved to people who actually know the patients concerned and are able to take decisions in the light of personal experience of their illnesses and needs. Thirdly, GPs constantly hear first-hand how patients perceive the secondary care services, and can therefore take patients' views into account when negotiating budgets. Fourthly, the fears about the use of emergency services were also voiced for specialists in physical medicine when fundholding began in 1990 and have not materialised in practice. Finally, general practice usually has better and more up-to-date (computerised) information than planners in purchasing authorities, so planning can be more relevant to patients' needs.

The theme of this book is partnership (see Introduction). It is essential that the good working relationships that have developed between psychiatrists and GPs in many areas are not threatened by these changes. It is an opportunity for relationships to develop to ensure the optimum treatment for our patients.

References

AUDIT COMMISSION (1986) *Making a Reality Out of Community Care*. London: HMSO.
GRIFFITHS, R. (1988) *Community Care: Agenda for Action*. London: HMSO.
—— (1993) Introduction. In *Countdown to Community Care* (ed. T. Groves). London: BMJ Publishing.
GROVES, T. (1993) What the changes mean. In *Countdown to Community Care* (ed. T. Groves). London: BMJ Publishing.
MORRIS, R. (1993) Community care and the fundholder. In *Countdown to Community Care* (ed. T. Groves). London: BMJ Publishing.
THORNICROFT, G. (1993) Care management and mental health. In *Countdown to Community Care* (ed. T. Groves). London: BMJ Publishing.

Part I. The context

1 General practice and psychiatry – a general practice perspective

DENIS PEREIRA GRAY

The needs of the population

The extent of the need

The psychiatric needs of the population have been well researched. The conditions that need inclusion are all those involving mental and emotional illness and all the range of fears and feelings which bring patients to their doctors.

The most important two facts are firstly the distress which people suffer, and secondly the vast quantity of such problems experienced by the population at large. As early as 1960, Ryle wrote:

> "That in the course of one year between 5 and 10 per cent of the population consult their doctor at least once with symptoms of neurosis, while a further 10 to 20 per cent present evidence of psychosomatic disorder."

The early studies by Shepherd *et al* (1966) were classic. About a third of the whole population experiences some significant suffering from some emotional problem each year.

In the national morbidity study 1981/82 (Royal College of General Practitioners *et al*, 1990), among the most common health problems for women, mental and emotional problems ranked second behind respiratory problems, while for men they ranked seventh. However, it is likely that a large proportion of poisonings and ''ill-defined conditions'' are manifestations of anxiety and depression. In this chapter the words 'mental' and 'neurosis' are avoided, as they are unsatisfactory terms for general practitioners, who can no longer use either comfortably with their patients. Similarly, the term 'mental illness service' is also avoided, as general practice is both the front line of the mental illness service in the British NHS and the part dealing with the largest numbers of patients. Instead, the words 'emotional problems' are used.

There are other aspects of emotional illness which have been found by research, and which point to the needs of patients.

Stigma

There is still a stigma about this kind of illness that is not present with physical illnesses. In particular, many people, even now, still feel that depression is blameworthy, that sufferers should 'pull themselves together', and that psychiatric treatment is shameful (Royal College of Psychiatrists, 1992). Stigma can prevent patients seeking help and also make them less ready to accept help or take treatment.

Somatisation *

The term 'somatisation' refers to patients who go to doctors believing that they have physical disease, but who do not, and do have emotional problems – commonly depression. Books have been written about this topic, which is special to general practice partly because it is the first port of call and partly because only GPs simultaneously treat physical and emotional problems. Grol's (1981) *To Heal or To Harm* was written from the Department of General Practice at Nijmegen, in The Netherlands. The Dutch school of general practice has been strong on emotional medicine (Lamberts & Riphagen, 1975; Dokter, 1978).

Somatisers are an important group, who may comprise up to 20% of all depressives (Goldberg *et al*, 1988). GPs researching somatisation, such as Wright (1990), have found a lower rate, which points to the possibility that in general practices where there is sensitive care of the emotionally ill, the rate of somatisation may fall as patients become more comfortable and able to present emotional problems more directly.

Somatisation is so common that it is logical for the doctors in primary care to be trained to deal with all the common forms of physical and emotional illness, and to be able to do the two together, that is, to diagnose, investigate, and treat in both modalities simultaneously. Generalist care is thus more cost-effective.

Yet a further need for this combination of skills in primary care arises because many chronic physical diseases make patients depressed, and the diagnosis of such depression may be more difficult (Freeling *et al*, 1985); the high rate of contact with their GPs by this group of patients makes the simultaneous diagnosis and treatment of both the physical and the emotional problem both logical and efficient.

Privacy of consulting

Stigma and somatisation, particularly together, both point to the need for the front line of any health service to be immediately accessible to patients.

They must be able to make an appointment without having to declare the problem and without having to tell friends, family, or employers what the problem is.

Women

Women consult more, and are more often diagnosed as having emotional problems. These sex differences are substantial and were known by the 1950s (Watts & Watts, 1952). The rate of such diagnoses in the third national morbidity survey in 1981/82 was more than 100% more for women than men (Royal College of General Practitioners *et al*, 1990).

Parental influences

Much has been written about psychiatric theory and research on the impact of parents and childhood on subsequent adult behaviour. The child is the father of the man (Weston, 1960). Psychiatrists encourage patients to describe their childhood experiences and especially their relationships with their parents, and psychoanalysis takes this to great depths. A health system where the doctors personally knew the parents would be an advantage in providing care, since the doctor could then use his/her own feelings and reactions to the parents as an additional source of information, and could gain other insights.

The development of general practice as a scientific discipline

The interpretation of the history of psychiatry in general practice is complicated, because its origins lie in the 1950/60s, when the first reports appeared. This was precisely the time when general practice emerged as a scientific discipline of medicine in its own right, which Pereira Gray (1989) dates to 1961. General practice shares much with psychiatry; both subjects are centrally concerned with the emotions and can claim in their own way to be 'the other half of medicine'.

General practice owes a special debt to psychiatry, as in the nine years 1957–66, four psychiatrists underpinned the then emerging new discipline of general practice with research which gave crucial new insights into the role of the medical generalist.

The first and greatest contribution came in 1957 from Balint, with his *The Doctor, His Patient and the Illness*. This book has become one of the most influential on general practice ever written. It threw new light on the complex presentations many patients make to GPs; it illuminated the role of the doctor's own personality with the ideas of the 'drug doctor' and the 'apostolic function'. It analysed the complexity of the doctor–patient relationship over years in the 'mutual investment company'. By describing the generalists' unique role at a time when specialisation in medicine was dominant, it changed the balance of medicine and gave general practice new insights and hope: "what Freud has become for psychiatry, Balint will become for general practice" (*Journal of the Royal College of General Practitioners*, 1972).

Secondly, Berne's (1964) *Games People Play* became required reading for all GPs who really want to understand their patients. Some of his 'games', which are complex patterns of behaviour with hidden meaning, are consulting-room behaviours, and a few of them, like the 'Yes but', are essential to know. Any doctor who consults in general practice or psychiatry without mastering this text will miss many nuances in the consulting-room.

Thirdly, Castelnuovo-Tedesco (1965) wrote *The Twenty-Minute Hour*. This book does not, like the other three, report original research, but it is the most practical of the four. It tackles two of the GP's central problems: the allocation of time, and the need for a more systematic approach to patients with emotional problems.

The fourth psychiatrist to transform thinking in general practice was Shepherd, in London. His earlier paper (Shepherd *et al*, 1959) recorded a prevalence rate in one practice for persons with "conspicuous psychiatric morbidity" of 11% in women and 7% in men in one year. His later book, *Psychiatric Illness in General Practice* (Shepherd *et al*, 1966), provided more facts from more practices, but the message was the same. There are large numbers of patients seeing GPs with such problems, with a preponderance of women. The implication was that their care would never all be a matter for referral and specialist services. GPs would simply have to learn, sooner or later, how to care for them in the words of the motto of their new College, "*Cum Scientia Caritas*" (science with compassion).

An ideal National Health Service for emotional illness

An ideal National Health Service would have the following characteristics:

(1) be used by the whole population
(2) provide easy, preferably same-day, availability to a highly trained doctor
(3) avoid any financial barrier, both to encourage access by the poor and because stigma may reduce help-seeking behaviour
(4) provide a front-line medical service which deals with most physical and emotional problems
(5) provide a service that relates to the whole person and avoids focusing on any particular disease, physical or emotional
(6) be a service which is available and frequently used by women
(7) be a service covering marital partnerships, cohabiting couples, and family groups, since so many problems are about behaviour in the family, bereavement, and other losses in life

(8) be rooted in the local environment and staffed by doctors and nurses familiar with local social problems, such as housing and unemployment

(9) provide for doctors and nurses visiting the homes of the patients to give the opportunity for making personal observations of the physical state of the home, and the style of living of the occupants; ideally, especially in the evenings and out of hours, the rare clinical experience of observing the family as a group interacting together in its own habitat in the face of stress can help the doctor to understand a problem

(10) provide a service continuously over many years, since many emotional problems are long term; continuity of care over decades is the ideal

(11) provide drugs, especially, where appropriate, antidepressants

(12) provide a service which can vary both the length of consultation and the frequency of contact (follow-up) easily

(13) provide easy access for referral, without financial expense, to specialists for the 5% who may benefit from referral

(14) provide relationships with secondary (specialist) services which are organised in accordance with the WHO system (Horder, 1983), so that secondary-care support does not compete with, duplicate, or dominate primary care; similarly, the tertiary (supraregional/ national) mental health services should be organised in support of the secondary services and as developmental centres, and should not duplicate or seek to control secondary care

(15) provide a multiprofessional primary health care team

(16) provide a service closely linked with other primary community services

(17) actively undertake research, especially on emotional medicine

(18) be actively involved in teaching undergraduate medical students, nurse students, vocational trainees, and general practitioners working for higher research degrees

(19) encourage specialists to work and train in primary care

(20) provide GPs with regular written reports on all patients referred to specialists

(21) for the rare few patients for whom compulsory admission is required, whether this takes place in hospital or the community, generalist and specialist doctors should work together and both sign the relevant documents

(22) the care of the emotionally ill should be audited by peer review in all settings where care takes place

(23) has high contact rates with children and adolescents, because these are the priority groups for prevention of emotional problems

(24) provide care for families over three or more generations

(25) ensure that no GPs qualify for independent practice without being trained and demonstrating competence in the detection and management of emotional problems, and ensure that no psychiatrists are allowed to qualify until they have been formally trained and demonstrated competence in general practice.

General practice in the British National Health Service

Given this specification for the ideal primary care service for the emotionally distressed, how does British general practice measure up?

Representativeness of research on general practice

In evaluating British general practice, it is necessary to be aware that the service is never as good or as bad as research suggests. This is because the best practice tends to be reported from enthusiastic and skilled GPs who enjoy their job and who derive great intellectual and emotional satisfaction from it. They often work in well organised practices with good staff and information systems. It is wrong simply to extrapolate from single practices to whole countries, although it is true that its history shows that the whole of general practice does consistently follow leading GPs and their performance. For example Eimerl (1960) described the diagnostic register and Tudor Hart (1975) first took the blood pressure of all his patients; 15 years later both were being followed by most general practices in the country. Thus such reports often predict national trends.

Equally, it is important not to accept uncritically the results of research carried out only in certain populations. Research is often conducted in general practice by specialists from teaching hospitals in big population centres. There is a long-standing inverse relationship in the resources committed to general practices around such hospitals. The conclusions from such studies equally cannot simply be extrapolated, and they may not be valid in other parts of the country.

How does British general practice measure up first as a system, and secondly in its performance as a system?

General practice as a system

The current general practice system may be judged according to the 25 ideal characteristics outlined above.

(1) A national system has been achieved – 98% of the population is registered.

(2) Availability. Access to the system does provide a same-day service for anything the patient describes as urgent, and in the teaching practices

in the South Western Region the commonest delay time for a routine appointment is the next day, so this objective is effectively achieved.

(3) No financial barrier. This has been achieved completely for the consultation with the doctor, but charges are made for prescriptions (£3.80 per item at the time of writing), and frequent prescriptions for depressives and antipsychotic medication can sometimes be a problem.

(4) Service handling physical and emotional problems. The system provides for this.

(5) Personal care. The NHS regulations place the adjective 'personal' first in the responsibilities of the GP.

(6) Women as users of the service. This has been achieved: over 72% of all adult women consult a general practitioner every year (Royal College of General Practitioners *et al*, 1972).

(7) Registration by couples and family groups. It is usual, but not invariable, for couples, whether married or not, to register with the same GP. Parent–child relationships are even easier to observe first-hand in family practice, and 99% of the time the child is registered with the mother's family doctor, and the GP has innumerable opportunities to see how the mother–child relationship is evolving.

(8) Local environment. Most GPs are, as described by Susser & Watson (1971), 'burghers'. That is to say, they do not expect, like 'spiralists', to keep moving to further their career. They live in the same community as their patients (except for a small minority of GPs in big cities) whom they meet in the street, in the shops, and at local public events. They know at first hand about local social issues, such as unemployment, and its effect on their patients (Beale & Nethercott, 1986). This objective is usually achieved.

(9) Home visiting. The *General Household Survey 1989* (Office of Population Censuses and Surveys, 1991) showed that about one-tenth of all consultations are still in the home. Furthermore these are focused, logically, on the housebound and the most dependent members of society, so that for patients over the age of 75 as many as half of all the average of seven contacts per year take place in the home.

(10) Continuity of care. Ritchie *et al* (1981) found that as many as 42% of patients had continuity of registration with their GPs 20 years or more since birth. In the author's practice in Exeter, in 1992 over 400 out of 1323 NHS patients had been registered with me for more than 20 years.

(11) Prescription of drugs. This objective has been achieved. All GPs can prescribe, and psychotropic medication is a common prescription in Britain.

(12) Varying length and frequency of consultations. The system in general practice gives the GP complete discretion to vary both of these as is clinically indicated.

(13) Referral to specialists is available throughout the NHS.

(14) Relationships with secondary care. The structure permits the relationship recommended by the WHO. The relationships are variable in practice.

(15) Multiprofessional team. Most GPs now work with nurses and in some counties like Gloucestershire every practice now has a practice nurse. In the provinces, attachment of both district nurses and health visitors is the norm, but this is less common in London. A minority of practices have counsellors (McLeod, 1988). In some health districts physiotherapists have been attached to every practice. Some community psychiatric nurses are attached. The general practice team is steadily growing both in numbers and in range of health professionals.

(16) Local community links. These are strong in rural areas but weak in big cities.

(17) Research in general practice. The opportunities are immense, especially with the defined age–sex register of the British system.

(18) Teaching. Medical students are now being taught more in general practice. All future GPs spend 12 months in a university-approved training practice. Teaching for nurses in primary care is variable and limited.

(19) More psychiatrists are working in primary care but virtually none have as yet been trained there by generalists.

(20) Regular reports. Good practice is clearly that specialists should report in writing to the referring GP.

(21) Compulsory admission. The ideal arrangement is possible and is usual for admissions, but rare for discharges.

(22) Medical audit. Medical audit is only just starting in the NHS. Structure permits audit in general practice, but no reports on emotional problems in general practice have yet been published.

(23) High contact rate with children and adolescents. The contact rate between British GPs and children under five is now as high as eight per year and rising on the *General Household Survey* figures based on random samples of the population (Office of Population Censuses and Surveys, 1991). The contact rate between adolescents and GPs is less than this but still high (three every year) as there are so many adolescent conditions treated in general practice, from acne to accidents.

(24) Family care over three generations. The system encourages this. High rates occur in general practice, although these are rarely published. In my practice in a personal list of 1323 patients, 72 were diagnosed as depressed in the previous 12 months, of which I had personally treated as a GP at some time 19 of their parents (26%) and an additional 15 (21%) had a parent currently registered with me and were well known. Thus in 1992 in about half of all depressive cases, the family doctor had personal knowledge of the personality and behaviour of at least one parent.

(25) Mutual training. Only about 40% of British GPs train formally in a psychiatric hospital post as part of their general practice training. However, teaching on half-day release courses and in the practice focuses heavily on

emotional problems, as it is these which trainees find the most difficult. Few psychiatrists yet train formally in general practice and only a handful of psychiatrists are members of the Royal College of General Practitioners. The educational system thus currently fails to meet this objective. The system is therefore well designed, but how does it perform in practice?

Strengths of general practice

Whole-population care

General practice is now probably the most widely used public service. It is used by 98% of the whole population.

Countering stigma

Since emotional problems are one of the commonest diagnoses made in general practice (Royal College of General Practitioners *et al*, 1972), it implies that general practice is reasonably accessible and that, to a considerable extent, the problem of stigma has been overcome.

Patient satisfaction

Given the relative responsibilities of primary care and secondary care, it is a considerable challenge for GPs to meet their patients' wants and needs. This is an open-access service provided day and night (more than half of all GPs get up at night for night calls and work the next day), in which a patient can bring any complaint, from a cough to cancer. Many symptoms, like weight loss, headache and fatigue, have both physical and emotional causes and whichever the cause is, the patient may be convinced it is the other.

Satisfaction levels are, however, one of the acid tests of any service – public or private. They will always continue as one element of quality of care. General practice comes out well in almost all surveys of consumer satisfaction (Jowell *et al*, 1990; Hawkins, 1992) and furthermore satisfaction is rising, not falling (Department of Health, 1991). The best-known of these is the regular *British Social Attitudes*; the seventh report (Jowell *et al*, 1990) concluded:

> "Overall dissatisfaction with the way the NHS is run has been steadily mounting. In 1983 only 26 per cent of the public expressed dissatisfaction; by 1986 this proportion had risen to 39 per cent, and by 1989 to 46 per cent. Overall satisfaction has accordingly dropped from 55 per cent in 1983 to 37 per cent in 1989. . . . Attitudes to primary health care services (especially to GPs) . . . have been stable and largely uncritical over the period."

TABLE 1.1
The percentages of patients expressing dissatisfaction with different services

	1983	1989
Local doctors/GPs	13%	12%
Being in a hospital as in-patient	7%	15%
Attending hospital as out-patient	21%	30%

The considerable effort made in vocational training schemes in trying to improve communication skills may be paying off. The figures in Table 1.1 included all hospital out-patients and in-patients and not any single specialty such as psychiatry. Nevertheless, the main conclusion is consistently greater satisfaction with GPs than with specialists.

Length of consultations

Detecting emotional distress, even by sensitive doctors, and exploring it, let alone treating it, takes time. Westcott (1977), when a trainee, showed that it was the patients with emotional problems who took the longest time. Given the frequency of such problems in the population, it is clear that providing time to listen, time to analyse, and time to explore feelings with patients is one of the major challenges for British general practice.

In the teaching practices in the south-west of England, the five-minute consultation was considered quite normal in the 1970s, but it has come under sustained attack (Pereira Gray, 1979; Donald, 1985). One of the unsung successes of British general practice during the last decade has been the steady lengthening of the time for the ordinary booked consultations. In 1991 in the same teaching practices in the South Western Region only one GP consulted faster than ten per hour, and about half consulted at eight per hour, and the other half at six per hour (ten-minute bookings).

The difference is critical for quality, and it has already been shown by Morrell *et al* (1986) that the difference of a few minutes in average booking rates makes a significant difference in the ability of the doctor to offer personal preventive medicine. The same is even more true for emotional problems; five minutes is too short, and a rate of six per hour with patients one knows well is possible. Twelve minutes is better. These are still average booking times and, whatever the booking rates, those with emotional problems will receive more time. General practice is increasingly adopting counselling skills, both by the doctors (*Journal of the Royal College of General Practitioners*, 1980) and in the team (McLeod, 1988).

A national survey, conducted by the Department of Health and the General Medical Services Committee (1990), found an average of just under nine minutes, while ten minutes is fast becoming the norm, and a minority of GPs are already booking at 12-minute intervals.

Undressing

Undressing by patients is common in general practice and getting commoner as so much personal preventive medicine, like cervical smears, breast examination and testicular examination, demands it. Pereira Gray (1986), in a chapter "Nakedness in medicine", argued that this represents a special privilege for the generalist, and many patients, having exposed their bodies, find it easier to expose their feelings.

Weaknesses of general practice

Despite these considerable achievements, there is good research evidence of serious weaknesses in general practice.

Missed diagnoses

General practice diagnosis rates do not match illness rates from community surveys, even when allowing for the fact that many of the emotionally ill do not consult. The consistent shortfall implies under-diagnosis. Freeling *et al* (1985) confirmed this by comparing interviews with patients in waiting-rooms before consultations, with GPs' diagnosis and awareness, and then with interviews with the same patients afterwards. In these London practices GPs missed about half of all the patients with depression, particularly those with significant chronic physical disease. Goldberg & Bridges (1987) showed that GPs were much worse than questionnaires in detecting depression, and Coyne *et al* (1991) showed the same in the USA.

Suicide rates

Mortality rates remain an objective measure. Suicide is important as one measure of the efficiency of general practice in diagnosing and treating depression. Suicide rates are a cause for concern and represent one important target for further reduction, in that they must be partially preventable. However, by international comparisons Britain comes out well, with one of the lowest rates in Europe, and well below the Scandinavian countries, which so often have the best health statistics in the world.

The reasons for this are unclear, but GPs in Britain prescribe more antidepressants than practitioners in other European countries, and these are known to be effective (Paykel *et al*, 1988; Hollyman *et al*, 1988). However, standardised mortality ratios for suicide, while declining in young women, are rising in young men (Department of Health, 1990) and general practice research here is urgently needed.

Many patients committing suicide have consulted a GP within the previous few weeks. While some suicides can never be prevented, the implication must be that some at least of those consultations represented a 'cry for help'. Only general practice research can fully determine whether that cry was recognised or recognisable. If so, was it treated and was it treated well? How many suicides could have been prevented or are at least in theory preventable? How many of these patients were abusing alcohol or drugs, or were psychotic?

Attempts at suicide

The majority of those arriving at hospital after an attempt have seen a GP within four weeks (Jones, 1977). Prospective controlled studies are needed to determine the optimum form of GP care.

Dearth of publications

There is a remarkable dearth of publications from general practice on emotional illness, and especially publications on depression, which are strikingly rare considering this is one of the commonest conditions seen in practice. After the pioneering work of Watts & Watts (1952) and Ryle (1960), and the substantial contribution made by GPs to the understanding of the doctor–patient relationship (Browne & Freeling, 1967; Balint *et al*, 1970), and a good deal on prescribing, surprisingly little has been published on diagnosis and care until the St George's group (Freeling *et al*, 1985; Wright & Perini, 1987), and Wright (1988, 1990) in his own practice.

Lack of information and audit

The rarity with which a diagnostic register is kept for depression and the rarity with which care of depression is audited in general practice compared with conditions like asthma, diabetes and hypertension, which are all less common, implies substantially less interest and less systematic care for the condition.

Remedies for the weaknesses

There are many possible remedies for these weaknesses.

Research

First and foremost, there needs to be more research in general practice. One remedy must be to encourage and fund more research so that practitioners reading the journals of general practice will be confronted with the subject more often.

Education

Secondly, there has been a deficiency in the vocational training courses. Emotional medicine has featured heavily in the release programmes, mainly through case analysis and much less in terms of theory and systematic history-taking.

Only a minority of vocational trainees have held senior house officer posts in psychiatry, and these do not seem always to transfer this experience into practice. There has been a similar lack of continuing education. Depression rarely features on week-long refresher courses, and when it does it is almost invariably presented by a specialist, and however excellent, this may not make the most impact. GPs learn much faster from fellow generalists. There is always a feeling that the findings of a specialist research worker operating with hour-long consultations are not transferable to day-to-day general practice. A talk by a psychiatrist presupposes psychiatry, whereas the educational need is to think emotional medicine in the presence of pathologically confirmed physical disease in general practice and in so-called 'social problems'.

These issues need to be presented by a GP using GP-type consultation material to show that depression on average appears in every surgery, wearing many different masks. The most successful model of changing behaviour in general practice, namely teaching by example through a competent and enthusiastic fellow GP, is common for almost every chronic disease except depression. It is encouraging that the Royal College of General Practitioners has just appointed a GP fellow with support from the Mental Health Foundation and the Department of Health.

Education for GPs can be effective. Johnstone & Goldberg (1976) began a long and fruitful series of studies on training techniques for family doctors (Goldberg *et al*, 1980). Pereira Gray (1977) described some interactive interpretative general practice group work. More recently the work on education of Gask (Kaaya *et al*, 1992) and Bowman *et al* (1992), all from Manchester, have proved effective.

The need for a systematic approach

General practitioners have a problem in being consistent and rigorous in identifying and recording information and being analytical enough in drawing conclusions. This puts them at a disadvantage in dealing with chronic diseases like asthma, depression, diabetes, and hypertension, in that quality of care increasingly consists of systematic, sensitive history-taking, and systematic follow-up. Of all these diseases, depression is different, as it has no physical sign and no instrument like a blood-sugar machine for diagnosis. Depression in general practice is best diagnosed, firstly by empathy and good listening skills, at which general practice is strong, but secondly by systematically asking a few key questions (see Chapters 3 and 5). The questions are the diagnostic instrument (Pereira Gray, 1987).

The value of the huge quantity of consultations over the years can be diminished if GPs allow repetitive short consultations to occur, with patients going over and over the same ground, and making no progress in tackling problems, gaining insight, or choosing between a series of options. The systematisation of consultations for emotional medicine is a high educational priority.

The most practical need is to equip GPs with a simple, quick, validated kit of key questions to ask whenever they suspect or detect emotional problems, especially depression. Here the work of Goldberg *et al* (1988) has been outstanding. Their dozen questions, all validated by research, asked against the background of a good doctor–patient relationship, can work wonders.

However, at present there is little evidence that many GPs are using systematic history-taking.

Practice organisation

(1) Personal factors

General practice and hospital medicine are in many ways complementary. The former is essentially personal, low-tech, low-key, and long-term, while hospital care is high-tech, high-profile, episodic, and less personal. The medical records should reflect these essential characteristics, but general practice has been slow to implement an appropriate record-keeping system. Even in the 1990s, many general practice notes are episodic and not biographical, and are weak in the very features where general practice is strong. Only a minority of general practice records yet contain a family/household chart (Zander *et al*, 1978). General practice records are surprisingly sparse, and referral letters are often weak in biographical information about the patient which GPs often know well and better than anyone else.

(2) Summaries

Summaries are one key. Hospital summaries are superior to the summaries in most general practice records. It was only in the mid-1980s that systematic summaries began to appear in general practice. Even now, these tend to be mechanistic and are strongly biased towards physical events rather than the story of the person's life. Appendicectomy is more likely to be recorded than divorce. The remedy is the biographical approach.

(3) Microcomputers

The advent of new and more flexible desk-top microcomputers is providing GPs with a unique potential to summarise the whole of their patient's lives in physical, psychological, and social terms (Royal College of General Practitioners, 1972). Computers which allow free text make it possible to record crucial patient insights, such as: "my husband says I always worry about little things", which may reveal the personality of the patient as much as the problem. It has been said that it is more important for the GP to know the nature of the patient who has the disease, than the nature of the disease the patient has. For the first time in the last few years, some general practice records are better than some hospital ones.

(4) The biographical approach to personal doctoring

Only those who have considerable personal experience can appreciate the biographical aspect of personal doctoring and teach it with enthusiasm. There are only five books of outstanding merit in conveying its essence to trainees and young principals, and no career GP's education is now complete without mastering the messages from all of them. These books are: Balint (1957), *The Doctor, His Patient and the Illness*; Fry (1966), *Profiles of Disease*; Lane (1969), *The Longest Art*; Berger & Mohr (1969), *A Fortunate Man*; Huygen (1978), *Family Medicine – A Medical Life History of Families*.

Although each of these books has some limitations, each illuminates continuity of care in general practice. They collectively convey the special significance of the biographical approach to primary care and the profound insights which many GPs do achieve. No one can teach the GP approach to emotional problems without incorporating this perspective. One remedy is to teach about these books and their message very much more.

So-called 'life events', like the death of a mother when young (Brown & Harris, 1978), are strongly associated with emotional problems, including for example depression in mothers. The continuity of British general practice often allows the GP to have personal knowledge of such events; it is then possible both to appreciate their significance and simultaneously to share the experiences in a real way with the patient.

One remedy is thus to record life events systematically, preferably on computer. The biographical approach means getting to know and understand the patient as a person and how their life has unfolded (Pereira Gray, 1978).

(5) Personal lists

In order to achieve understanding of patients as people, repeated contact over long periods of time is essential. One of the great advantages of the personal-list system (Pereira Gray, 1979) of practice organisation is that it systematically encourages the same patients to see the same doctors over long periods of time, and so encourages mutual understanding to develop.

The alternative, combined-list system has advantages in offering patients a wider choice of doctor and gives doctors greater flexibility. The price, however, is that inevitably personal contact between any given patient and any given doctor is reduced. Freeman & Richards (1990) have measured this, and shown that with the personal-list systems up to 83% of consultations may be with the same doctor, compared with say 50% in combined-list practices. The key difference, as far as emotional medicine is concerned, is that personal lists strongly favour continuity of care, a personal orientation to the whole patient, through the biographical approach to medicine.

However, personal lists are in a minority in Britain, so they need to be researched more.

(6) Alternative carers

The latest problem is that some leading experts, having studied the research evidence of failure of diagnosis by GPs in big cities, have lost confidence in GPs' ability to provide a high-quality service, and are now constructing alternative sources of care for patients. These can take the form of alternative carers within the primary health care team or alternative sources of care, such as mental health centres, outside the team altogether.

In the short term, in areas where general practice is weak, these may lead to useful improvements, but in the long term numerous prices will be paid, particularly as somatisers are not likely to go to mental health centres since they deny that their symptoms are emotional in origin, and mental health centres will inevitably miss those patients with the early signs of serious physical disease like cancer, who can present with depression.

Conclusions

The care of those with emotional problems in Britain is in question. This chapter suggests that in terms of the ideal specification for a comprehensive NHS, British general practice is excellently placed to meet patients' needs. The evidence, however, is that GPs, particularly in big cities, are for a variety of reasons not taking advantage of the enormous potential of their role. About half of those clinically depressed are missed, although substantial numbers of these on patient satisfaction surveys report that they are satisfied wih their GP.

The reasons for this weakness lie in the origins of the specialty of general practice, and in its tendency to continue traditional ways of working rather than use methods more logical and appropriate for long-term personal care in the community.

A lack of awareness about research, a lack of professional leadership, and a superficial approach to practice organisation have done much to diminish the immense potential of the average of 12-year continuity which the average patient still has with the average GP in the NHS.

By helping working GPs to apply a more systematic approach to this important part of their work, it should soon be possible to improve the quality of care received by patients with emotional problems. Probably at the same time the job satisfaction of the GPs and the primary health care team will be substantially enhanced.

More research, more teaching of GPs by GPs, and more analysis of general practice methods of organisation, especially personal lists, should open up major opportunities for better care. The potential of new ways of working more systematically and using teams and microcomputers augurs well for the future.

References

BALINT, M. (1957) *The Doctor, His Patient and the Illness.* London: Pitman.
——— , HUNT, J., JOYCE, D., *et al* (1970) *Treatment or Diagnosis.* London: Tavistock.
BEALE, N. & NETHERCOTT, S. (1986) Job loss and health – the influence of age and previous morbidity. *Journal of the Royal College of General Practitioners*, **36**, 176–177.
BERGER, J. & MOHR, J. (1969) *A Fortunate Man.* London: Penguin.
BERNE, E. (1964) *Games People Play.* London: Penguin.
BOWMAN, F. M., GOLDBERG, D. P., MILLAR, T., *et al* (1992) Improving the skills of established general practitioners: the long-term benefits of group teaching. *Medical Education*, **26**, 63–68.
BROWN, G. W. & Harris, T. (1978) *The Social Origins of Depression.* London: Tavistock.
BROWNE, K. & FREELING, P. (1967) *The Doctor–Patient Relationship.* Edinburgh: Livingstone.
CASTELNUOVO-TEDESCO, P. (1965) *The Twenty-Minute Hour.* Boston, Little Brown. (Republished (1986) by the American Psychiatric Press.)
COYNE, J. C., SCHWENK, T. L. & SMOLINSKI, M. (1991) Recognizing depression: a comparison of family physician ratings, self-report, and interview measures. *Journal of the American Board of Family Practice*, **4**, 207–215.
DEPARTMENT OF HEALTH (1990) *Health and Personal Social Services Statistics for England* (1990 edn), Table 1.5, p. 12. London: HMSO.
——— (1991) *Survey of Patients' Opinions.* London: Department of Health.
——— & GENERAL MEDICAL SERVICES COMMITTEE (1990) *Workload Survey for the Review Body on Doctors' and Dentists' Remuneration.* London: Department of Health.
DOKTER, H. J. (1978) Department of General Practice at the Erasmus University of Rotterdam. *Journal of the Royal College of General Practitioners*, **28**, 349–351.
DONALD, A. (1985) Oasis or beachhead? James Mackenzie Lecture 1985. *Journal of the Royal College of General Practitioners*, **35**, 558–564.
EIMERL, T. S. (1960) Organised curiosity. *Journal of the Royal College of General Practitioners*, **3**, 246–252.
FREELING, P., RAO, B. M., PAYKEL, E. S., *et al* (1985) Unrecognized depression in general practice. *British Medical Journal*, **290**, 1880–1883.
FREEMAN, G. & RICHARDS, S. (1990) How much personal care in four group practices? *British Medical Journal*, **301**, 1028–1230.
FRY, J. (1966) *Profiles of Disease.* Edinburgh: Livingstone.
GOLDBERG, D., SMITH, C., STEELE, J. J., *et al* (1980) Training family doctors to recognise psychiatric illness with increased accuracy. *Lancet* ii, 521–523.
——— & BRIDGES, K. (1987) Screening for psychiatric illness in general practice: the general practitioner versus the screening questionnaire. *Journal of the Royal College of General Practitioners*, **37**, 15–18.
——— , DUNCAN-JONES, P., *et al* (1988) Detecting anxiety and depression in general medical settings. *British Medical Journal*, **297**, 897–899.
GROL, R. (ed.) (1981) *To Heal or To Harm.* Nijmegen, Department of General Practice, University of Nijmegen. (Reprinted (1988) by the Royal College of General Practitioners.)

HAWKINS, C. (1992) *Letter to District Health Authorities and Family Health Services Authorities.* Bristol: South Western Regional Health Authority.

HOLLYMAN, J. A., FREELING, P., PAYKEL, E. S., *et al* (1988) Double-blind placebo-controlled trial of amitriptyline among depressed patients in general practice. *Journal of the Royal College of General Practitioners*, **38**, 393–397.

HORDER, J. (1983) Alma Ata Declaration. *British Medical Journal* **286**, 191–194.

HUYGEN, F. J. A. (1978) *Family Medicine – A Medical Life History of Families.* (Republished (1990) by the Royal College of General Practitioners.)

JOHNSTONE, A. & GOLDBERG, D. (1976) Psychiatric screening in general practice. *Lancet*, i, 605–608.

JONES, D. R. (1977) Follow-up of self-poisoned patients. *Journal of the Royal College of General Practitioners*, **27**, 717–719.

JOURNAL OF THE ROYAL COLLEGE OF GENERAL PRACTITIONERS (1972) Michael Balint (editorial). *Journal of the Royal College of General Practitioners*, **22**, 133–135.

―――― (1980) Is counselling the key? (editorial). *Journal of the Royal College of General Practitioners*, **30**, 643–644.

JOWELL, R., WITHERSPOON, S. & BROOK, L. (eds) (1990) *British Social Attitudes. The 7th Report.* Aldershot: Gower.

KAAYA, S., GOLDBERG, D. & GASK, L. (1992) Management of somatic presentations of psychiatric illness in general medical settings: evaluation of a new training course for general practitioners. *Medical Education*, **26**, 138–144.

LAMBERTS, H. & RIPHAGEN, F. E. (1975) Working together in a team for primary health care – a guide to dangerous country. *Journal of the Royal College of General Practitioners*, **25**, 745–752.

LANE, K. (1969) *The Longest Art.* London: George Allen and Unwin. (Reprinted (1992) by the Royal College of General Practitioners.)

MCLEOD, J. (1988) *The Work of Counsellors in General Practice. Occasional Paper 37.* London: Royal College of General Practitioners.

MORRELL, D. C., EVANS, M. E., MORRIS, R. W., *et al* (1986) The five minute consultation: effect of time constraint on clinical content and patient satisfaction. *British Medical Journal*, **292**, 870–873.

OFFICE OF POPULATION CENSUSES AND SURVEYS (1991) *General Household Survey 1989.* London: HMSO.

PAYKEL, E. F., FREELING, P. & HOLLYMAN, J. A., *et al* (1988) Predictors of therapeutic benefit from amitriptyline in mild depression: a general practice placebo-controlled trial. *Journal of Affective Disorders*, **14**, 83–95.

PEREIRA GRAY, D. J. (1977) *A System of Training for General Practice. Occasional Paper 4.* London: Royal College of General Practitioners.

―――― (1978) Feeling at home. James Mackenzie Lecture 1977. *Journal of the Royal College of General Practitioners*, **28**, 6–17.

―――― (1979) The key to personal care. *Journal of the Royal College of General Practitioners*, **29**, 666–678.

―――― (1986) Nakedness in medicine. In *The Medical Annual 1986.* Bristol: Wright.

―――― (1987) Editor's preface. In *The Presentation of Depression: Current Approaches. Occasional Paper 36* (eds P. Freeling, L. J. Downey & J. C. Malkin). London: Royal College of General Practitioners.

―――― (1989) The emergence of the discipline of general practice, its literature, and the contribution of the College Journal. McConaghey Memorial Lecture, 1988. *Journal of the Royal College of General Practitioners*, **39**, 228–233.

RITCHIE, J., JACOBY, A. & BONE, M. (1981) *Access to Primary Health Care.* London: HMSO.

ROYAL COLLEGE OF GENERAL PRACTITIONERS (1972) *The Future General Practitioner – Learning and Teaching.* London: British Medical Journal.

――――, OFFICE OF POPULATION CENSUSES AND SURVEYS & DEPARTMENT OF HEALTH AND SOCIAL SECURITY (1972) *Morbidity Statistics from General Practice 1970–71. No 46.* London: HMSO.

――――, ―――― & ―――― (1990) *Morbidity Statistics from General Practice 1981–82.* London: HMSO.

ROYAL COLLEGE OF PSYCHIATRISTS (1992) *Attitudes Towards Depression. Research Study Conducted for the "Defeat Depression Campaign"*. London: Royal College of Psychiatrists.

RYLE, A. (1960) The neuroses in a general practice population. *Journal of the College of General Practitioners*, **3**, 313–328.

SHEPHERD, M., FISHER, M., STEIN, L., *et al* (1959) *Proceedings of the Royal Society of Medicine*, **52**, 269.

SHEPHERD, M., COOPER, B., BROWN, A. C., *et al* (1966) *Psychiatric Illness in General Practice*. London: Oxford University Press.

SUSSER, M. W. & WATSON, W. (1971) *Sociology in Medicine* (2nd edn). London: Oxford University Press.

TUDOR HART, J. (1975) The management of high blood pressure in general practice. *Journal of the Royal College of General Practitioners*, **25**, 160–192.

WATTS, C. A. H. (1966) *Depressive Disorders in the Community*. Bristol: Wright.

——— & WATTS, B. (1952) *Psychiatry in General Practice*. London: J. & A. Churchill.

WESTCOTT, R. H. (1977) The length of consultations in general practice. *Journal of the Royal College of General Practitioners*, **27**, 552–555.

WESTON, T. E. T. (1960) The child is father of the man. Butterworth Gold Medal Essay. *Journal of the Royal College of General Practitioners*, **3**, 160–171.

WRIGHT, A. F. (1988) Psychological distress in a general practice: outcome and consultation rates. *Journal of the Royal College of General Practitioners*, **38**, 542–545.

——— (1990) A study of the presentation of somatic symptoms in general practice by patients with psychiatric disturbance. *British Journal of General Practice*, **40**, 459–463.

——— & PERINI, A. (1987) Hidden psychiatric illness: use of the General Health Questionnaire in general practice. *Journal of the Royal College of General Practitioners*, **37**, 164–167.

ZANDER, L. I., BERESFORD, S. A. A. & THOMAS, P. (1978) *Medical Records in General Practice. Occasional Paper 5*. London: Royal College of General Practitioners.

2 Psychiatry and general practice – a psychiatric perspective

GERALDINE STRATHDEE

This chapter is written from the perspective of a community psychiatrist involved in the development of primary mental health care. Firstly, the extent and nature of the psychiatric morbidity are examined. Secondly, the profile of service provision and the effect the movement to develop community care has had on both specialties are identified. Thirdly, models of collaboration and service development are discussed. Finally, the challenges to service provision are also discussed.

Nature and extent of psychiatric morbidity

In Britain, the extent of psychiatric morbidity presenting to primary care was established by Shepherd *et al* (1966). In a study of London general practices, they found that among a population of 15 000, in any year, 14% consulted at least once for a condition entirely or largely psychiatric in nature. Later studies found that a further 10–12% of the population suffered similar disorders, but that these went unrecognised by doctors.

Between one-fifth and one-quarter of the workload of the average GP concerns mental health problems (Goldberg & Bridges, 1987; Sharp & Morrell, 1989). The majority of such patients have either neurotic disorders or personality problems, and 9% of both these and psychotic patients suffer chronic disability, with symptoms continuously present for at least a year, or requiring prophylactic treatment.

General practitioners are the point of first contact for most of those with acute psychological disorders (World Health Organization, 1983), deal with those in crisis, are the gate-keeper to assessment services, and look after those in need of continuing care.

The relationship between the primary and secondary services

The traditional relationship

General practitioners used to have relatively few options available to them in the treatment of the mentally disordered: to treat the patient themselves using a limited armamentarium of drugs and some psychotherapeutic techniques, such as those inspired by the Balint movement (Balint & Norrell, 1973), or to refer to the hospital-based specialist (Kessel, 1963).

The relationship between primary care and psychiatry has been fraught with many tensions. These have included the problems caused by the geographical distance to the hospital, differences in the philosophy of care, and conflicts caused by the hierarchical specialist–generalist relationship (Horder, 1988). Historically, contact between the two services was almost exclusively between the doctors, usually by the referral letter, and seldom involved other members of the primary or secondary care teams. Domiciliary consultations formed one of the few opportunities for face-to-face contact between the doctors, but Sutherby *et al* (1992) found that the practice of joint visits has now almost disappeared.

Parkes *et al* (1962), in a study of schizophrenic patients living in the community, concluded that while the hospitals and out-patient clinics were responsible for initiating most of the treatment required for maintaining the patients' health, it was the GPs who dealt with the frequent crises and relapses. Where the psychiatric team has involved itself in the provision of emergency services, this has been through domiciliary visits (Littlejohns, 1986), casualty departments in general hospitals (Johnson & Thornicroft, 1992), or, in a very few areas, dedicated emergency clinics. There has been little substantive evaluation of either outcome or satisfaction among GPs with these services.

Until the advent of community care, assessment and consultation services were provided almost exclusively in hospital out-patient clinics. Studies across three decades have shown that general practitioners are dissatisfied with many aspects of these psychiatric services, including: long waiting-lists; disappointment with assessments; lack of clarity about management; and concern about the outcome of the consultations (Kaeser & Cooper, 1971; Johnson, 1973; Strathdee, 1990). Communication between GPs and hospital-based doctors has been a particular difficulty (Pullen & Yellowlees, 1985). Hansen (1987) found primary care teams to be dissatisfied with a hospital-based system of care. The main reasons included too little contact with mental health professionals for consultation on difficult cases, too few possibilities for direct referral to specialist services, and too few in-patients discharged back to primary care.

Changes to service provision

Since the 1960s, there have been rapid changes in both specialties. Psychiatry has seen the development of a growing range of treatment techniques, including psychopharmacology, behavioural and cognitive techniques, and family, marital, and other psychotherapeutic interventions. These in turn have accorded well with, and facilitated the movement to, the closure of the large psychiatric hospitals, and the development of local community-based care (Department of Health and Social Security, 1975). Within the specialty there has been a growth in multidisciplinary methods of working, later somewhat diluted by the gradual movement out of the hospitals of autonomous practitioners such as Community Psychiatric Nurses (CPNs).

Within medicine, general practice as a specialty has gained respect and acceptance, and has since introduced its own Royal College training and examination system. As in psychiatry, the development of a primary care team, rather than a uni-disciplinary approach, has advanced rapidly. This has expanded to include the sessional attachment of other disciplines, including nurses and psychologists, and has been facilitated by the organisation of primary care into the larger health centre and the development of sessional payments of such services, independent of the mental health services (Goldberg, 1991).

The development of community mental health services

Much of the development of British community psychiatric services has taken the form of an uncritical replication of the American model, with the establishment of community mental health centres and teams in parallel with, rather than integrated with, primary care teams. In such centres, unlike mental health services based in primary care clinics, there has often been a drift away from care of the seriously ill towards the so-called 'worried well' (Patmore & Weaver, 1990).

There are those who argue that the strength of the primary care infrastructure in Britain offers a unique resource, which should be the focus for community care (Tyrer, 1985). This view concords with the World Health Organization's declaration (1973) "that the primary care physicians should form the cornerstone of community psychiatry", as they "are best placed to provide long-term follow-up and be available for successive episodes of illness". The Royal College of General Practitioners (1984) likewise considers that GPs are particularly well placed to practise prevention.

However, there is little consensus on the best way in which to organise district mental health services (Kingdon, 1989), or even on a common planning strategy. Community mental health services have districts with an average of 200 000–250 000 population as the commonest unit of planning. Even when these are divided into sectors of 40 000–60 000 population, this still represents a very different scale of need from the average size of a general practice. More recently, and perhaps fuelled by the controversy over the role of psychiatric nurses, debate has begun to diversify into an examination of the appropriate deployment of mental health resources.

Important questions that are largely unanswered include which client groups are most appropriately treated by which specialty and in what setting. For example, should most people with neurotic disorders be seen by counsellors, psychologists, nurse therapists, or other practitioners employed by GPs and working in primary care? Have the secondary services, in the form of psychotherapy units and mental health teams, any expertise to contribute to such a service? With the relatively recent appearance of a wide range of self-help groups, such as Relate for people with relationship problems and CRUSE for bereavement counselling, to what extent should the medical profession, with its connotations of illness and ill health, remain involved in such 'problems of life'? Where should the primary responsibility for the long-term mentally ill rest? What is the quality of care offered to residents of sheltered homes in the community?

What should be the roles of GPs and of the specialist services? While it is clear that primary care teams will often have the larger role in the care of psychiatric patients, should the mental health services continue to establish services which parallel primary care, or should they integrate their care with that provided uniquely by the British primary care system?

General practitioners and the care of people with severe and long-term mental disorders

The implementation of community care has altered clinical practice and the organisation of services in primary care, which has been involved in the care of the severely chronically ill at least since the 1960s. Parkes *et al* (1962), following up a cohort of schizophrenic patients discharged from London mental hospitals, found that almost three-quarters had seen their GP in the year after discharge, more than half consulting over five times; just under 60% had attended hospital out-patient clinics in the same time, and, of these, over half had been seen fewer than five times. Johnstone *et al* (1984) likewise found that one-quarter of a similar group of patients saw *only* their GP over a five-year follow-up. Pantellis *et al* (1988) in the South Camden Schizophrenia Study found that only three-fifths of the known schizophrenics in the area were in contact with the psychiatric services. Lee & Murray (1988), studying the long-term outcome of depressed patients, found that over half had lost contact with the hospital services. Meltzer *et al* (1991) again demonstrated that even when day-care or rehabilitative facilities were lacking, patients in the community found their GPs an easily accessible source of care.

In their review of deinstitutionalisation, Thornicroft & Bebbington (1989) delineated the effects of transferring the functions of the psychiatric hospital to the community. Those which have a particular effect on primary care are: the decrease in bed numbers resulting in the locus of treatment being transferred to homes; the decrease in respite facilities, with subsequent increase in burden of care for relatives; and lack of hospital staff to undertake physical assessment and treatment. Length of stay in hard-pressed district in-patient units (50% of patients stay less than one month) has led to patients remaining with carers or relatives, who look to their family doctors for support and intervention. The growth of group homes, hostels, and other forms of sheltered accommodation inevitably lead to more demand for both physical and psychiatric care from local GPs (Horder, 1990).

While patients reside in the community, whether or not they have contact with the secondary services, the demand on GP services for crisis intervention will rise. Primary care teams are also likely to see patients with more severe and longer-term disorders than they would have previously.

In a survey of 500 GPs in the South West Thames Region, Kendrick *et al* (1991) found that while 90% of the doctors were happy to undertake the physical care of patients with long-term mental illnesses, most were reluctant to accept full responsibility for their psychiatric care. Three-quarters wanted the psychiatric services to maintain primary responsibility, and four-fifths believed that the CPN should be the key worker. However, almost all were willing to share responsibility with the secondary services.

Horder (1990), studying the establishment of three hostel and group homes for patients discharged from a long-stay psychiatric hospital, found that the residents were sick more often and consulted their GP more often than the population at large (an average of 7–8, compared with the population norms of 4 a year). Despite this, the unanimous opinion of the GPs involved was that the work had not been unduly arduous or difficult, and that off-duty work was minimal. Three-quarters of the doctors had no regrets about taking clinical responsibility for the patients, and several spontaneously commented on its interest and value. She concluded that the amount of work devolved to GPs in community facilities depends on such factors as age and health of residents, staffing levels, training, experience, and morale in the homes and the standard of local community psychiatric services.

Crisis and assessment services

Although seldom producing substantive, objective measures of outcome on the mental health of patients, a wave of audit studies have begun to elicit the methods of working which GPs believe would better meet the needs of their mentally ill patients. One hundred and fifty-four GPs in the district of Camberwell (Strathdee, 1990) were consulted to obtain their views on the development of crisis and assessment services in the planning of a new community-oriented service. The format of emergency services were a particular concern of the GPs. There was a consensus that new services should offer provision of immediate access to a specialist opinion, personal contact with a senior psychiatrist, and the assessment of patients in their own homes, with, if possible, the provision of out-reach facilities such as a crisis intervention team. Ferguson (1990), in an audit of GPs in Bassetlaw, also found a preoccupation with obtaining rapid response to crisis, and Stansfeld (1991) was advised that this should be on a 24-hour basis.

With regard to assessment services, the Camberwell doctors believed better communication and more information was essential. They believed out-patient facilities would be improved by: having shorter waiting-lists, the introduction of information packs (for both GPs and patients) explaining the treatments available (e.g. cognitive therapy), and guidelines as to which cases are appropriate for referral, with named personnel to contact. Particularly for chronic patients, the doctors stressed the need for a statement of the objectives and rationale of treatments, and an estimation of their length and possible side-effects and complications. Open access to CPNs and psychologists was regarded as useful by the doctors, who were less convinced of the need for professionals such as psychiatrists and psychologists to hold regular sessions in the surgeries.

Community psychiatry and the neuroses

While most psychiatrists consider that a significant proportion of scarce resources must be husbanded for the care of the most seriously ill patients, with mental health teams concentrating on this group, the position with regard to other disorders is less clear. A number of initiatives have been taken to extend the choice of psychological interventions in primary care. Most of this work has concentrated on the neurotic disorders (Paykel *et al*, 1982; Catalan *et al*, 1984; Marks, 1985; Johnstone & Shepley, 1986), particularly depression (Blackburn *et al*, 1981; Teasdale *et al*, 1984). The role of CPNs remains contentious, as they tend to work with neurotic rather than psychotic patients, and with the acutely rather than the chronically ill (Wooff *et al*, 1988; Paykel, 1990).

Of interest has been initiatives to train GPs themselves to undertake and apply psychological treatments (France & Robson, 1986). With the plethora of sessional workers in primary care, concern has been expressed that the primary care team should be strengthened in its role rather than de-skilled by the ease of referral. Horder (1988) identified the needs of individual practitioners as requiring help with interview technique, and the recognition of early symptoms, signs and life events most likely to contribute to illness. He asserts that personal contact between psychiatrist and GPs is of fundamental importance to clinical work, education, and organisation.

Models of collaboration between psychiatry and primary care

In planning community services, organisational structures are crucial. As Tansella (1989) counsels, ''what is important in community care is not only the number and characteristics of various services but the way in which they are arranged and integrated.'' Jones *et al* (1986) also caution that ''unless attention is given to finding administrative solutions to the repeated official exhortations (DHSS, 1975, 1978, 1981; Griffith, 1988) for collaboration and co-operation with GPs we will fail to provide the mix of services needed''. A number of authors (Lindholm, 1983; Tyrer *et al*, 1989; Strathdee & Thornicroft, 1992) consider that, for better working practices between specialists and generalists, the delineation of small, geographically defined areas or sectors as the unit of service provision is essential.

A number of service models have been developed which integrate psychiatric and primary services to varying degrees. Five of these are described below.

Primary care clinics

At the most basic level has been the devolution of out-patient clinics from hospital sites and the establishment of consultation clinics in primary care. Nineteen per cent of all consultant general adult psychiatrists in England and Wales (Strathdee & Williams, 1984) and half the Scottish psychiatrists (Pullen & Yellowlees, 1988) have worked in this way since the late 1970s. Although the initiative was warmly welcomed by the primary care teams, the impetus had come from grass-roots psychiatrists dissatisfied with the lack of coordination of care imposed by the geographical separation of primary and secondary services (Strathdee, 1988).

These clinics have a variety of formats (Strathdee & Williams, 1984; Mitchell, 1985; Strathdee *et al*, 1992). GPs have expressed a preference for the 'consultation' style, wherein the psychiatrist and referrer jointly make an assessment, and the GP undertakes the treatment with supervision. In the 'shifted out-patient model', the specialist sees patients in the local surgery to provide crisis intervention and perform assessment and short-term treatment. In longer-standing arrangements, the liaison-attachment model evolves, with the management of patients integrated between the specialist and primary care teams. This model is cost-effective, in that the psychiatrists can contribute to the care of more patients by providing advice on patients not seen, treating others through supervision, and enhancing the skills of the primary care team (Creed & Marks, 1989; Darling & Tyrer, 1990).

An early criticism of the clinics was that specialists in primary care would inevitably, as with the American community mental health centres, drift towards seeing the 'worried well'. However, the proportion of patients with serious and long-term mental illness seen is at least equal to that encountered in hospital out-patient clinics (Tyrer, 1984; Brown *et al*, 1988; Tyrer *et al*, 1989). In fact there is evidence to suggest that the clinics provide for the previously unmet need of chronic patients reluctant to attend hospital follow-up clinics, especially women, schizophrenics, those with paranoid illnesses (Brown *et al*, 1988), and the homeless (Joseph *et al*, 1990).

The Tyrer 'hive' model

A model in which the primary care liaison clinics form an important component of a total district service is the 'hive' model described by Tyrer (1985). He suggests that comprehensive care can only be achieved by a system which integrates community psychiatric care with hospital care. The hospital should be sited within easy reach of all parts of the catchment area, and day hospitals, community clinics, and mental health centres ('subunits' of care) should be located where there is the greatest psychiatric morbidity. Links can then be made with all the actual and potential psychiatric services, including the primary care teams, in the locality. In Nottingham, where the 'hive' model has been developed, Tyrer (1985) found that with GP clinics incorporated into the subunit structure, there was a 20% fall in admissions to hospital. He perceived additional benefits to be the earlier detection of psychiatric illness and a greater ability to prevent relapse in those patients who traditionally are poor attenders at hospital clinics, such as the young and those who feel stigmatised by psychiatric intervention.

Ferguson *et al* (1992) by rating social and clinical functioning and satisfaction, found that this model of service was at least as good as, and on some measures superior to, hospital-based care. The service facilitated rehabilitation of patients whose use of day-hospital facilities increased.

The Greenwich sector model

In less well developed and resourced districts, mental health teams have tried pragmatic strategies to move closer to their primary care colleagues. The Greenwich sector model is an example of how a hospital-based service was reorganised in order to integrate with primary social as well as health services (Strathdee, 1992).

Five strategies were used: (a) the replacement of a hospital out-patient clinic by a regular session in the largest health centre, serving almost one-third of the patients; (b) all members of the mental health team, including CPNs, the occupational therapist, and the psychiatrist, held concurrent 'clinics'; (c) a similar service was planned with the second largest health centre; (d) both new referrals and follow-up patients were seen at the 'clinic'; (e) and face-to-face discussions with the GPs enabled joint working with many patients.

Previously the rehabilitation services had been based in a large psychiatric hospital outside the district, and so a second follow-up clinic was replaced with a peripatetic system of 'care coordination clinics' (a pragmatic form of case management) at the local day centre and area social services office. In these, all the agencies and professionals involved (including GPs and other members of the primary care team) met with the user and carer to review progress, agree actions, and designate clear responsibility for patients with severe and long-term mental health disorders. This system is described in detail elsewhere (Strathdee, 1992).

Although there was agreement that all professionals in the team had at least 70% of their case load constituted by the care of the most severely ill, two of the CPNs and the community occupational therapist held additional regular consultation sessions in the health centres. Relaxation, anxiety management, social skills, carer support, education, and other group sessions were undertaken. There were no practice counsellors, but there was sessional input from the local Relate group.

For patients resettled in sheltered accommodation, the most 'psychologically minded' GP in the nearest practice involved with patients in each home was identified. Through planned contacts, efforts were made to improve communication and offer professional support and training in the care of the residents.

A series of joint audit meetings was held between the psychiatric team and GPs to discuss aspects of service delivery – for example, crisis intervention, the development of treatment, and good practice pro formas.

The Falloon model

An approach focusing on family and carer education and support has come from Falloon (1989; Falloon *et al*, 1984), who has developed an effective, family-based treatment package for schizophrenia. The patient-oriented management combines optimal neuroleptic drug therapy, rehabilitation, counselling, problem-solving psychotherapy, crisis intervention, and practical assistance with problems such as finances and housing. The approach seeks to reduce stress in the individual and family through better understanding of the illness, and training in behavioural methods of problem-solving. Falloon *et al* (1990) advocate the application of this approach in primary care, with referrals processed initially by CPNs based in general practices.

The Norwegian integrated model

Hansen (1987) experimented with a model which involves even more integration with primary care, including not only primary health care but also social and other agencies. The community psychiatric service was organised separately from the hospital service; the psychiatric teams were based at the same location as primary care agencies, and met with the primary care teams. Referrals from both community and hospital agencies were accepted only if a primary care agency assumed responsibility for continuity of care. Both day and night emergencies were dealt with by the primary care teams, who had rapid access to the psychiatric services if they felt this to be necessary. Referrals for admission were always undertaken by the primary care coordinator, even when the judgement that it was necessary had come from the psychiatric team.

The three main aims formulated for the service were that it should: replace admissions with consultation and treatment within primary care; provide access to consultation for all primary care workers and agencies, regardless of profession; and execute ambulatory treatment without the patient being disconnected from the primary care provider. An 18% reduction in admissions was achieved over two years. Hansen, commenting on the experiment, considered that the role of primary care was at the core of any attempt to shift the emphasis of psychiatric treatment from an institution to the community.

Challenges for the future

Recent legislation and government policies (Secretaries of State, 1987, 1989, 1990; NHS Management Executive, 1991) have sought to increase the influence of primary care on the secondary services. Morley (1992) considers that it is necessary to recognise the interdependence of primary and secondary care, develop a shared understanding of needs and priorities, and by consultation reach agreement about quality and resources. Scott & Manintun (1992) believe that the contracting of services may improve planning, so that it takes account of cost–benefit, opportunity–cost, performance indicators, explicit standards, compliance, conformity and controls, and accountability. Their concern, however, is that the attention to the characteristics of groups may distract GPs from the assessment of, and response to, the needs of individual patients.

Challenges for the future include: how to effect the optimal liaison, if not integration, of primary and secondary mental health services; determination of the funding structure of mental health professionals in primary care, particularly nurse therapists and CPNs; whether to develop a system of *GP specialists*, with particular partners taking the lead in the planning and implementation of service developments in mental health.

Challenges to the effective provision of clinical services include: how to disseminate treatment techniques, such as cognitive and behavioural therapies; how best to involve primary care with social, housing, and other primary agencies in the implementation of legislation which aims at ensuring the priority of care for the long-term mentally ill; and the development of simple, reliable outcome measures of the effectiveness of interventions. Organisations such as the Mental Health Foundation have funded GPs in research in this area, resulting in pragmatic yet innovative suggestions to improve practice and organisation.

Kendrick (1990; Kendrick *et al*, 1991) proposes the establishment of practice policies for the care of patients with long-term mental disorders. He advocates registers of the 20–30 long-term mentally ill patients on each practice list. As with the successful implementation of such registers in the fields of care for diabetic and asthmatic patients (Wood, 1990), this improves the quality of clinical care. Horder (1990) has set out guidelines for the functioning of community hostels, including that they should be within easy access of shops, sports facilities, cinemas, day centres, workshops, and pubs. In the areas of clinical duties and responsibilities, emergencies, prescribing, and communication between mental health and primary services, plans for medical cover should be discussed before the admission of residents.

The profile of secondary and tertiary prevention as well as primary prevention is receiving attention by the funding bodies. The distinction between health promotion and disease management for chronic disorders is a fine one. For their more stable population, GPs are well placed to practise prevention, as they can use their frequent contacts with patients to recognise changes in behaviour or consultation habits (Widmer & Cadoret, 1979). Over time, they can play a key role in working with patients, carers, and relatives in recognising patterns of relapse and enabling timely, tested, and appropriate medication to be instituted (Birchwood *et al*, 1989).

Primary care is now in a position to influence the direction of community services for the next decade. As Morley (1992) concludes, primary care is becoming a partner in the mainstream, rather than at the margins of the health service. While developments over the next five years will be facilitated by the integration of district health authorities and family health services authorities, my belief is that the currency most used by primary care – committed practitioners working together locally – will have the larger influence.

References

BALINT, E. & NORRELL, J. (1973) *Six Minutes for the Patient: Interactions in General Practice Consultation*. London: Tavistock.

BIRCHWOOD, M., SMITH, J., MACMILLAN, F., *et al* (1989) Predicting relapse in schizophrenia: the development and implementation of an early signs monitoring system using patients and families as observers, a preliminary investigation. *Psychological Medicine*, **18**, 649–656.

BLACKBURN, I. M., BISHOPS, S., GLEN, A. I. M., *et al* (1981) The efficacy of cognitive therapy in depression: a treatment combination. *British Journal of Psychiatry*, **139**, 181–189.

BROWN, R., STRATHDEE, G., CHRISTIE-BROWN, J., *et al* (1988) A comparison of referrals to primary care and hospital outpatient clinics. *British Journal of Psychiatrists*, **153**, 168–173.

CATALAN, J., GATH, G., EDMONDS, G., *et al* (1984) Effects of non-prescribing of anxiolytics in general practice. 1. Controlled evaluation of psychiatric and social outcome; 2. Factors associated with outcome. *British Journal of Psychiatry*, **144**, 593–610.

CREED, F. & MARKS, B. (1989) Liaison psychiatry in general practice: a comparison of the liaison-attachment scheme and the shifted outpatient clinic models. *Journal of the Royal College of General Practitioners*, **39**, 514–517.

DARLING, C. & TYRER, P. (1990) Brief encounters in general practice: liaison in general practice psychiatry clinics. *Psychiatric Bulletin*, **14**, 592–594.

DEPARTMENT OF HEALTH AND SOCIAL SECURITY (1975) *Better Services for the Mentally Ill*, cmnd 6233. London: HMSO.

—— (1978) *Collaboration in Community Care. Central Health Services Council*. London: HMSO.

—— (1981) *Care in Action*. London: HMSO.

FALLOON, I. R. H. (1989) Behavioural approaches in schizophrenia. In *Scientific Approaches on Epidemiological and Social Psychiatry. Essays in Honour of Michael Shepherd* (eds P. Williams, G. Wilkinson & K. Rawnsley). London: Routledge.

——, BOYD, J. L. & MCGILL, C. W. (1984) *Family Care of Schizophrenia*. New York. Guilford Press.

——, SHANAHAN, W., LAPORTA, M., *et al* (1990) Integrated family, general practice and mental health care in the management of schizophrenia. *Journal of the Royal Society of Medicine*, **83**, 225–228.

FERGUSON, B. (1990) Clinical audit – a proposal. *Psychiatric Bulletin*, **14**, 275–277.

——, COOPER, S., BROTHWELL, J., *et al* (1992) The clinical evaluation of a new community psychiatric service based on general practice psychiatric clinics. *British Journal of Psychiatry* **160**, 493–497.

FRANCE, R. & ROBSON, M. (1986) *Behaviour Therapy in Primary Care*. London: Croom Helm.

—— & BRIDGES, K. (1987) Screening for psychiatric illness in general practice: the general practitioner versus the screening questionnaire. *Journal of the Royal College of General Practitioners*, **37**, 15–18.

GOLDBERG, D. (1991) Integrating mental health into primary care. In *Evaluation of Comprehensive Care of the Mentally Ill* (eds H. Freeman & J. Henderson). London: Gaskell.

GRIFFITH, R. (1988) *Community Care: An Agenda for Action*. London: HMSO.

HANSEN, V. (1987) Psychiatric service within primary care. Mode of organisation and influence on admission rates to a mental hospital. *Acta Psychiatrica Scandinavica*, **76**, 121–128.

HORDER, E. (1990) *Medical Care in Three Psychiatric Hostels*. London: Hampstead and Bloomsbury District Health Authority, Hampstead and South Barnet GP Forum, and the Hampstead Department of Community Medicine.

HORDER, J. (1988) Working with general practitioners. *British Journal of Psychiatry*, **153**, 513–521.

JOHNSON, D. A. (1973) An analysis of out-patient services. *British Journal of Psychiatry*, **122**, 301–306.

JOHNSON, S. & THORNICROFT, G. (1992) *A Survey of Mental Health Emergency Services in England and Wales*. Unpublished research report, Institute of Psychiatry, London.

JOHNSTONE, A. & SHEPLEY, M. (1986) The outcome of hidden neurotic illness treated in general practice. *Journal of the Royal College of General Practitioners*, **36**, 413–415.

JOHNSTONE, E. C., OWENS, D. G. C., GOLD, A., *et al* (1984) Schizophrenic patients discharged from hospital – a follow-up study. *British Journal of Psychiatry*, **145**, 586–590.

JONES, K., ROBINSON, M. & GOLIGHTLEY, P. (1986) Long-term psychiatric patients in the community. *British Journal of Psychiatry*, **149**, 537–540.

JOSEPH, P., BRIDGEWATER, J. A., RAMSDEN, S. S., *et al* (1990) A psychiatric clinic for the single homeless in a primary care setting in inner London. *Psychiatric Bulletin*, **14**, 270–271.

KAESER, A. C. & COOPER, B. (1971) The psychiatric out-patient, the general practitioner and the out-patient clinic; an operational study: a review. *Psychological Medicine*, **1**, 312–325.

KENDRICK, A. (1990) The challenge of the long-term mentally ill. In *The Royal College of General Practitioners Members' Reference Book*. London: Sterling Publications.

——, SIBBALD, B., BURNS, T., *et al* (1991) Role of general practitioners in care of long term mentally ill patients. *British Medical Journal*, **302**, 508–511.

KESSEL, N. (1963) Who ought to see a psychiatrist? *Lancet*, i, 1092–1095.

KINGDON, D. (1989) Mental health services: results of a survey of English district plans. *Psychiatric Bulletin*, **13**, 77–78.

LEE, A. S. & MURRAY, R. M. (1988) The long-term outcome of Maudsley depressives. *British Journal of Psychiatry*, **153**, 741–751.

LINDHOLM, H. (1983) Sectorised psychiatry. *Acta Psychiatrica Scandinavica*, **67** (suppl. 304).

LITTLEJOHNS, P. (1986) Domiciliary consultations – who benefits? *Journal of the Royal College of General Practitioners*, **36**, 313–315.

MARKS, I. (1985) Controlled trial of psychiatric nurse therapists in primary care. *British Medical Journal*, **240**, 1181–1184.

MELTZER, D., HALE, A., MALIK, S., *et al* (1991) Community care for patients with schizophrenia one year after hospital discharge. *British Medical Journal*, **303**, 1023–1026.

MITCHELL, A. R. K. (1985) Psychiatrists in primary health care settings. *British Journal of Psychiatry*, **147**, 371–379.

34   Strathdee

MORLEY, V. (1992) The future of primary health care. *British Medical Journal*, **304**, 1582–1583.

NHS MANAGEMENT EXECUTIVE (1991) *Integrating Primary and Secondary Health Care*. London: Department of Health.

PANTELLIS, C., TAYLOR, J. & CAMPBELL, P. (1988) The South Camden schizophrenia survey. *Bulletin of the Royal College of Psychiatrists*, **12**, 98–101.

PARKES, C. M., BROWN, G. W. & MONCK, E. M. (1962) The general practitioner and the schizophrenic patient. *British Medical Journal*, **1**, 972–976.

PATMORE, C. & WEAVER, J. (1990) *A Survey of Community Mental Health Centres*. London: Good Practices in Mental Health.

——, MANGEN, S., GRIFFITH, J., *et al* (1982) Community psychiatric nursing for neurotic patients: a controlled trial. *British Journal of Psychiatry*, **140**, 573–581.

PAYKEL, E. (1990) Innovations in mental health in the primary care system. In *Mental Health Service Evaluation* (eds I. Marks and R. Scott). Cambridge: Cambridge University Press.

PULLEN, I. M. & YELLOWLEES, A. (1985) Is communication improving between general practitioners and psychiatrists? *British Medical Journal*, **290**, 31–33.

—— & —— (1988) Scottish psychiatrists in primary health-care settings. A silent majority. *British Journal of Psychiatry*, **153**, 663–666.

ROYAL COLLEGE OF GENERAL PRACTITIONERS (1984) *Combined Reports on Prevention. Reports from General Practice, 18–21*. London: Royal College of General Practitioners.

SCOTT, M. & MANINTUN, M. (1992) Imposed change in general practice. *British Medical Journal*, **304**, 1548–1550.

SECRETARIES OF STATE SOCIAL SERVICES, WALES, NORTHERN IRELAND AND SCOTLAND (1987) *Promoting Better Health. The Government's Programme for Improving Primary Health Care*. London: HMSO.

—— (1989) *Working for Patients*. London: HMSO.

—— (1990) *Working for Patients*. London: HMSO.

SHARP, D. & MORRELL, D. (1989) The psychiatry of general practice. In *Scientific Approaches on Epidemiological and Social Psychiatry. Essays in Honour of Michael Shepherd* (eds P. Williams, G. Wilkinson & K. Rawnsley). London: Routledge.

SHEPHERD, M., COOPER, B., BROWN, A., *et al* (1966) *Psychiatric Illness in General Practice*. Oxford: Oxford University Press.

STANSFELD, S. (1991) Attitudes to developments in community psychiatry among general practitioners. *Psychiatric Bulletin*, **15**, 542–543.

STRATHDEE, G. (1988) Psychiatrists in primary care: the general practitioner viewpoint. *Family Medicine*, **5**, 111–115.

—— (1990) The delivery of psychiatric care. *Journal of the Royal Society of Medicine*, **83**, 222–225.

—— (1992) The interface between psychiatry and primary care in the management of schizophrenic patients in the community. In *Schizophrenia in the Community* (eds R. Jenkins, V. Field & R. Young). London: HMSO.

—— & WILLIAMS, P. (1984) A survey of psychiatrists in primary care: the silent growth of a new service. *Journal of the Royal College of General Practitioners*, **34**, 615–618.

——, FISHER, N. & McDONALD, E. (1992) Establishing psychiatric attachments to general practice: a six stage plan. *Psychiatric Bulletin*, **16**, 284–286.

—— & THORNICROFT, G. (1992) The principles of setting up mental health services in the community. In *Principles of Social Psychiatry* (eds J. Leff & D. Bhugra). Oxford: Blackwell Scientific.

SUTHERBY, K., SRINATH, S. & STRATHDEE, G. (1992) The domiciliary consultation service: outdated anachronism or essential part of community psychiatric outreach? *Health Trends* (in press).

TANSELLA, M. (1989) Evaluating community psychiatric services. In *Scientific Approaches on Epidemiological and Social Psychiatry. Essays in Honour of Michael Shepherd* (eds P. Williams, G. Wilkinson & K. Rawnsley). London: Routledge.

TEASDALE, J. D., FENNELL, M. J. V., HIBBERT, G. A., *et al* (1984) Cognitive therapy for major depressive disorder in primary care. *British Journal of Psychiatry*, **144**, 400–406.

THORNICROFT, G. & BEBBINGTON, P. (1989) Deinstitutionalisation: from hospital closure to service development. *British Journal of Psychiatry*, **155**, 739–753.

TYRER, P. (1984) Psychiatric clinics in general practice: an extension of community care. *British Journal of Psychiatry*, **145**, 9-14.

—— (1985) The 'hive' system: a model for a psychiatric service. *British Journal of Psychiatry*, **146**, 571-575.

——, TURNER, R. & JOHNSON, A. (189) Integrated hospital and community psychiatric services and use of inpatient beds. *British Medical Journal*, **299**, 298-300.

WIDMER, R. B. & CADORET, R. J. (1979) Depression in family practice: changes in pattern of family visits and complaints during subsequent developing depressions. *Journal of Family Practice*, **9**, 1017-1021.

WOOD, J. (1990) A review of diabetes care: initiatives in primary care settings. *Health Trends*, **22**, 39-43.

WOOFF, K., GOLDBERG, D. & FRYERS, T. (1988) The practice of community psychiatric nursing and mental health social work in Salford: some implications for community care. *British Journal of Psychiatry*, **153**, 30-37.

WORLD HEALTH ORGANIZATION (1973) *Psychiatry and Primary Medical Care*. Copenhagen: WHO Regional Office for Europe.

—— (1983) *First Contact Mental Health Care*. Copenhagen: WHO Regional Office for Europe.

3 Epidemiology of mental disorder in general practice

DAVID GOLDBERG

Goldberg & Huxley (1991) have suggested a framework for understanding the pathway by which individuals become defined as mentally ill and eventually reach mental illness services. This framework serves to organise epidemiological data about mental illness into groupings which depend upon how far along this pathway individuals have reached, and draws our attention to the 'filters' through which patients must pass in order to receive specialised treatments. In many countries most patients are referred to the mental illness services by other professionals, so that one can postulate a filter between the community and the referring professional, as well as between that professional and the mental illness service.

The framework consisted of five levels at which survey data could be considered, each one corresponding to a stage on the pathway to psychiatric care. A set of four filters were postulated between these five levels, and these are shown in Table 3.1, which gives the most recent estimates of the number of people who will suffer an episode of a mental disorder lasting at least two weeks during a calendar year, expressed as a rate per 1000 population at risk (Goldberg & Huxley, 1991). The most recent British estimate of morbidity in primary care comes from the third national study (Her Majesty's Stationery Office, 1986), which gives an annual period prevalence of 101.4/1000 for episodes of mental disorder diagnosable by ICD-9 criteria (World Health Organization, 1978); this figure is strikingly similar to Shepherd's earlier estimate of 102/1000 in 1966, or the annual rate of 94/1000 in Groningen calculated by Giel and his colleagues (Shepherd *et al*, 1966; Giel *et al*, 1990).

Many studies have been conducted on consecutive attenders, without calculating population risks. Ormel & Giel (1990) review 16 well-conducted studies in primary-care settings, in which over half show rates of mental disorder according to the GP in the 20–39% range, but the spread is wide, so that it is clear that physicians vary widely in their diagnostic practices. By and large, recent surveys have confirmed earlier findings: in consulting

TABLE 3.1
Five levels and four filters, with estimates of annual period prevalence rates at each level (from Goldberg & Huxley, 1991)

Level	Rate/1000/year
Level 1. The community	260–315
First filter: illness behaviour	
Level 2. Total mental morbidity – attenders in primary care	230
Second filter: ability to detect disorder	
Level 3. Mental disorders identified by doctors ('conspicuous psychiatric morbidity')	101.5
Third filter: referral to mental illness services	
Level 4. Total morbidity – mental illness services	23.5
Fourth filter: admission to psychiatric beds	
Level 5. Psychiatric in-patients	5.71

settings, patients with diagnosable psychiatric disorders most commonly consult for physical symptoms, and it is useful to use classifications of complaint which take into account the relationship (if any) between their presenting complaint and the psychiatric disorder found by standardised assessment.

Bridges & Goldberg (1985) used an expanded version of an earlier classification, and produced an operational definition of illnesses in which there is a psychiatric disorder present, but the patient is seeking help for somatic symptoms. Four conditions have to be satisfied in order to describe a patient as a 'case' of 'somatisation':

(a) the patient must be seeking help for somatic symptoms
(b) the patient must attribute these symptoms to some physical disorder
(c) a specific mental disorder as defined by research criteria must be present
(d) the somatic symptoms are not due to physical disease, but can be thought of as part of the mental disorder.

The majority of the mental disorders satisfying criterion (c) in consulting settings are depressive illnesses and anxiety states, and these also make up the majority of cases presenting as psychological complaints. However, in the case of somatisation, patients do not consider that they have such a disorder: they are seeking help for the somatic symptom which is part of the mental disorder.

It can be seen from Table 3.2 that almost one-third of patients with new illnesses have a mental disorder, but the majority of these do indeed satisfy criteria for 'somatisation'. Most of the 'hidden psychiatric disorders' – that is to say, those that are present but are undetected by the doctor – are either cases of somatisation or are disorders that are in fact unrelated to the disorder for which help is being sought.

TABLE 3.2

Relationship of mental disorder to reason for consultation in 590 new onsets of illness in primary care in Manchester (from Bridges & Goldberg, 1985)

	All patients (n = 590)	Psychiatric cases only (n = 195)
Not mentally ill	67%	N/A
Physical illness with secondary mental disorder	1%	3.2%
Unrelated physical and mental disorder	8%	24.0%
Somatisation	20%	57.0%
Entirely mentally ill	5%	15.0%
Total	100%	100%

It is possible to compare the morbidity in primary care with that seen by the specialised services by examining data from the Morbidity Statistics in General Practice for 1981–82 (HMSO, 1986) and data prepared from the Salford Case Register in 1983 (Table 3.3). It can be seen that the period prevalence of mental disorders is approximately five times higher in primary care, but the distribution of the various diagnostic groups is very different. Only depressive illnesses are equally common in the two settings, and these comprise about a quarter of all cases seen. However 'other neuroses' (mainly anxiety disorders and somatic presentation of affective illnesses) and adjustment disorders together make up well over 60% of the cases seen in primary care, but only 20% of those seen by mental illness services. By contrast, about one-third of cases seen by mental illness services are schizophrenias and dementias, to be compared with only 4% in primary care: furthermore, the rates per 1000 treated by mental illness services are even higher for these disorders, implying that some patients with these disorders are not in contact with their family doctors, but are treated by the specialist services.

TABLE 3.3

Rates per 1000 population at risk per year, by diagnosis for primary care (Morbidity Statistics in General Practice, 1981–82; HMSO, 1986) and mental illness services (Malcolm Cleverly of the Salford Case Register; data for 1983)

Services	Primary care		Mental illness: all patients	
Organic, dementia	2.2	(2.2%)	2.75	(13.2%)
Schizophrenia	2.0	(2.0%)	4.08	(19.6%)
Affective psychosis	3.0	(3.0%)	1.47	(7.0%)
Depression	28.0	(27.6%)	5.35	(25.6%)
Other neurosis	35.7	(35.2%)	2.46	(11.8%)
Alcohol, drugs	2.7	(2.7%)	1.37	(6.6%)
Personality disorder	1.1	(1.1%)	1.62	(7.8%)
Adjustment, other diagnoses	26.7	(26.3%)	1.74	(8.4%)
All diagnoses	101.4	(100.0%)	20.87	(100.0%)

However, it can also be seen that nearly all the cases of adjustment disorders and neuroses, and about three-quarters of all cases of depression, are in fact treated in primary care. It is clear that GPs therefore need to have available a classification which is adapted for these special groups, but which will also enable them to diagnose and manage those with severe mental disorders – since the period prevalence of the top three diagnoses in Table 3.3 is approximately similar in the two settings. Finally, staff in primary care are constantly seeing patients who have both physical and psychological disorders, and they will need to have a classification available which takes account of this fact.

Research diagnoses versus clinical diagnoses

Studies where independent assessments have been made by research psychiatrists typically show two sorts of discrepancy – patients deemed to have mental disorders by their GPs who do not meet standard diagnostic criteria for mental disorders; and those thought mentally ill by the researchers but treated for physical symptoms by their GPs (Goldberg & Huxley, 1991). Little harm comes from the first sort of discrepancy other than unnecessary prescription for psychotropic drugs: the fact that the disorder has been recognised, together with the active therapeutic stance of the GP, probably speeds resolution of symptoms. It must also be admitted that not all of those who are found to be mentally unwell by the researchers actually want their GP to see them as mentally ill. Many know that they have transient disorders; some do not wish to have treatment for symptoms such as panic attacks even when it is offered, while others are mainly concerned to have their doctor exclude serious physical causes for the somatic symptoms which are troubling them. Failure to detect disorder can therefore be a collusive phenomenon between a reluctant patient and a GP who is unsure what to do about any disorder that is detected.

Despite the exceptions mentioned, it is important that staff in primary care are able to detect psychological disorders, since several different surveys have shown that detected disorders have a better outlook than those that remain undetected.

Alternative classification of mental disorders seen in primary care

One of the pioneers of 'moral' treatment for the mentally ill, Dr Tuke, observed that "a classification is a fiction, that will discharge its function if it proves to be the most apt for its time". Different professional groups quite legitimately need classifications for different purposes, and it is most unlikely that the purposes of psychiatrists working in private practice will be remotely the same as those of primary care physicians working for a National Health Service.

Where family doctors are concerned, there seem to be three major official choices which they can make when they are confronted by a mentally ill patient. They can use what are essentially classifications designed by psychiatrists (such as ICD–10 or DSM–IV); they can use adaptations of these classifications produced by their colleagues (such as the ICPC classification (Lamberts & Wood, 1990) of the World Organisation of National Colleges, Academies & Academic Associations of GPs – WONCA); or they can use triaxial classifications, with separate assessments of physical health, psychological adjustment, and social adjustment.

Classifications designed by psychiatrists such as ICD–10 or DSM–IV are generally found to be overcomplicated for use in general medical settings. GPs do not really need to recognise 26 varieties of major depressive episode, or 31 different kinds of mood, anxiety and somatoform disorder. However, the simplified version of the predecessor of this classification produced by WONCA has troubles of its own, since the 21 conditions recognised are sometimes overinclusive, and at other times do not allow recognition of important syndromes. For example, dementia and delirium are included together as 'organic psychoses', and all childhood disorders are grouped together, while chronic neurosis, fatigue syndromes, and even chronic psychosis are nowhere to be found. Nor is the user given any advice concerning treatment. An important British research study showed that triaxial classifications – using psychological illness, physical illness, and social circumstances as the axes – produced better agreement between observers than use of the official classifications (Jenkins *et al*, 1988). However, the obstinate fact is that GPs will not use formal triaxial systems in their routine work, so that they seem destined for use by researchers.

Faced with these unappealing alternatives, many GPs try to avoid classification wherever possible, and to do this because they wish to remain 'patient centred'. Doctors who do this will only diagnose depression by *agreeing with the patient*. They tend to use vague umbrella terms like 'emotional distress' to cover the multiplicity of psychological disorders which confront them. There is, of course, no necessary antithesis between being patient centred and finding out what is actually wrong with the patient, but there is a real risk that such taxophobic doctors may miss, and therefore undertreat, many cases of emotional distress.

The 10th revision of the International Classification of Disease

The 10th revision of the ICD (ICD–10) has some important differences from its predecessor where mental disorders are concerned. The traditional dichotomy between 'psychosis' and 'neurosis' is no longer recognised; the user is provided with clear diagnostic criteria for use in research projects; and special versions of the classification are available for use in specialised settings.

The special version of the mental disorders section of ICD–10 for use in primary care

The designers of ICHPCC–2 were clearly correct to focus their classification down onto a couple of dozen disorders that are commonly encountered in primary care, but it seems likely that the borders between the various disorders could be drawn in a more useful way, and it would be of great importance to ensure that primary-care workers were given assistance in recognising disorders for which there are treatments.

The WHO has therefore produced a new classification for use in primary care, to be called ICD–10 (PHC). Twenty-four conditions have been identified for use in primary care settings on the grounds that they are reasonably common, and each has a clear management plan associated with it. The classification has initially been presented to primary care doctors in the form of a set of 24 cards, one for each condition. The front of each card has details of the presenting complaints, the diagnostic features and the differential diagnosis of the disorder, while the back has detailed plans about the management of the condition.

The cards will be accompanied by a choice of other supporting materials: a glossary giving definitions of all technical terms used; advice on the way in which psychological inquiries should be fitted into the course of the usual medical consultation, and the circumstances which should act as 'triggers' for the GP to focus upon psychological adjustment; and a diagnostic flowchart showing how the various diagnoses logically relate to one another.

The conditions which have been suggested for inclusion in ICD–10(PHC) is shown below. It is likely that this list will be modified in the light of experience gained in field trials, and it is the intention of the WHO to produce a classification which is reliable and is found to be useful by workers in general medical settings.

(a) *F0 Organic disorders*
     F00   Dementia
     F05   Delirium
(b) *F1 Psychoactive substance abuse*
     F10   Alcohol use disorder
     F11   Drug use disorder
     F17.1 Tobacco use

(c) *F3 Psychotic disorders*
    F20   Chronic psychotic disorder
    F23   Acute psychotic disorder
    F31   Bipolar disorder
(d) *F4 Mood, stress-related and anxiety disorders*
    F32   Depression
    F40   Phobic disorders
    F41.0 Panic disorder
    F41.1 Generalised anxiety
    F41.2 Mixed anxiety and depression
    F43   Adjustment disorder
    F44   Dissociative disorder
    F45   Unexplained somatic complaints
    F48   Neurasthenia
(e) *F5 Physiological disorders*
    F50   Eating disorder
    F51   Sleep problems
    F52   Sexual disorders
(f) *F7 Developmental disorders*
    F70   Mental retardation
(g) *F9 Disorders of childhood*
    F90   Hyperkinetic disorder
    F91   Conduct disorder
    F98   Enuresis

Specimen card for major depressive episode

On the front of the card the user is reminded that depression frequently presents with one or more physical symptoms, although further enquiry will reveal depression or loss of interest. The diagnostic features of the disorder are then described, and the primary worker is reminded that symptoms from anxiety are frequently also present (see Fig. 3.1(a)).

On the back of each card (Fig. 3.1(b)) the primary care worker is provided with management guidelines, always gathered under four headings: essential information for patient and family; specific counselling to be given; medication; and indications for specialist consultation. SRI items are picked out in bold type – these are essential. However, the main value of the card is probably the information that is not in bold type – since this is less likely to be well known to staff in primary care.

The assessment of ICD–10(PHC)

The adequacy of the list of 24 categories described so far is being tested in field trials in 14 countries. The first trials are concerned with the inter-rater

DEPRESSION - F32* Management Guidelines

Essential Information for Patient and Family

1) Depression is common and effective treatments are available.
2) Depression is not weakness or laziness; patients are trying their hardest.

Specific Counselling to Patient and Family

1) **Ask about risk of suicide.** Can the patient be sure of not acting on suicidal ideas? Close supervision by family or friends may be needed.

2) Plan short-term **activities which give enjoyment or build confidence.**

3) **Resist pessimism and self-criticism.** Do not act on pessimistic ideas (e.g. ending marriage, leaving job). Do not concentrate on negative or guilty thoughts.

4) If physical symptoms are present, **discuss link between physical symptoms and mood** (see card on Unexplained Somatic Complaints F45*).

5) After improvement, discuss signs of relapse, plan with patient action to be taken if signs of relapse occur.

Medication

1) **Consider** antidepressant drugs if sad mood or loss of interest are prominent for **at least 2 weeks and 4 or more of these symptoms are present:**

- Fatigue or loss of energy — Disturbed sleep
- Guilt or self-reproach — Poor concentration
- Thoughts of death or suicide — Disturbed appetite
- Agitation OR slowing of movement and speech

If good response to one drug in the past, use that again.
If older or medically ill, use newer medication with fewer side effects.
If anxious or unable to sleep, use more sedating drug.

2) **Build up to effective dose** (e.g. imipramine starting at 25 to 50 mg each night and increasing to 100-150 mg by 10 days) - lower doses if older or medically ill.

3) **Explain how medications should be used:**
- Medication must be taken every day.
- Improvement will build over 2-3 weeks.
- Mild side effects may occur and usually fade in 7-10 days.
- Check with the doctor before stopping medication.

4) **Continue** antidepressant at least 3 months after symptoms improve.

Specialist Consultation

1) If **suicide risk** is severe, consider consultation and hospitalization.
2) If **significant depression persists,** consider consultation about other therapies.
3) More **intensive psychotherapies** (e.g. cognitive therapy, interpersonal therapy) may be useful for acute treatment and relapse prevention.

ICD-10 PHC
MNH/MND/93.1

DEPRESSION - F32*

Presenting Complaints

May present initially with one or more physical symptoms (fatigue, pain). Further inquiry will reveal depression or loss of interest.

Sometimes presents as irritability.

Diagnostic Features

LOW OR SAD MOOD

LOSS OF INTEREST OR PLEASURE

Associated symptoms are frequently present:
- Disturbed **sleep**
- **Guilt** or low self-worth
- **Fatigue** or loss of energy
- Poor **concentration**
- Disturbed **appetite**
- **Suicidal** thoughts or acts

Movements and speech may be slowed, but may also appear agitated.

Symptoms of anxiety or nervousness are frequently also present.

Differential Diagnosis

If hallucinations (hearing voices, seeing visions) or delusions (strange or unusual beliefs) are present, see also see card on Acute Psychotic Disorders F23* about management of these problems. If possible, consider consultation about management.

If history of manic episode (excitement, elevated mood, rapid speech) is present, see card on: Bipolar Disorder F31*.

If heavy alcohol use is present, see card on: Alcohol Use Disorders F10*, Drug Disorders F10*.

Fig. 3.1 Specimen card showing on the front (a) diagnosis of depression according to ICD-10(PHC), and on the back (b) management guidelines.

reliability of the assessments and how well the classification fits with the problems encountered by participating primary care doctors, as well as the acceptability and usefulness of the classification. The classification is expected to be modified further in the light of the field trials, and is to be made available towards the end of 1994.

The success of the new classification will probably depend upon the perceived usefulness of the management plans provided: it has the potential greatly to improve both the detection and management of disorders in primary care.

Acknowledgements

The work of WHO's new classification for primary care is reported by kind permission of Professor Norman Sartorius and Dr Bedirhan Ustun. Other members of the working party include: Dr D'A. Busnello (Brazil); Dr J. Cooper (UK); Dr N. Dedeoglu (Turkey); Dr Deva (Malaysia); Dr Gureje (Nigeria); and Dr N. Wig (India).

References

BRIDGES, K. & GOLDBERG, D. (1985) Somatic presentations of DSM–3 psychiatric disorders in primary care. *Journal of Psychosomatic Research*, **29**, 563–569.

GIEL, R., KOETER, M. & ORMEL, J. (1990) Detection and referral of primary care patients with mental health problems: the 2nd and 3rd filter. In *The Public Health Impact of Mental Disorder* (eds D. Goldberg & D. Tantam). Bern: Hogrefe-Huber.

GOLDBERG, D. & HUXLEY, P. (1991) *Common Mental Disorders – A Biosocial Model*. London: Routledge.

HER MAJESTY'S STATIONERY OFFICE (1986) *Morbidity Statistics from General Practice*. London: HMSO.

JENKINS, R., SMEETON, N. & SHEPHERD, M. (1988) Classification of mental disorder in primary care. *Psychological Medicine* (monograph suppl. 12).

LAMBERTS, H. & WOOD, M. (1990) *ICPC: International Classification of Primary Care*. Oxford: Oxford University Press.

ORMEL, J. & GIEL, R. (1990) Medical effects of non-recognition of affective disorders in primary care. In *Psychological Disorders in General Medical Settings* (eds N. Sarotorius, D. Goldberg, G. de Girolamo, *et al*). Bern: Huber, Hogrefe.

SHEPHERD, M., COOPER, A. B., BROWN, A. C., *et al* (1966) *Psychiatric Illness in General Practice*. Oxford: Oxford University Press.

TUKE, D. H. (1858) *A Manual of Psychological Medicine*. Edinburgh: Livingstone.

WORLD HEALTH ORGANIZATION (1978) *Mental Disorders: Glossary and Guide to their Classification in Accordance with the Ninth Revision of the International Classification of Diseases* (ICD–9). Geneva: WHO.

——— (1990) *ICD-10, Chapter V. Mental & Behavioural Disorders: Diagnostic Criteria for Research*. Geneva: WHO.

4 Law and ethics

DEREK CHISWICK

The management of patients with serious psychiatric disorders in general practice requires consideration of legal and ethical issues. Psychiatric disorders commonly produce abnormalities of function and behaviour of such severity that they may have serious implications, not only for the patient, but also for the patient's family, friends, and perhaps colleagues. In these circumstances doctors necessarily take a broad view of the patient and the need for treatment. For nearly 200 years, successive governments in Britain have decided that certain aspects of the treatment of mentally ill people by doctors should be subject to legislation. In no other branch of medicine have special powers been given to doctors whereby some patients may be admitted to hospital and treated against their will.

In this chapter there is discussion of: the application of the law to psychiatry in the setting of general practice; some common ethical problems encountered in treating psychiatric disorder, including confidentiality, the management of suicide risk, and coercive treatment; the effects of psychiatric disorders on functions such as driving, making a will, and the capacity to manage one's affairs; and contemporary issues concerning the treatment of mentally disordered offenders. No attempt has been made to provide authoritative legal opinion or a gold standard of ethical practice. Few problems in this area have clear-cut legal or ethical answers. In cases of particular difficulty advice should always be sought from colleagues, and from medical defence and other appropriate professional organisations.

Psychiatry and the law

Purpose and ethics of mental health legislation

Psychiatric disorders may affect the judgement and reasoning of patients such that they lack the capacity to recognise the effects of the illness upon themselves and others. Where these effects threaten the safety of patients or those about them, mental health legislation makes possible compulsory admission to hospital for treatment. Legislation is enabling rather than directive; it enables action to be taken but does not direct that it should do so. Mental health law must provide a balanced safeguard, protecting the interests of the patient, family, professional carers, and society at large.

Three civil rights underpin mental health legislation:

(a) the right to freedom and liberty
(b) the right to be protected from the dangerous consequences of another person's mental disorder
(c) the right to receive compulsory treatment against one's wishes but in one's own interest.

The third of these is often forgotten. If as a consequence of serious mental disorder a person is jeopardising his/her own safety or that of the family, then in a civilised society he/she may reasonably expect others to intervene and take action.

Requirements for compulsory admission

There are three essential components in any compulsory admission:

(a) the presence of a mental disorder
(b) risk to the health or safety of the patient or of others
(c) no alternative to compulsory admission to hospital as a means of safeguarding the risk.

It cannot be overemphasised that these components are matters for clinical judgement. Few have been tested in court. In general, doctors are more likely to be challenged for failing to implement compulsory admission than for doing so.

In this chapter the legislation principally discussed is the Mental Health Act 1983, which is applicable in England and Wales. The general thrust of the Mental Health (Scotland) Act 1984 and the Mental Health (Northern Ireland) Order 1986 is similar, although there are some important differences in detail. Readers should refer to the Acts and the codes of practice which Departments of Health have been obliged to produce. Definitions and explanations of some of the legislation are contained in the Appendix at the end of this chapter.

Mental disorder

Mental disorder is a generic term defined in the Mental Health Act as "mental illness, arrested or incomplete development of mind, psychopathic disorder and any other disorder or disability of mind".

This broad definition could include within its ambit just about every psychiatric disorder known to mankind. However, some disorders are specifically excluded, for example dependence on alcohol or drugs and sexual deviancy. In general, sections concerning shorter periods of compulsory detention simply specify 'mental disorder', whereas detention for longer periods requires the clinician to state the subcategory of mental disorder from which the patient suffers. GPs are most likely to implement the Act in cases of 'mental illness', a term that is undefined except in the Northern Ireland legislation.

Sections 2, 3 and 4 (see Appendix)

It is recommended policy, as far as possible, to avoid the use of emergency admission under section 4. Local factors, particularly the availability of doctors approved under section 12, often dictate procedure. Emergency admission is easy to implement and requires one medical recommendation. Longer detention (admission for assessment and admission for treatment) is more complex to apply; it requires two medical recommendations. All compulsory admissions require an application by the nearest relative or an approved social worker to the managers of the hospital. The Mental Health Act does not specify any lower age limit; its use for children under 16 is uncommon.

Effecting admission to hospital

A recommendation by a GP for the compulsory admission of a patient to hospital is a clinical decision which should be reached after consultation with other professional staff. A broad perspective must be taken concerning a variety of factors:

(a) the nature of the mental disorder and the appropriateness of compulsory admission to hospital
(b) alternative measures, including voluntary admission, and their implications
(c) the implications of compulsory admission for the patient
(d) the attitudes of relatives or carers
(e) the practical task of organising admission to hospital.

Roles of approved social worker and nearest relative

Making an application is likely to be distressing for a relative, and it is recommended that an approved social worker should normally perform the function. Disagreement between medical practitioner and social worker on the need for compulsory admission may be difficult to resolve. Alternatives should be explored and, if necessary, other professional staff (e.g. a community psychiatric nurse) involved; the patient should not be abandoned. Facts should be recorded in the notes.

Practical aspects of admission to hospital of detained patients

Practical arrangements for the admission of patients under the Mental Health Act vary across regions. The GP in effecting admission must have due regard for the safety of the patient, relatives, professional staff, and him/herself. Advice should be obtained from the local psychiatric service; in some areas community psychiatric nurses may be involved. At times it may be necessary to involve police. Ideally there should be a procedure laid down in advance, particularly for emergencies occurring out of hours.

Treatment in hospital

Consent

The treatment of psychiatric disorders in hospital is not the responsibility of GPs. However, the Mental Health Act 1983 introduced in Part IV of the legislation important measures in relation to consent to treatment which are of interest to all doctors. The Act lays down entirely novel procedures, but these apply only to detained patients (with one significant exception), and only to medical treatment for mental disorder. The Act therefore has nothing to say about treatment for physical disorders except insofar as a physical disorder (e.g. pneumonia) may cause a psychiatric disorder (e.g. delirium) for which a patient is detained in hospital. In effect, treatments have been divided into three categories; for this discussion they are given the unofficial descriptions 'irreversible', 'causing concern', and 'other'.

Irreversible treatments. In this category (section 57) only two psychiatric treatments are presently included. These are psychosurgery, and surgically implanted hormones given to reduce male sex drive. These treatments are exceedingly rare. Between 1989 and 1991 there were 56 psychosurgical operations carried out in England and no surgical implantations of anti-male sex hormones for mental disorder. Section 57 requires that the patient is able to, and gives, consent. It also requires three people appointed by the Mental Health Act Commission to satisfy themselves that the patient has given valid consent and that the treatment should be given. Section 57 is of significance in that it applies to *all* patients whether detained or informal. In Scotland similar provisions apply only to detained patients.

Treatments causing concern. At present the only treatments in this category (section 58) are electroconvulsive treatment (ECT), and medicines given for mental disorder for more than three months during compulsory detention. These treatments can only be given if either the patient gives consent, or a doctor appointed for the purpose by the Mental Health Act Commission has examined the patient and certified that the treatment should be given. These provisions are in common use; between 1989 and 1991 there were over 7000 second opinions under section 58 obtained from the Mental Health Act Commission.

All other treatments for mental disorder. This includes all treatments not referred to above and, in particular, medicines for mental disorder given for up to three months during compulsory detention. For these treatments no consent under the Act is necessary.

Part IV of the Act deals with consent to treatment and is commonly applied in relation to the use of ECT and neuroleptic medication or prophylactic lithium. Part IV of the Act provides protection not only for the clinician, who may provide treatment without consent, but also for the patient, who obtains the benefit of an independent second opinion. In former years it was not uncommon for severely depressed and retarded patients who were unable to give consent, but who did not actively refuse treatment, to be given ECT after discussion with a relative and perhaps after obtaining an informal second opinion from a colleague. This practice is becoming increasingly uncommon because of the advantages obtained by treatment under Part IV. The latter does of course require detention under the Act.

Compulsory treatment in the community

There are two aspects of compulsory treatment in the community which warrant discussion. Firstly, there are the practical aspects of its administration. Patients with schizophrenia who remain well when on medication but who relapse after defaulting from treatment are common in practice. Can such patients receive medication in the community against their will? In short the answer is no. It may be possible to persuade them, but they cannot be forced. It would be unthinkable for a community psychiatric nurse, or practice nurse, to administer an intramuscular injection in the patient's own home and against the patient's will.

The second problem is the legal issue. In theory, patients on leave of absence in the community under section 17 are still subject to Part IV of the Act and may therefore receive treatment without consent under section 58. However, when the period of leave expires, and if they have not previously been recalled to hospital, then the authority to administer treatment lapses. In an important legal case, a judge ruled that patients may not be admitted to hospital simply for an overnight stay in order to reinstitute leave of absence. Compulsory admission to hospital must be for the purpose of receiving treatment *in hospital* (Dyer, 1987).

At the end of 1992, a man suffering from schizophrenia climbed into the lions' cage at London Zoo and was badly mauled. The incident was recorded on amateur video and the subsequent wide television coverage raised public and political awareness of the problems of providing proper care for patients with schizophrenia. Proposals for a community supervision order were put forward by the Royal College of Psychiatrists (1993). This would apply to a previously detained patient and would consist of an agreement to accept treatment and supervision in the community. A patient who subsequently defaulted could be liable to recall to hospital.

The Department of Health (1993) conducted a review of compulsory care in the community. It rejected the College proposal and instead suggested widening the powers of guardianship, removing the six-month limit on leave of absence and introducing what it calls 'supervised discharge' for detained patients. Legislation is likely to follow. Many observers feel that improved care in the community cannot be obtained by legislation and that the provision of adequate resources is more important than new laws.

Guardianship

Guardianship (section 7) provides a framework for compulsory care in the community but does not necessarily effect it. It can be made only in respect of a person aged over 16. It confers on a nominated guardian the power to require the patient to reside at a specified place and to attend for medical treatment and appropriate occupational or educational training. It does not provide authority for the administration of medication without consent, and the place of residence may not be a hospital. In practice it may be useful in the management of some people with learning disabilities. However, the requirement that they must suffer from either mental impairment or severe mental impairment (see Appendix) excludes from its provisions the great majority of people with learning disabilities.

A crucial component is that the patient must recognise "the authority" of the guardian and be prepared to work with the various agencies concerned. Without such voluntary agreement on the part of the patient, guardianship is of little value.

Discharge of detained patients

There has been serious concern over the discharge of psychiatric patients to the community in the absence of proper plans for their continuing care. The codes of practice lay down procedures which should be adopted before such patients are discharged. Discharge-planning case conferences have become common practice and are frequently attended by GPs. The importance of a discharge plan which identifies measures to be taken and the persons responsible for them cannot be overemphasised.

Statutory bodies involved in the care of compulsory patients

Mental Health Act Commission

The complexity of overseeing certain aspects of the Mental Health Act was recognised by Parliament. The Mental Health Act Commission (MHAC) is a statutory body constituted as a special health authority. It consists of 90 part-time members, including lawyers, doctors, nurses, social workers, and laymen. It is required to inspect the manner in which hospitals implement the provisions of the Mental Health Act, to visit and interview detained patients, to provide second opinions for the purposes of Part IV of the Act, and to produce a biennial report (Mental Health Act Commission, 1991). The MHAC has taken an interest in various aspects of treatment of the mentally disordered, including care in the community. Broadly analogous functions are carried out by the Mental Welfare Commission for Scotland, and the Mental Health Act Commission for Northern Ireland.

Mental health review tribunals

Rights of appeal against detection are specified in the Mental Health Act. Virtually all patients, other than those detained under emergency powers, may apply to have their case considered by a mental health review tribunal. A tribunal consists of three members: a legally qualified chairman, a medical member, and a lay member. The decisions of a tribunal are limited to refusing or directing discharge. However, they may make recommendations concerning leave of absence or transfer to another hospital. These powers are often applied in the cases of patients detained in secure hospitals. A mental health review tribunal is not a court, but procedure in the last ten years has become increasingly legalistic. In many instances patients are represented by counsel.

Ethical problems in practice

When clinicians refer to ethical problems in psychiatry, they are usually considering a complex case in which clinical, legal, and ethical dilemmas overlap. It is often impossible to consider any of these aspects in isolation, and rarely is the key to a problem provided solely by a legal or ethical solution. In practice decisions have to be made about treating real people. The balancing of conflicting interests, to which previous reference has been made, is not easy. In psychiatric practice most dilemmas involve issues of coercive treatment in its various forms, or confidentiality. The following discussions are based on examples.

Case 1

A 30-year-old man with a history of hospital treatment for schizophrenia lives alone in his flat. He has defaulted from out-patient contact and has refused to allow a community psychiatric nurse into his home. His mother normally contacts him by telephone and visits weekly. On her visit she knows that he is in the flat, but he does not answer the door or the telephone. His mother contacts the GP for advice.

The first issue is a clinical one of establishing whether the man is ill, and if so ill enough to warrant assessment or treatment in hospital. It will take time and detective work to answer these questions. Involvement of an approved social worker and community psychiatric nurse to make inquiries locally may be helpful. There are ethical requirements to protect the interests of the patient and to address the concerns of his mother. Forced entry to the flat may have to be considered (under section 135 – see Appendix). Any removal of the patient from his flat to hospital must be carried out legally, safely, and professionally.

Case 2

A 45-year-old woman with chronic schizophrenia lives in hostel accommodation. She is socially impaired but is for the most part unobtrusive and self-absorbed. Her sister remains in close contact. The staff bring to the attention of her GP an ulcerating lesion of the skin of her left breast. She is referred to a consultant surgeon, and clinical examination strongly suggests carcinoma of the breast. The patient refuses to discuss surgery and speaks about people trying to kill her. The surgeon confirms that without surgical treatment the patient will develop an invasive fungating lesion of her chest wall.

Surgery is essential in the best interests of the patient. It would be necessary to discuss the situation with the patient's sister. She cannot give consent for the patient (no person can 'give consent' for another adult to have treatment) but to have her involvement is good clinical practice. Subject to the agreement of the surgeon and anaesthetist, treatment could go ahead without the patient's consent on the basis of the duty of care owed towards the patient. The latter was established by the House of Lord's decision in *Re F* (Gunn, 1990). The patient may passively accept admission to hospital; if not, much time and effort will be necessary to effect her admission in a sensible and professional manner. The Mental Health Act is not of great relevance unless she requires treatment for her psychiatric disorder in hospital. Even if she were detained in hospital, operating on her without her consent would derive from the surgeon's duty of care and not the provisions of the Mental Health Act.

Case 3

A GP is telephoned by the police, who are making inquiries about one of his patients. The patient, a 35-year-old man with a mild learning disability, has been reported to the police by some local children. They say he has offered to show them some bird nests, and has given them sweets and lemonade. The police want to discuss him with you. In particular they want to know whether he has any history of sex offending and whether he has received any treatment. They suggest that if you refer him to a psychiatrist they would probably not take any further proceedings.

The over-riding ethical obligation is that of confidentiality to the patient, although there are also ethical obligations to the general public. Confidentiality can be breached in exceptional cases in order to protect the public. However, this case does not seem to be of that order. It would be inappropriate to enter into any discussion of the patient with the police. In those rare and exceptional cases where some discussion may be appropriate, then the doctor should make a considered, rather than instant, response. Preliminary discussion with a colleague or advice from a professional organisation may be necessary. The doctor should insist that any discussion is with a senior police officer in person, and should be satisfied that the medical information being requested is of material significance in preventing serious harm to a member of the public.

Case 4

The wife of a 40-year-old self-employed builder visits her GP concerned by her husband's behaviour. In the last two months he has been behaving strangely. He has been unusually loud and overactive in his behaviour, has been sleeping less and less, has been ordering vast quantities of building supplies, and has been telephoning distant relatives at all hours of the day and night. He insists he feels on top of the world and has refused to see a doctor.

The description by the wife strongly suggests a psychiatric disorder, namely hypomania. In any event, the husband clearly warrants assessment by the general practitioner and is likely to require admission to hospital. There are ethical obligations to prevent the patient putting himself and his family in jeopardy. The mechanics of effecting medical intervention are difficult in such cases. Examination by doctors and assessment by an approved social worker is necessary if section 2 is to be implemented. If emergency admission under section 4 is to be used, the groundwork should be prepared in advance so that safe and speedy admission to hospital takes place. Often these cases reach a crisis point, which provides an opportunity for implementing the Mental Health Act and arranging admission.

Case 5

A 70-year-old widow has been consulting her GP for the previous 12 months with symptoms of clinical depression. She has failed to respond to conventional antidepressant medication. Her daughter expresses her concerns to the GP, saying that her mother has been speaking of suicide; she describes her mother as manipulative. When you see the patient she denies any suicidal ideation but says her daughter does not care about her and would be happy to see her dead.

The most important task is clinical, and consists of proper assessment of her clinical condition and the risk of suicide or self-harm. Strained intrafamily relationships are frequently the result, rather than the cause, of psychiatric disorder; they can easily distract the clinician from making a proper diagnosis. The over-riding ethical obligation is to provide proper medical treatment for the patient. This will follow normal clinical lines. If, ultimately, compulsory admission becomes necessary, the advantages of involving an approved social worker rather than the nearest relative are self-evident.

Legal implications of psychiatric disorder

The presence of a psychiatric disorder may have serious legal implications for certain tasks a patient may wish to discharge.

Driving

In accordance with the Road Traffic Act 1972, an applicant for a driving licence is required to disclose any relevant disability. A relevant disability is one prescribed in the 1972 Act, or any other disability that is likely to cause the driver of a vehicle to be a danger to the public. A licence will be refused if the authorities are satisfied that a relevant disability exists. Although the only mental disorder prescribed in the Act is severe mental handicap, other disorders may be relevant. A history of mental disorder must be disclosed by an applicant for a driving licence, and it is now routine for the licensing authority to seek further information from relevant doctors. The dangers of psychotic patients, or those with depressive disorders, driving have probably been underestimated.

Managing property and affairs

The capacity of patients with a psychiatric disorder, particularly the elderly (see Chapter 10), to manage their own affairs may cause serious problems to the patients, relatives, creditors, and business associates. It is assumed that patients are capable of managing their affairs until it is proven otherwise. People can elect to have a third party manage their affairs by appointing them power of attorney; or their affairs can be compulsorily taken out of their hands by the appointment of a receiver by the Court of Protection.

Power of attorney is an instrument that can be authorised only by a person who understands its meaning and implications. An ordinary power of attorney ceases to have effect when such capacity is lost. Under the Enduring Powers of Attorney Act 1985, a person can make an enduring power of attorney which gives instructions to be implemented in the event of actual or impending incapacity.

Court of Protection

The Court of Protection is an office of the Supreme Court, which may appoint a receiver to manage the property and affairs of a person who is incapable of doing so by reason of mental disorder. In Scotland a curator bonis appointed by the Court of Session or a sheriff court has similar powers. Doctors, including GPs, may be asked to assess the mental condition of patients and their capacity to manage their affairs. The powers of the Court of Protection are described in Part VII of the Mental Health Act 1983, and its proceedings are governed by the Court of Protection Rules 1984.

Any doctor may certify mental disorder. For the purposes of the Court of Protection, mental disorder is given a broad definition which includes "any other disorder or disability of mind". In assessing patients for this purpose, it is important to ascertain whether the patient understands the obligations of owning property or assets. Doctors should therefore brief themselves with some knowledge of a patient's property and affairs. Their opinions should be given in simple language.

Making a will

A valid will can be made if a person has the capacity to understand the nature and effects of the task. This is referred to as 'testamentary capacity', and it requires the testator to be of "sound disposing mind". Sometimes wills are challenged, often after death, on the grounds that the testator lacked testamentary capacity. Doctors may be called upon to assess testamentary capacity in relation to a patient who wishes to make a will. They should be satisfied that the patient (a) understands the nature and implications of making a will, (b) appreciates the extent of the estate, (c) appreciates the people who may reasonably expect to be beneficiaries – even though the patient may choose to exclude them. A valid will can be made by a mentally disordered person during a lucid interval, and by a person whose affairs are being managed by the Court of Protection. It is not uncommon for doctors to be involved in post-mortem reconstructions of a patient's mental state to assess testamentary capacity in a disputed will. It is easier to establish testamentary capacity in a live patient than a dead one!

Cautionary note

Doctors should exercise caution when they are asked to 'witness a document'. Any person known to the signatory can act as a witness. The involvement of the doctor as a witness may imply that the signatory is of sound mind when signing the document. It is safer for doctors not to act as an ordinary witness but to provide, if appropriate, a medical statement in response to a specific request concerning the mental capacity of the signatory for the particular task.

Contemporary issues concerning mentally disordered offenders

Mentally disordered patients commonly come to the attention of the police. Disturbed behaviour in a public place may lead to apprehension by the police, and sometimes desperate relatives telephone the police rather than the doctor for assistance. The nature of the relationship between psychiatric disorder and criminal behaviour is too complex to be discussed here. Suffice it to say that offences by psychiatric patients are likely to be minor rather than major. More significantly, whether or not the patient remains 'a patient' or becomes 'an offender' depends to a great extent on variables that have little to do with his or her mental condition. The criminalisation of psychiatric disorder is often a reflection of the quality of primary-care and secondary-care arrangements for psychiatric patients and the sophistication of services provided by other agencies, for example social work and housing departments.

Case 6

A 25-year-old single man has had two admissions to hospital for schizophrenia and has defaulted from out-patient care. After increasingly volatile behaviour at home, his elderly mother has excluded him from the house. He returns home at 10.30 p.m. having taken some drink. He attempts to gain entry and shouts abuse from the road. Eventually be breaks a window. His mother calls for the police and he is taken to the local police station.

What happens next will depend largely on the services that are available. If there is good liaison between the police, GP, local psychiatric service and an approved social worker, immediate admission to hospital can take place. If any of these elements are absent, then it is likely that the patient will be charged by the police with malicious damage and even remanded in prison for a psychiatric report. The latter has sadly become increasingly common.

The ranks of mentally disordered prisoners have been swollen by the large reduction in the numbers of psychiatric beds that has occurred in the last 40 years, particularly in England and Wales. Precise relationships are difficult to establish. Another significant factor may be a change in the style of practice in acute psychiatric admission wards; disturbed and offender patients who present problems in management are often rejected by psychiatric services. Psychiatric wards in district general hospitals may lack adequate resources and staff to manage such patients. There is good evidence to suggest that eventually these patients only receive treatment through the intervention of the criminal justice system.

In an effort to deal with these and other problems related to mentally disordered offenders, a recent government review has made sweeping recommendations for change (Chiswick, 1992). These have implications for primary care, psychiatric services, and other agencies involved in the care of mentally disordered patients. For primary-care services there is a particular need to ensure that services for psychiatric patients are available 24 hours a day, even when the patient is in police custody.

Appendix

Mental Health Act 1983

Section 2: Admission for assessment

Application by nearest relative or approved social worker; mental disorder; two doctors (one approved under section 12, one preferably the patient's general practitioner); up to 28 days; Part IV (consent to treatment) applicable.

Section 3: Admission for treatment

Application by nearest relative or approved social worker; specified category of mental disorder; two doctors (one approved under section 12, one preferably the patient's general practitioner); up to six months, renewable; Part IV (consent to treatment) applicable.

Section 4: Emergency admission for assessment

Application by nearest relative or approved social worker; mental disorder; one doctor (preferably a doctor who already knows the patient, usually the general practitioner); up to 72 hours, but may be extended to section 2 by second doctor; Part IV (consent to treatment) not applicable.

Section 7: Guardianship

Application by nearest relative or approved social worker; specified category of mental disorder; two doctors (one approved under section 12); up to six months, renewable; appointment of guardian who can require patient to reside at a specified place and attend for treatment; Part IV (consent to treatment) not applicable.

Section 135: Warrant to search for and remove patients

Application by an approved social worker to a justice of the peace for a warrant to be issued to a police constable; person believed to be suffering from mental disorder and is ill-treated, neglected or is unable to care for himself and is living alone; constable to be accompanied by approved social worker and a doctor; detention at a place of safety for up to 72 hours.

Relative

Defined in section 26 together with order of precedence for determining *nearest* relative; husband or wife may be 'cohabiting partner' if living together for not less than six months; partner of either sex who has lived with patient for five years or more may be considered a relative, though is last in list of precedence.

Mental disorder

"Mental illness, arrested or incomplete development of mind, psychopathic disorder and any other disorder or disability of mind."

Mental impairment

"A state of arrested or incomplete development of mind (not amounting to severe mental impairment) which includes significant impairment of intelligence and social functioning and is associated with abnormally aggressive or seriously irresponsible conduct."

Severe mental impairment

"A state of arrested or incomplete development of mind which includes severe impairment of intelligence and social functioning and is associated with abnormally aggressive or seriously irresponsible conduct."

Psychopathic disorder

"Persistent disorder or disability of mind (whether or not including significant impairment of intelligence) which results in abnormally aggressive or seriously irresponsible conduct."

Mental Health (Scotland) Act 1984

Section 18: Application for admission

Application by nearest relative or mental health officer; specified category of mental disorder; two doctors (one approved under section 20); approval by a sheriff; up to six months, renewable; Part X (consent to treatment) applicable.

Section 24: Emergency admission

Recommendation by a doctor; consent of relative or mental health officer where practicable; mental disorder; up to 72 hours; may be converted to section 26; Part X (consent to treatment) not applicable.

Section 26: Short-term detention

Extension of section 24; report by doctor approved under section 20; mental disorder; consent of nearest relative or mental health officer where practicable; up to 28 days; Part X (consent to treatment) applicable.

Section 37: Guardianship

Application by nearest relative or mental health officer; mental disorder; two doctors (one approved under section 20); approval by sheriff; up to six months, renewable; appointment of guardian who can require a patient to reside at a specified place and attend for medical treatment; Part X (consent to treatment) not applicable.

Section 117: Warrant to search for and remove patients

Application by a mental health officer or a mental welfare commissioner to a justice of the peace for a warrant to be issued to a police constable; person believed to be suffering from mental disorder and is ill-treated, neglected or is unable to care for himself and is living alone; constable to be accompanied by a doctor; detention at a place of safety for up to 72 hours.

Mental disorder

"Mental illness or mental handicap however caused or manifested."

Categories of mental disorder for section 18

Mental illness *or* a persistent mental disorder manifested only by abnormally aggressive or seriously irresponsible conduct *or* mental impairment *or* severe mental impairment.

Mental Health (Northern Ireland) Order 1986

Article 4: Admission for assessment

Application by nearest relative or approved social worker; mental disorder; one doctor (usually general practitioner); up to 7 days, renewable, can be converted to Article 12; Part IV (consent to treatment) applicable.

Article 12: Detention for treatment

Mental illness or severe mental impairment; doctor appointed by Mental Health Act Commission; up to six months, renewable; Part IV (consent to treatment) applicable.

Article 129: Warrant to search for and remove patients

Application by an officer of a health and social services board or a police constable to a justice of the peace for a warrant to be issued to a police constable; person believed to be suffering from mental disorder and is ill-treated, neglected or is unable to care for himself and is living alone; constable to be accompanied by a doctor; detention at a place of safety for up to 48 hours.

Mental disorder

"Mental illness, mental handicap and any other disorder or disability of mind."

Mental illness

"A state of mind which affects a person's thinking, perceiving, emotion or judgement to the extent that he requires care or medical treatment in his own interests or the interests of other persons."

Mental handicap

"A state of arrested or incomplete development of mind which includes significant impairment of intelligence and social functioning."

Severe mental handicap

"A state of arrested or incomplete development of mind which includes severe impairment of intelligence and social functioning."

Severe mental impairment

"A state of arrested or incomplete development of mind which includes severe impairment of intelligence and social functioning and is associated with abnormally aggressive or seriously irresponsible conduct."

References

CHISWICK, D. (1992) What mentally ill offenders need. *British Medical Journal*, **304**, 267–268.
DEPARTMENT OF HEALTH (1993) *Legal Powers on the Care of Mentally Ill People in the Community*. London: Department of Health.
DYER, C. (1987) Compulsory treatment in the community for the mentally ill? *British Medical Journal*, **295**, 991–992.
GUNN, M. (1990) Consent to treatment. *Journal of Forensic Psychiatry*, **1**, 81–87.
MENTAL HEALTH ACT COMMISSION (1991) *Fourth Biennial Report 1989–1991*. London: HMSO.
ROYAL COLLEGE OF PSYCHIATRISTS (1993) *Community Supervision Orders*. London: Royal College of Psychiatrists.

Further reading

BLUGLASS, R. & BOWDEN, P. (1990) *Principles and Practice of Forensic Psychiatry*. Edinburgh: Churchill Livingstone.
GUNN, J. & TAYLOR, P. J. (1993) *Forensic Psychiatry: Clinical, Legal and Ethical Issues*. Oxford: Butterworth Heinemann.

Legislation

DEPARTMENT OF HEALTH & WELSH OFFICE (1993) *Code of Practice. Mental Health Act 1983* (2nd edn). London: HMSO.
DEPARTMENT OF HEALTH & SOCIAL SERVICES (1992) *Code of Practice. Mental Health (Northern Ireland) Order 1986*. Belfast: HMSO.
SCOTTISH HOME & HEALTH DEPARTMENT (1990) *Mental Health Act (Scotland) 1984. Code of Practice*. Edinburgh: HMSO.

Part II. Clinical problems

5 Loss, grief and psychosocial transitions

COLIN MURRAY PARKES

On both scientific and humanitarian grounds, the provision of proper care for people who are faced with major losses in their lives must be a matter of concern to members of the primary care team.

There is now good evidence, from the study of bereavement and other types of loss, that major life events of this kind carry an increased risk to physical and mental health (Parkes, 1986). Profound effects on the immune response as well as on other physiological systems have been demonstrated and, in certain circumstances (notably those of the older widower), loss is associated with an increased risk of mortality.

Bereavement is the best known and most thoroughly researched type of loss, and intuition tells us that it is also one of the most traumatic, but many other types of loss can be included among the "slings and arrows of outrageous fortune", and many of these bring people into contact with their GPs. Physical illness and disablement bring in their train a succession of losses, as do major surgery and other drastic treatments. Birth, as well as death, can be a time of loss and there are, in fact, many life changes which cause both loss and gain. At each stage of the life cycle, turning points are reached which, for good or ill, will play an important part in determining the health, happiness, and social adjustment of each member of society.

Nobody supposes that GPs should take responsibility for guiding people through all of these events, but the members of the primary care team are often in a position to assess the need for help at such times and, if it is needed, to steer people towards the best sources of help available to them.

Of course, the most appropriate and effective source of help for most of people is the family. The family exists in order to support its members, and doctors must beware of interfering with this important function. But there are many situations in which families find it difficult to support their members, perhaps because they are too widely scattered or because the family itself has become dysfunctional. At times of bereavement all are grieving, and it may be difficult for any member to ask for help from or offer help to the others. The family doctor may be in a position to evaluate the family as a whole and to see that help is given when needed.

Fortunately there is also good reason to believe that appropriate counselling given by people with proper training to the minority of bereaved people who are at special risk can substantially reduce that risk. This does not imply that every bereaved person needs counselling, or that only expensive, professional psychologists or psychiatrists are qualified to give it. The random-allocation studies on which these conclusions are based indicate that bereaved people at special risk get the most benefit from counselling, and at least one study has shown that this counselling can be successfully given by volunteers who have been carefully selected and trained for the job (Raphael, 1977; Parkes, 1981). Organisations such as Cruse[1] can now provide the requisite standard of counselling in most parts of the UK, but it is important for general practitioners and other referrers to have a good knowledge of the indicators of risk if the best use is to be made of their services.

What is true of bereavement is often true of other types of loss. Counselling has been shown to reduce the psychological risks associated with major surgery and with complicated pregnancies; it may also reduce the morbidity which results from these events and from myocardial infarctions. The fine reputation of the hospices rests largely on their success at providing psychosocial support to patients with life-threatening illnesses and to their families. It follows that a proper understanding of the reactions to loss, of the circumstances that increase risk, and of the counselling that can reduce that risk, are essential to every member of the primary care team.

Reaction to loss

This chapter focuses mainly on bereavement, since this remains the prime example of the reaction to loss. The reader who wishes to extend this model to a wider range of losses and critical life events is recommended to read *Psychological Problems in General Practice* (Markus *et al*, 1989).

Grief is the prime component of the physiological reaction to loss, and pining for the lost object the *sine qua non* of grief. Without this painful feeling of missing the lost person, grief cannot truly be said to be present, and there must be serious doubt whether a real loss has taken place. So painful is the pining that we refer to 'pangs' of grief, which are often associated with all the psychological accompaniments of severe anxiety and fear.

These pangs can best be understood as a deeply felt urge to cry and to search for the lost object, an urge which is present in most social animals and which has evident survival value when the loss is only temporary. When, however, the loss is permanent, the urge to cry and to search is immediately

---

1. Cruse: Bereavement Care (126 Sheen Road, Richmond, Surrey TW9 1UR) is the foremost national organisation in the UK for people bereaved by death. Volunteer counsellors who are carefully selected and trained provide support through approximately 200 local branches.

opposed by the intellectual awareness that such unrestrained expression of emotion is not only pointless but likely to evoke embarrassment and disapproval. The bereaved are, therefore, in a state of conflict.

How they resolve this conflict varies greatly. Some, who pride themselves on their self-control, will keep a 'stiff upper lip' and keep busy in order to distract themselves from the need to grieve; others will 'break down', giving unrestrained vent to their anguish. Religious and cultural traditions have a strong influence.

Another component of the reaction to loss, which is more evident as time passes, is the urge to review and revise one's internal model of the world. This occurs whenever a set of assumptions about the world is invalidated by change, and it has been termed 'psychosocial transition'. Just as an amputee must discover the many habits of thought and behaviour which must be revised if he is to learn to live as an amputee, so the widow must discover the implications of that change of state. For a while, both of them will tend to cling to their old view of the world. Amputees frequently find themselves going to tread on a leg that is not there (sometimes with disastrous consequences), and the widow, out of habit, lays the table for two and refers, in conversation, to the dead husband as if he were still alive. Illusions of the presence of the lost object can occur as the phantom limb and the sense of the presence of a dead partner which are reported by most amputees and most widows.

This transition takes a long time. At first the sufferer will feel lost and bewildered. The possession of an accurate internal model of the world is a source of security, and its invalidation makes people lose confidence and causes the familiar world to feel unfamiliar ('My world has been turned upside down').

The concept of 'grief work', the process of review by which each memory, each link with the lost world, must be brought into consciousness and examined in terms of its continued relevance, recognises the cognitive task which we all face at times of major change.

Of course, the old model of the world does not cease to exist when a new one has been built; it remains, like an unused railway line, alongside the new track and, at any time, a reminder of the past can trigger an outdated and obsolescent chain of thought. Perhaps for this reason the bereaved will often remind us that 'It doesn't end, you don't forget'. Having said that, there is, if all goes well, a tendency for people to spend increasing periods of time thinking and behaving in ways that accord with their new life.

Unfortunately, all may not go well and a number of complications can interfere with the course of grieving. These have been classified as follows.

Classification of reactions to loss

 (a) Normal or uncomplicated grief
 (b) Non-specific stress reactions
   (i) Anxiety state and panic reactions
   (ii) Post-traumatic stress disorders

        (iii) Depressive reactions
        (iv) Other psychiatric and psychosomatic disorders triggered by loss
   (c) Morbid grief reactions
        (i) Delayed or inhibited grief
        (ii) Chronic grief
        (iii) Identification reactions
        (iv) Compulsive care-giving
        (v) Conflicted grief.

These categories, while they have some diagnostic value, should not be regarded as exclusive. There is a great deal of overlap between them, and individuals will often be found to have features of more than one category of loss reaction.

Non-specific stress reactions are among the commonest to come to the notice of the GP. Since they arise from many circumstances other than loss events, they are covered elsewhere in Chapter 8.

Morbid grief reactions are more specific to loss itself. The first to be described and still, in many minds, the epitome of pathological grief are the *delayed or inhibited reactions*. After a period of delay which may last for months or years, the partial or full expression of grief may take place in a form which is then seen as abnormal. Once initiated, delayed reactions sometimes become chronic.

Chronic grief is severe from the start, but instead of moving towards resolution it persists. Sufferers tend to remain withdrawn and preoccupied with their loss. This is the commonest form of pathological grief to be seen in psychiatric clinics.

Identification with a lost person is not uncommon. Sons may take on the mannerisms of their fathers, etc. Identification becomes pathological when it is the symptoms of the illness of a dead person that are adopted. These hypochondriacal conditions may so closely resemble the symptoms of a real illness that they are misdiagnosed.

Other psychosomatic disorders are usually self-perpetuating somatic expressions of the physiological reaction to minor ailments. Thus, insomnia, palpitations and anorexia are all common symptoms during the first month after a major loss – they are most likely to persist if they themselves cause further anxiety. The bereaved lose the sense of invulnerability that enables most of us to cope with the minor upsets of life without undue fear. They easily become over concerned about their own health and about that of their dependents and other close relatives.

Compulsive care-giving may be one way of handling this anxiety. The bereaved, having failed to ward off one disaster, may spend their lives preventing others. In other cases the care-givers will care for people who remind them of the dead persons, or they may offer to counsel people in a similar situation to themselves as if by looking after others they can make up for the care which they have not received.

There are plenty of people who, having come through a loss, find themselves motivated to help others. It only becomes problematic when the emotional charge which belongs properly to the person's own bereavement distorts perception of the needs of others. Such people may overwhelm the person for whom they are caring with excessive displays of sympathy; they will often be blind to the other's true needs, and may find it hard to encourage the development of autonomy and to let go when help is no longer needed.

Anger and guilt are not uncommon following losses, and there are circumstances in which they are perfectly justified. When severe and persistant they give rise to *conflicted grief*, from which recovery may take a long time. Some focus their anger on a search for someone to punish, as if by finding the culprit and achieving retribution they could undo the damage that has been done. Doctors are often the victims of unjustified complaints in such cases, and even those complaints that are justified are sometimes exaggerated. Counselling may lead to more rational behaviour.

Others blame themselves for what has happened. Grief then becomes a duty to the dead as if, by punishing themselves, the bereaved could make restitution for what they have done. In some cases these reactions may give rise to delusions of guilt and worthlessness, resembling major depressive illness (see Chapter 5). Differential diagnosis is not easy, and a course of antidepressant medication should be considered.

Assessment of risk and the prevention of problems

Longitudinal studies have made it possible to identify, before or at the time the loss takes place, many of the factors which are likely to cause problems later. This opens the door to prevention, since it enables us to offer help to those most in need of it and also suggests the kind of help likely to be needed. Whether or not this information is used as a means of selecting people for counselling, it is likely to be of use to all who set out to help people faced with major losses in their lives.

There are two types of risk factor: those which indicate particularly traumatic situations, and those which indicate characteristics of persons at risk:

(a) Situational factors
  (i) lack of preparation (e.g. sudden, untimely bereavement)
  (ii) mutilation or other horrific circumstances
  (iii) magnitude of loss (e.g. loss of spouse or child)
  (iv) culpability for loss (e.g. driver in a road traffic accident)
  (v) other incidental trauma (e.g. multiple losses)
  (vi) family or culture discourage expression of grief or other negative emotions

(b) Vulnerability factors
  (i) problems of attachment
    (1) grief prone
    (2) learned fear
    (3) learned helplessness
  (ii) problems of coping
    (1) substance abuse
    (2) avoidance
  (iii) dysfunctional families.

Situational factors

Unexpected, untimely, and multiple losses are sufficiently traumatic to induce psychiatric disturbance, even in the absence of vulnerability factors. The reaction often takes the form of a post-traumatic stress disorder (see p. 125), in which high levels of anxiety and tension coexist with conscious efforts to avoid reminders of the loss and a tendency to experience feelings of panic when confronted by such reminders. Horrific memories or fantasies of the imagined traumatic events may come to 'haunt' the survivor by day and in nightmares.

The greater the loss, the greater is the grief. Those people who have put all their eggs in one emotional basket, be it an only child or the partner in a childless marriage, will react severely when the person in whom they have invested so much is taken away. The loss of a child to a woman is sometimes cited as the most severe form of loss but, although it gives rise to severe grief, it is ultimately likely to be less destructive to the life plan than is the untimely death of a young partner or spouse.

When losses are attributable to human agency (e.g. suicide, murder, or a road traffic accident for which the survivor holds himself to blame) special problems arise in the management of anger and guilt. Conflicted grief often follows such losses.

Multiple losses often seem to overwhelm the individual's capacity to respond emotionally. At other times a person may grieve for one loss while apparently ignoring others. Often one loss will cause another: the loss of a husband may lead to the consequent loss of home, income, etc. Grief for one of these losses may impair the survivor's ability and motivation to cope with the others.

Some events, such as man-made disasters, may involve all of these risk factors, and it is no surprise therefore to find that disasters are severely disruptive of the lives of the survivors, whose need for counselling is likely to be greater than that of most bereaved people.

The social situation in which loss occurs and in which the survivors remain afterwards also plays a significant part in determining the outcome of bereavement. Lack of a family, or, worse still, the presence of a family which is seen as unsupportive, increases the likelihood of problems. Often it is the family who cannot tolerate grieving. Repeated injunctions to 'stop crying', 'be brave', 'pull yourself together', and the concomitant expectation that, if the sufferer does not maintain a strict control he/she will 'break down', places a considerable burden on the bereaved.

Such pressures are not confined to the family: patients and staff on surgical wards, members of the police or armed services, and other occupations whose heroic image must be maintained, tend to produce 'superior labial sclerosis' (stiff upper lip). Although denial of the need to grieve can sometimes enable people to get through an emergency without becoming upset, they also tend to produce delayed and inhibited reactions. In the care-giving professions, repeated exposure to loss, without appropriate opportunities being provided for staff to share the griefs they face, can cause 'burn-out', an insidious form of disillusionment and depression which accounts for many losses to these professions and demoralised teams.

Personal vulnerability

This interacts with situational factors to increase risk and to colour the form of the reactions to loss. Most of the factors which increase vulnerability to other psychiatric disorders also increase vulnerability to loss.

Of special interest are the disturbances of attachment which play an important part in the development of trust in oneself and others. Attachments are the bonds which hold people together. They arise early in childhood and are greatly influenced by the type of parenting the child receives. Research in the field of child development has shown clearly that it is insecure attachments rather than deliberate neglect that lie at the root of most later attachment problems. Insecure parents regularly pass on their insecurity to their children, who then grow up with little trust in themselves or others. When these children leave home and make new relationships, the patterns of clinging or ambivalence which bedevilled their relationship with their parents are repeated. When, in time, these relationships come to an end, whether through death or other separation, then grief is likely to be chronic or conflicted. (For a summary of recent work in the field of attachment and a more detailed explanation of the influence of attachments on subsequent grief, see Parkes *et al*, 1991.)

Learned fear and learned helplessness are other types of insecurity which can result from insecure parenting and which predispose people to pathological anxiety and depression at times of loss later in life.

Each person learns ways of coping with problems, most of which are effective in the short term. Long-term solutions are often more difficult to achieve, and those people whose personal experience of life has left them with little reason to believe in their own ability to control events are unlikely to have much faith in them. When major losses occur such people often resort to short-term solutions, such as alcohol or other drugs, avoidant behaviour, or hyperactivity (which is a form of distraction), which only succeed by postponing the work of grieving. These solutions create their own problems either directly, as a side-effect, or indirectly, by delaying the process of grieving.

Families can become dysfunctional for a number of reasons. Sometimes the security of the family rests on one senior person. If that person is lost, the whole family may be undermined. Reserves of money, power, status, time, energy, etc., can be depleted by events affecting entire families. Just when they need each other most, the family may find it impossible to obtain or give the resources needed by its members. Splits within a family may occur when individuals, under some stress, find themselves expressing their bitterness against others who are in no frame of mind to ignore it. At such time, minor antipathies can explode and the "Never darken my door again" syndrome divide the family. These splits and failures of function are particularly likely to follow losses affecting more than one family member.

Management by the primary care team

At its best, the primary care team can become an extended family to the nuclear families that are its patients (Chapter 1). Both by accident and in the other transitions which take place between birth and death, losses will occur, and the primary care team is likely to be involved. These contacts provide the team with opportunities to monitor, assist the process of transition and, at the same time, to reduce the risks which attend them. Contacts may be made before, during, or after the loss: if before, they enable help to be given to people to prepare themselves for the loss; during the course of the loss such contact may mitigate its impact and to evaluate the need for further support; after the loss, further monitoring and ongoing support becomes possible. In the long term, a small proportion of survivors will require treatment for a psychiatric or psychosomatic disorder which has arisen as a result of the loss. The measures proposed here aim to minimise that proportion.

Preparation for loss

Even the most eagerly anticipated life transition may contain an element of loss. The birth of the first baby, promotion, retirement, or even recovery from a long-standing illness can bring in their train changes in the life plan which are unwanted, difficult and, often, unexpected. Yet most major transitions do cast their shadow before, and members of the primary care team are often aware of the likely outcome of illnesses and their treatments long before these implications are apparent to the victims.

To most care-givers the most unpleasant task they have to perform is to break bad news. This is, perhaps, the nearest we come today to performing surgery without an anaesthetic, and it is undertaken reluctantly. Doctors often report that their medical training has done little to prepare them for this task, and they feel anxious and inept. Their anxiety may be communicated to the patient, who will then feel unsupported at a time when support is desperately needed.

To communicate effectively, emotional support has to be combined with information. Emotional support should create a calm and secure base from which the patient can explore the frightening and insecure realm which she/he is entering. This means paying attention to the setting in which the communication takes place, as well as to the way in which this is done. Privacy is essential, and a softly furnished room is much better than a busy ward or a treatment room lined with instruments. For most people the presence of a close relative is welcome at such times, but there are a few who prefer to face their problems alone rather than involve others who are themselves seen as fragile. Within a family, some are likely to have more awareness of the true situation than others. They can be our allies in gently bringing home the truth.

Doctors learn their own ways of putting people at their ease, and skills need to be used to the full, in a leisurely and unpressured way. The GP must appear to have all the time in the world and be prepared to stay with the situation for as long as needed. This may sound like a counsel of perfection for busy doctors, but there is no way to speed up emotional support. Set aside a reasonable time to break bad news in order to do the job properly.

The information imparted must be true (lies will soon be discovered and destroy trust), but couch it in terms which the patient will understand, and deliver it in 'bite-sized chunks'. Telling too much too soon can be as harmful as telling too little too late. Try to deliver the information at the rate and time when the patient is ready receive it. Some secure people will want to be told the whole truth at a sitting, and will indicate by their response that they have understood its implications. Other, less secure people, may need to take 'several bites at the cherry'.

The best way to decide what the recipient is ready to hear is to invite questions. Few people will ask a question unless they are ready to hear the answer. It is not a bad idea to start off by finding out how much the person already knows. This will soon tell us how big an information gap has to be bridged. At times the patient's expectations are worse than reality, in which case the news may be good rather than bad. Words like 'cancer' and 'death' often have special or inaccurate meanings to patients, and it is worth exploring what they mean if they use such words. A question like "Have you known anyone else with cancer?" will often elicit the family horror story, which may have little resemblance to the patient's illness.

It is often possible to find positive things to say, but one should not be absurdly optimistic or encourage the patient to cling to hopes that are unrealistic.

Perhaps the most difficult interactions are those that arise when the outcome is uncertain. Patients and relatives may press for a prognosis when none is possible (and even with terminal illness the ability to predict the length of survival is very inexact). In such cases it may be helpful to discuss the alternative outcomes, so that contingency plans can be made for all eventualities.

Support in the course of loss

If patient and family have been kept informed of developments throughout the illness, large gaps between expectation and reality are less likely, and they will be better able to cope with the event of loss when it takes place. At such moments the professionals take on a parental role, giving comfort by non-verbal means. Intuition usually tells us how to behave, and there is nothing wrong in crying with the person we are helping as long as it is our shoulder that they are crying on rather than vice versa.

When someone has died, the family will often seek guidance about whether or not to view the body. Since this may be their last chance to say goodbye and to take in the reality of the death, it is usually best to encourage it. The state of the body is relevant here – some people will be haunted by the memory of physical mutilation. In such cases it is important that there be no surprises, and people should be warned what to expect. The comment ''He'll feel very cold'' is often helpful if the body has been refrigerated, as this can come as a shock to someone whose last contact was with the warmth of life.

Further support

Whether or not the doctor intends to provide counselling, a single visit to a bereaved family from the family doctor is almost always appreciated. This will enable an assessment to be made of the need for further counselling and provide the family with the opportunity to ask questions about any aspects of the illness or death which continue to trouble them. It reassures the family of the doctor's continuing care, and this in itself may reduce the need for such care.

In the event that further counselling is needed (the risk factors outlined above will enable this decision to be made), the doctor will have to decide who should give it. A knowledge of local resources will usually indicate whether it should be a member of the primary care team, from Cruse, or from some other organisation. There is no harm in introducing a stranger at this time, since bereaved people often find it therapeutic to explain themselves and to go over the events of the loss to someone who is not already acquainted with the facts.

In counselling the bereaved, as in all counselling, it is important to choose a setting in which the bereaved person will feel secure enough to talk and express their feelings about what has happened. Ideally this should be the person's home, but a GP surgery or other private place will often suffice.

Most bereaved people will have a number of pressing problems to discuss and it is sometimes necessary to interrupt if you begin to feel overwhelmed. Nobody, the bereaved included, can cope with more than one problem at a time. We may have our own ideas about what the bereaved person ought to be talking about, but it is wise to let them decide the priorities and to avoid intensive questioning. Only as time progresses is it justifiable to become a little more active in moving the conversation gently into important areas that seem to have been omitted. Even here, never go more than one step ahead of the patient.

It is useful to highlight feelings by asking such questions as "What did (do) you feel about that?" when a traumatic event is described. This implicitly gives the other person permission to get upset and indicates that there is nothing wrong with having feelings. Bereaved people will often be ashamed and embarrassed if they cry, and they should be reassured that tears are quite natural at this time.

Because the physiological accompaniments of grief can themselves create further anxiety, some explanation of the nature of grief, in language which the bereaved can understand, can be reassuring. While, in the early stages of bereavement, a doctor may often try to facilitate the expression of grief and reducing avoidance, there will come a time when people need to stop grieving and get on with their lives. Just as some have needed permission to grieve, they may now need to be reassured that it is not a duty to the dead to grieve for them forever.

The temptation to tell bereaved people how to run their lives must be avoided, for in the long run, they must stand on their own feet; show respect for their opinions and encourage them to make decisions and take responsibility, and help them to move towards an autonomous existence. This may be done by progressively reducing the frequency of the counselling sessions.

Sometimes the bereaved will have become attached to the counsellor. In such cases, the ending of counselling can be another bereavement. There is nothing wrong with this, but it does imply that ending should be planned well in advance, so that the bereaved have the opportunity to grieve for this loss while it is still possible for the counsellor to help them. Counsellors may also need support at this time.

Treatment of pathological grief

The treatment of pathological grief is described more fully in Parkes (1986).

When grief has been inhibited, delayed or avoided, the aim must be to help the bereaved to express the repressed emotions. Linking objects which bring the dead person into the room (e.g. photographs, mementoes, etc.) will often help, as will a form of role play in which an empty chair is imagined to be occupied by the dead person and the bereaved are encouraged to speak to that person.

In cases of chronic grief, when the problem is not so much in the expression of grief as in the resumption of normal activity, it is helpful to negotiate with the bereaved the tasks which they can undertake in order to move towards a more satisfactory life.

Conflicted grief, which often coexists with chronic grief, requires a close examination of the roots of the anger and guilt which complicate the course of mourning. Rather than negating the patient's anger or guilt, no matter how irrational its mode of expression may be, it is usually more effective to challenge the bereaved to find some more creative way of expressing their feelings. It is, after all, a pity to waste such powerful forces. The Taj Mahal is not the only great thing to have come out of the discontents occasioned by bereavement.

Hardest of all to help are the compulsive care-givers – people who find it easier to offer help than to accept it. In working with such people it is essential to remember that the sympathetic emotions that they express for the objects of their care properly belong to themselves. If we are not afraid to make this connection, we may find that the bereaved person can make it too.

Despite all efforts, a bereaved person will sometimes get 'stuck'. Over several months, nothing seems to be changing, the therapy is getting nowhere. There are three useful questions to consider in such cases. Is there an underlying depressive illness? Is there some earlier loss which has never been expressed, and thoughts of which have been rekindled by this more recent loss? Is there some lack of trust, perhaps due to a long-standing prejudice, which makes it impossible for the counsellor to be seen as a source of security rather than a threat?

In such cases, referral to a psychiatrist is a reasonable option. The psychiatrist will take a detailed psychiatric history, covering the events and circumstances before the loss, and this in itself may uncover earlier losses and help the patient to achieve a new perspective. Psychologists have also been taking an interest in bereavement in recent years, and have developed their own approaches to anxiety reduction and cognitive reappraisal of life at points of loss and change.

Social workers, particularly those trained in crisis intervention, are of special value where a loss may be part of a larger family problem. In such cases, referral for family therapy is also an option. Finally, there is the full range of child psychiatric, child guidance and educational psychology services to be considered if bereaved children are at risk.

Whatever action is taken, it is important to remember the needs of the helpers for support. Counselling at times of loss can be stressful for counsellors as well as clients, perhaps because it sparks off feelings about losses in their own lives, or because the sharing of other people's grief can drain time and energy which may already be depleted. Organisations such as Cruse expect all of their counsellors to be supervised, and it is illogical for GPs or other members of the primary care team to carry out counselling without some form of supervision or support. This can be individual or in groups, such as the type developed by Balint (see Chapter 1).

The distinction between bereavement counselling and other types of counselling is, of course, more theoretical than practical. In practice, bereaved people need help with a range of problems that may have little to do with loss. Conversely, people with a wide range of psychiatric and other problems will be found to have suffered losses of one sort or another. GPs and their practice teams are in the front line of all of this work, and will find their own lives enriched if they take an active interest in counselling.

Outcome and prognosis

Since every love relationship is different, it would be surprising if every grief followed the same course. Normal grief often seems to go on longer than expected by friends and family, perhaps because their own grief is so soon over. Following a major loss, as of a husband or wife in middle life, the pangs of grief tend to reach a peak in 5–14 days, but will still be quite frequent a year later. The appetite for food is lost by many during the first month, but by three months any weight loss will usually have been regained. Other appetites may take longer to return. Most widows report that they begin to feel that they are recovering in the course of the second year but they are also likely to say, years later, that grief does not end. Anniversaries and other reminders continue to evoke pangs of grief, and memories of the lost person remain vivid. Older bereaved people usually show less extreme grief than younger, but this grief can be protracted and loneliness is the besetting problem of old age. Children fluctuate in the intensity of their grief and seem to be more easily distracted from it than adults. Lasting problems are most likely to occur in very young children when no satisfactory substitute for a lost parent is available. The progress of adolescents towards autonomy can also easily be disrupted by the death of a parent.

Women, on the whole, show more emotional disturbance after bereavement than men and are more likely to be referred for psychiatric help. Men, on the other hand, take longer to adjust to unmarried life, and widowers have a much higher death rate than widows.

On the whole, treatment of the psychiatric complications of bereavement is rewarding and a good prognosis can be expected in most instances.

Exceptions are mostly elderly people with a known previous psychiatric
history, poor physical health, and limited social support.

References

MARKUS, A. G., PARKES, C. M., TOMSON, P., *et al* (1989) *Psychological Problems in General
Practice.* Oxford: Oxford University Press.
PARKES, C. M. (1981) Evaluation of a bereavement service. *Journal of Preventive Psychiatry*, **1**,
179–188.
—— (1986) *Bereavement: Studies of Grief in Adult Life* (2nd edn). London: Tavistock and Pelican;
New York: International Universities Press.
——, STEVENSON-HINDE, J. & MARRIS, P. (eds) (1991) *Attachment Across the Life Cycle.*
London: Routledge.
RAPHAEL, B. (1977) Preventive intervention with recently bereaved. *Archives of General Psychiatry*,
34, 1450–1454.

6 Family and marital relationships

DENIS PEREIRA GRAY

Life is about people and people all have relationships with each other. Human relationships are central to the understanding of human behaviour and pervade and affect every aspect of society. Most of history has been influenced by relationships. Much of the greatest literature and drama describes and portrays on page, stage, or screen the infinite subtleties of human relationships.

The way people live their lives and behave in the face of stress, including illness, will be immensely affected by the relationships they have in their lives, especially in their families, in their work, and with those professionally concerned with them.

General practice and psychiatry stand together in having identified the special significance of the doctor–patient relationship, and the psychoanalytical school has illuminated it in depth. Balint (1957), as a psychoanalyst, initiated a whole series of analyses on the doctor–patient relationship in general practice. The theory of parent figures and the complexities of transference are but particular aspects of this. General practice texts such as Browne & Freeling's (1976) have been written entirely on this subject.

However, most of the recent theory on family relationships has been derived more from social work and child psychiatry than from general practice, which has contributed relatively little, considering the unique perspective on families which family doctors have. Indeed, they have a ring-side seat in the formation and development of many, if not most, family relationships.

Features of general practice relevant to family relationships

(a) Family-planning care means that GPs see the majority of young women as they begin a sexual relationship, and they often hear their feelings about the man during contraceptive check-ups – over two-thirds of all family planning is provided through general practice (Department of Health, 1990).

(b) General practitioners meet the male partner in about four-fifths of family units, and the men or women who are 'missing' partners become patients in about three-quarters of family units.

(c) Over 90% of GPs provide antenatal care and so get to know a woman going through a pregnancy and see her perhaps six to ten times, with two to three postnatal visits and a postnatal examination as well (General Medical Services Committee, 1992).

(d) The average duration of registration, even in cities, is at least 12 years (Difford, 1990, personal communication), and in 1981 Ritchie *et al* reported that 42% of all NHS patients had a relationship for 20 or more years since birth.

(e) Children are registered with the mother's family doctor in the NHS over 95% of the time.

(f) The contact rate between patients and their GPs is great and growing. The national average is now as high as five per patient per year, and for children under five years it is as high as eight consultations per child per year (Office of Population Censuses and Surveys, 1991). A British baby is seen every six to seven weeks on average, almost always with a parent, usually the mother, by the GP. A unique opportunity is provided for professional observation of child-rearing practices and the developing parent–child relationships.

(g) On home visits, especially out of hours, the whole family is often seen interacting together under anxiety and stress.

(h) If difficulties in child behaviour arise, the GP is the first port of call (shared in many practices with health visitors) and the familiar day-to-day problems ('won't eat', 'won't sleep' and 'won't obey') are all reflections of parental attitudes and the emerging parent–child relationship. These therefore emerge in the consulting-room as specific problems.

(i) Child-care surveillance as an integral part of general practice has been the policy of the Royal College of General Practitioners since September 1978 (*Journal of the Royal College of General Practitioners, 1978*) and *Healthier Children – Thinking Prevention* was published by the College in 1982 as a statement of the importance of this work and the case for the child's environment was defined there as the home and family.

(j) Life-long care is a special feature of general practice rarely described or discussed, but is commoner than is realised. In the author's practice in Exeter, a city of about 100 000 population, more than half of all patients attending the antenatal clinic at the time of writing this chapter had been born in the practice. (Four patients with life-long care have married another of the author's patients, giving three-generational relationships on both sides of the family at once.)

(k) Multiple family relationships are also commoner than is realised. The author, at the time of writing, has as patients one or more grandparents of more than half of all the children under five years on his personal list. More than 60% of the children registered have a grandparent registered in the same practice (on another partner's list, but with the records accessible to the author), and in half of all the children, he has personally treated at some time or other a great-grandparent, of whom 5% are still his patients.

(l) Multiple family relationships greatly enhance the doctor's understanding of what is happening in families as grandparents, especially grannies and great-grannies, talk – "I tell you doctor, she's spoiling that child!" or "It worries me the way she leaves him with teenage baby sitters!".

Difficulties for general practice

There has been a relative dearth of research on counselling about human relationships by GPs or their teams. Those that do it, and do it well, often are teachers (trainers) rather than researchers and have not written down their techniques.

In medical schools, on vocational training courses, and in continuing education for established principals, the speakers tend to come from psychiatry, and often consciously or subconsciously convey the skills of the specialist and do not teach the psychiatric skills of the generalist. They frequently convey the message that the doctor should refer, as they often simply cannot actually comprehend how skilled counselling and psychiatric care can be done in ordinary day-to-day general practice, because they do not have the long-term and multiple family relationships and the flexibility of follow-up which the GP does.

The need is to teach GPs by GPs how to capitalise on the unique strengths which the NHS gives them. The special advantages are not often portrayed, and the techniques for capitalising on them are rarely taught.

The generalist approach

Against this background, the first need for general practice is for a simple, practical working approach which makes sense of the majority of relationships, and which can be used in the timeframe of general practice, that is, repeated ten-minute consultations.

Encouragement

It is first necessary to support new GPs, who often fear that this work will be hugely time consuming and unproductive.

People as people

The first principle to grasp is that understanding people is the very essence of general practice. People are the name of the game. In the words of Drucker's (1977) management theory, this is the business GPs are in. People provide GPs with their greatest job satisfaction, and the continuing contact means that each succeeding year in general practice becomes progressively more interesting as the rich variety of life in families unfolds before the doctor's very eyes.

Furthermore, a deep understanding of people, although slow to build up, is of equal use in managing the physical problems of the illnesses of general practice. For example, much of the advice about common health problems like asthma, hypertension, depression, and hyperlipidaemia involves discussion and often changing ways of living. The doctor who understands his/her patients is at a huge advantage in these negotiations.

Personal lists

Group practices are growing in size (Department of Health, 1990) and partnerships are getting bigger all the time. Combined-list systems are in the majority, thus constantly diluting the precious repeated contact between patients and doctor. Freeman & Richards (1990) found that the proportion of consultations with the patient's personal doctor in practices with combined-list systems was about 50% but was over 80% in personal-list practices.

Personal lists also foster personal relationships between patient and doctor, and foster interest in personality and family issues. The research question of the value of personal lists looms larger every year as groups get bigger. They are "the key to personal care", and the personal list system is one of the greatest organisational issues in British general practice (Pereira Gray, 1979).

Shortage of texts

The oral tradition of general practice has been about personal care, long-term care, and families and their relationships. This is what trainers teach and is demonstrated by the succession of James Mackenzie Lectures at the Royal College of General Practitioners. Much less has been more formally published, although the texts that do exist deserve to be better known (Lane, 1969; Berger & Mohr, 1969; Browne & Freeling, 1976; Huygen, 1978).

All the effort and emphasis at present is on disease: asthma, depression, diabetes, hypertension. The biographical approach to medicine in general practice and the implications of Pereira Gray's (1978) claim that general practice can be seen as a behavioural science in its own right have not received their proper share of attention. Analysis and research on these are urgently needed. Two of the most valuable starting pieces, one by a psychiatrist (Berne, 1964) and one profound analysis of the work of a GP (Berger & Mohr, 1969), are now both about 25 years old.

Records

Record-keeping systems need to be organised to reflect the special characteristics of GPs, especially family household charts (Zander *et al*, 1978) and household relationships.

The long-term view

General practitioners have a perspective not over months or even years, but decades. What is the pattern in this family over the last 25 years? What is the likely position in ten years' time?

Time

Time is the most precious resource in general practice, which has much more of it than it realises, but it does not always use it well. Each patient averages 3.2 consultations per year (Royal College of General Practitioners *et al*, 1990), and the Department of Health (1991) found that the average consultation in general practice lasts "just under nine minutes". There is therefore $3.2 \times 8 = 26$ minutes a year available, that is, about half an hour per patient per year.

As those with relationship problems feature among the high consulters rather than the low ones, as they have longer rather than shorter consultations (Westcott, 1977), there is more time in practice for these patients, and there is time with partners, husbands, and parents as well. The challenge is not to find the time, which is how the problem is often perceived, but how to use it – and the answer, as so often in general practice, is analysis and a systematic approach and systematic recording.

Furthermore, three or four productive consultations can save time and prevent patients endlessly returning and repeatedly going over the same ground unproductively.

Understanding the home/household

The essential key is to take a proactive approach and to build up systematically a picture of the patients and to accept that it can sometimes take years to fit all the bits of the jigsaw together. For example, GPs are becoming clearer about the patterns of consulting associated with women who have been abused in childhood, yet it may take these patients years to broach the subject, although when it is at last discussed a flood of light may be thrown on years of work and hundreds of consultations in both hospital and general practice.

As Pereira Gray (1978) said in the 1977 James Mackenzie Lecture, one challenging model for the doctor is to be able to visualise what the patient is feeling at home. Can the doctor call to mind the home, where it is, what it is like, who is in it, and how they are getting on together?

Parallels with counselling

General practitioners can adopt the counselling philosophy, but not all the techniques of counselling. Thus it is helpful to accept that the aims of relationship work are to inform patients, to help patients to acquire insight, to make up their own minds, and to make their own choices about their lives.

Counselling techniques are, however, not always appropriate, and general practice needs to evolve its own techniques, using the special features of the doctor–patient relationship, for example, doing physical examinations as well, relating to partners, spouses, and parents, and capitalising on the special authority of the doctor. Thus, while the ends of traditional counselling are much the same, the means may be different in the consulting-room, and the main differences are in the use of time, the length of the process over years, and the doctor's use of authority to speed work along.

Critical to relationship work in general practice is the use of time. Psychoanalysis has dominated thinking, with its long consultations and the idea of working in units of time of 60 minutes. There is nothing sacred about 60 minutes, and this is not an appropriate model for general practice, which needs to use its hour (6 times 10 minutes) in a different and more flexible way.

Family structure

A key step in counselling is to set out the family structure, starting with whoever is in the household at the time. Zander *et al* (1978) showed a simple way to chart this. GPs can easily evolve their own amendments – mine include using arrows to show pressurising relationships, where one member of the family feels under pressure from another, and red lines and arrows to show family violence. It is surprising and sad how few general practice records show family/household charts and how few GPs realise how much time they save in subsequent consultations. They also act as an *aide-mémoire*, so that, for example, the family doctor when seeing a mother or adolescent is instantly reminded of the names of all the children in the family and their ages and the birth order.

Colour, culture, creed, class, and customs

To understand people, one has to understand the framework in which they live their lives. None of these five variables may be crucial, but each and all can be important factors in the lives of many people. It is how the patient sees it that matters.

Colour

Colour is visible but hard to discuss. Most family doctors working with patients of different colour, provided they engage in regular frequent talks and do not narrow the consultation down (Byrne & Long, 1976), will soon become aware whether their patients feel at odds with the society in which they live and work. If they do, many apparent relationship problems, especially some at school, at work, and with authorities in society, especially local government and the police, may be better understood.

Culture and creed

One of the unmet needs in training is to help GPs understand the cultures of different groups of patients in society. One of the important contributions of the book *The Future General Practitioner* (Royal College of General Practitioners, 1972) was to list a framework for the whole of general practice, one section of which was entitled ''Medicine in society''. This outlined the GP's role in society. Many medical decisions and much medical advice have quite a different impact if the patient and doctor have different cultural or religious perspectives. The Abortion Act 1968 created immediate difficulties for doctors in general or hospital practice who are Roman Catholics and for some other Christians. The ramifications of relationships in households simply cannot be understood if the doctor does not understand the main principles of the culture and religion.

Fortunately there are a growing number of texts available, and some are specifically medical, such as Qureshi's (1989) *Transcultural Medicine*. Most patients from minority cultures are usually only too pleased to talk to their doctor about their way of living and their religion, and this is not only usually of great interest, but listening does wonders for the patient–doctor relationship.

A common cultural issue is the health and relationships of a foreign wife. It is a common experience in general practice that such women may face special tensions in accommodating to a new culture and bringing children up in ways different from those of their own childhood.

Culture and creed and the relationships they engender can dominate and swamp consultations in general practice, as when I was once called to a teenage girl crying hysterically on a late evening visit. She was from an ethnic minority group, but had been brought up in England at an English school. She was to be married the next day to a man she had never seen, chosen in accordance with her culture by relatives. She faced that night a clash between Eastern and Western values and culture, and the stakes were high. She risked losing her family, her home, her religion, and all her cultural supports. Her family doctor was white, male, middle aged, and Christian. The lengthy consultation which ensued amounted to emotional first aid only, as cultural factors were over-riding.

The computer record

The medical record can be of value if it shows key facts about culture and creed, and they are more easily remembered and used if they are easily available during consultations. Most computer systems do not yet accommodate this easily, so free text entries are an advantage.

Class

Social class in Britain remains important, with sharply different health statistics between the classes. Here, class matters mainly when there are class differences within the home or when the practice is insensitive to class issues in the consulting-room.

One element of social class is the attitude to education. It is sometimes possible to give encouragement to teenagers or young adults and help them to grow, although the doctor may have to take a very long-term view. For example, I have a patient brought up in a big family on a council estate with an alcoholic parent in a home with little interest in education and no books. Through repeated encouragement, one young man, after leaving school without examinations, took evening classes, and is now at university.

Customs

Customs are the most general and interesting category. How does this household work? What do they see as a normal way of life? What are their values? Much of this is commonsense, but analysis can help GPs, particularly in responding to the needs of adolescents. Are there any books in the house? If not, does this point to problems for an older teenager trying to study with no room to work in.

Do the parents value them, let alone their work? Did both parents or an older child go to a university, is a younger sibling under pressure to follow? How much of a girl's anorexia is a reflexion of a parent–child relationship or school relationship? GPs, after years of talking with people as they go through their lives, are good at understanding family codes and customs, but are less good at classifying them and using the understanding more formally in consulting. A taxonomy is the first need and is likely to be a fruitful area for research.

Personality

'Personality' has been defined by the *Oxford English Dictionary* as the "distinctive character or qualities of a person". As such, personality analysis becomes a central subject of interest to those who want to be personal doctors.

Simple personality characteristics, like introvert and extrovert, have passed into everyday language. The use of more formal tests is steadily growing in general practice, but so far almost entirely in educational or academic settings. Freeling used the Myers–Briggs on the first Nuffield course for general practitioner educationalists (*Journal of the Royal College of General*

Practitioners, 1975) and Lewis & Bolden (1989) used the Learning Styles Questionnaire (LSQ) of Honey & Mumford (1986) in relation to general practitioner learning. The Exeter Department of General Practice also uses the FIRO-B and Belbin instruments.

Relationship problems essentially consist of clashes between personalities. Advice must therefore rest on analysis and understanding of the two or more people concerned. General practitioners are usually people-oriented people and often do these assessments naturally; the need remains to categorise and codify common scenarios in primary care, so that they can be studied and alternative interventions examined.

Parent–child relationships

The family doctor has a rare set of privileges in understanding parent–child relationships. First he/she is one of the few people, and sometimes the only person, outside the family who knows whether the pregnancy was intended and, if not, how much the mother regretted it or considered abortion. Secondly, he/she is one of the few often to know whether the father is, in the mother's view, the husband/cohabitee or not.

Then, seeing the mother perhaps six or seven times through the pregnancy for antenatal care, and then two or three times postnatally and doing the postnatal examination, it is easy to learn how the mother views the arrival – which can vary from excitement to continuing regret. Bonding is observed first-hand, as is the knowledge about breast-feeding. Indeed, even the style of breast-feeding predicts how far any mother will defer to the wishes of the child (demand versus regular feeding). By the time of the six-week postnatal examination and the asides when family planning is being discussed (''I hope to have another in a year or two'' or ''I could never go through all that again!''), the family doctor should have a reasonable picture of how that family is functioning at home (Pereira Gray, 1978).

The introduction of child health surveillance into general practice has strengthened the already good links between children and their family doctors. Seeing the children regularly, in health as well as sickness, gives an excellent opportunity, as do the numerous contacts for illness, which alone run to an average of one consultation or visit every eight weeks right up to the age of five (Office of Population Censuses and Surveys, 1991). An important part of child health surveillance is inquiring about and systematically thinking about the emerging and developing parent–child relationship. This is why many GPs interested in personal care rejected (*Journal of the Royal College of General Practitioners*, 1978) the Court concept of the GP paediatrician (Committee on Child Health Services, 1976), as they wanted to see personally the way their children were growing up in the practice. Nowadays there are earlier opportunities to intervene, with health visitors in the practice, when these go awry, and to intervene at an earlier stage than used to be possible in the past.

The 'won't do' syndromes

Nevertheless, however comprehensive the child health surveillance, there will always be a group of problems presented by a parent, usually the mother, which can be summarised as the 'won't do' syndromes. These can take many forms, but three of the commonest are: "he won't sleep, doctor", "he won't eat", or "won't obey". All these represent tensions in the parent–child relationship, but can best be understood and managed as tensions in the family relationships. As a simple *aide-mémoire* they can be caused by the three 'f's: fear, failure, and friction.

The fear is parental fear, and is commonest in feeding problems. Insecure, especially young, mothers fear the child will starve or die if it does not eat enough. Meal-time battles ensue when the amount of food thought appropriate by the mother does not match the child's wishes or needs. Careful reassurance by the family doctor or the health visitor, coupled with a judicious use of centile growth charts and advice, to remove all pressure and let the child eat what it wants, while sitting at the table, with no food between meals, will usually restore good relations.

The 'won't sleep' syndrome is similar, and often reflects the fear of one parent that the neighbours will complain. But this is the overt reason – the real reasons are usually deeper and to do with family feelings and behaviour. Amazingly elaborate rituals can ensue, with the child commonly ending up in the parent's bed. It is always valuable for the family doctor to get the parents to describe in detail exactly what happens in the household and how often. Intense unhappiness can occur. There are often sexual overtones, and it has been well said that the child in the bed may be another form of contraception.

The 'f' for friction is often the friction between the new parents, who need to agree the rules of the house; many children sense and exploit differences in parental views, especially about discipline. Behavioural problems ensue; parental friction then prevents a consistent parental response. The management is usually to see the two parents together and help them agree a common policy.

The 'f' for failure is the inability of a parent to say no to a child in such a way that it is meant, so the child finds successful rebellion pays and then continues. The 'won't do' is usually presented as a 'won't obey', and the mother's unhappiness can represent clinical depression. Careful discussion with the mother, building up her confidence in herself, and helping her to think through to adolescence and what self-gratification with drugs, for example, can mean, is usually possible within the context of day-to-day general practice.

Several forms of criminal behaviour, especially stealing in children, can be associated with emotional disturbance, the so-called 'cry for help'. It is always worth exploring the relationships in the household and school, and often the child is reacting to lack of love or, more commonly, lack of quality time with one or both parents.

Sibling relationships

Sibling relationships get much less attention than parent–child or marital ones, but deserve much more. They can be marvellous and loving, but have a latent tension which can easily erupt in jealousy, especially between siblings of the same sex.

Scapegoating

Scapegoating is a destructive form of group behaviour which can occur in families. It can apply to children or any family member. The child gradually starts to attract all the criticism and all the sins are heaped upon him/her. It is a serious condition, with danger of emotionally scarring, and it is an important diagnosis for a family doctor to make as such children are vulnerable.

One useful question is to ask the parent what is good about the child, and a prolonged silence or, as I received in one instance, "Nothing!", clarifies the feelings quickly.

Marital or man–woman relationships

Marital partnership relationship problems are common in primary care. In the author's practice, as many as one-eighth of all adults have at some time consulted for such problems. They are coded as an item on the computer diagnostic record and so can be analysed.

They appear most often via the woman, as women are far higher consulters in most Western countries, and marital issues then emerge, particularly in depression. Indeed, marital problems are a potent cause of depression.

Description

The first step is simply to legitimise the discussion. Most people feel guilty about talking about their marriages and relationships even to their doctor, and the subject may only come up when patients are at the end of their tether or generally overwrought or depressed. The doctor can help by providing an empathic ear and simply listening. A follow-up appointment can then be made.

The presenting patient's experience

Next, it is necessary to summarise the patient's description of the problem, capturing, essentially, what are the important things the patient feels. Exactly who is doing what to whom and how often? In particular it is important to clarify if there has ever been any physical or sexual violence, and if so how often and when.

Throughout the consultations the GP has to achieve a difficult balance in being gently sympathetic, without taking sides. He/she may be the husband's/spouse's doctor too, and one loose word can be relayed at home as ammunition in a verbal battle.

The patient's perception of cause

At about the third consultation it is worth clarifying exactly why the patient thinks the other person is acting as described. General comments: "Because he is a brute!", should not be left, but be gently probed further with questions like: "How do you think this began?" or "Why should he be a brute?" (Reflecting the exact term used has three advantages: firstly it reassures the patient that she is being listened to carefully; secondly, it helps rapport; and thirdly, it facilitates further information.)

It is always important to see how far the presenter sees the partner as being under pressure and from what. It is common for reference to be made to chronic unemployment and its debilitating effects, often to pressures at work, and sometimes to ill health (not always reported). Alcohol consumption should always be explored.

Issues to clarify are the element of control in the marriage. Does the woman have her own money and bank/savings account? Who takes what kind of decisions? It is always necessary to find out if either partner has, or thinks the other has, another relationship, and if so whether it is thought to be sexual.

Questions about the relevance and influence of the other partner's parents may be useful. Broad, open-ended questions work best. Do you think he/she is like his/her parents? Do you think his/her childhood was important? Is he/she at all like his/her parents? A ten-minute consultation on this alone is usually well worthwhile.

Patient–doctor synthesis

At some point it is necessary to summarise the problems and to be sure there is agreement with the patient that it is a correct summary. Saying "Is there anything more you would want to add?" can help. It is then necessary to start to help the patient to do something about them. There are many options, and the skill lies in helping patients to appreciate the choices and to decide for themselves. It is important to move the consultation on past the summary, as otherwise an endless and unproductive series of complaints can continue for years.

Planning

The next step is to establish that there needs to be a plan, and that it is the patient's responsibility to make it, while the doctor will offer some thoughts and possibilities. Asking "Have you got a plan of what to do?" usually leads to a negative reply, especially if the depression questionnaire is being used and the patient has answered 'yes' to having feelings of hopelessness. The doctor now needs a menu of practical proposals which can be quietly discussed, the process being rather like offering a patient family-planning advice. The following options exist.

Telling the partner about consulting

Commonly the patient consulting does not tell the partner the marriage is being discussed. Discussing the discussion is worthwhile in itself, although many patients will not feel able to talk at home to their partner, which is a bad prognostic sign. Offering another agency for marriage guidance advice such as 'Relate' both gives the patient a choice and may sometimes be more acceptable to the other partner, especially if not registered with the practice. This, or referral to a practice counsellor, may be the end-point if the doctor does not wish to continue.

Seeing the partner

The main issue is to find an opportunity to see the couple together. This is the crossing point between background advice and specific formal counselling. The ways the interview is arranged are important. Asking patients to bring the spouse with them is one. Writing to the spouse and asking them to come is another. Telephoning is a third possibility.

Waiting until the spouse comes of their own accord for something else is a possibility. Engineering a three-year check a little early is a new variant. Each method has its own advantages and disadvantages. The main complication of asking the presenter to ask the partner is that the partner may feel 'dragged in', or start with the impression that the doctor is on the other person's side. This is less likely to occur if the doctor approaches the spouse directly.

Counselling couples

Counselling couples is not to every practitioner's taste, and is best done by those with a strong interest in behavioural medicine and with experience of interactive small groups. Some training or formal experience is highly desirable.

The first step is for the doctor to say that he/she is the doctor to both and will not take sides.

Then the second partner can be given the chance to explain their point of view, and a parallel process follows of listening and asking questions until synthesis has again been agreed. This is usually quicker and easier with the second partner alone, but it can be done as a three.

The most important phase is the joint discussion with the two partners together, at which they are encouraged to listen to each other and find their own solutions. In general practice this phase is usually intense and short lived. Couples rarely need many interviews, since they either make progress or one partner drifts away.

One way of maintaining this work in ordinary general practice surgeries is to recognise a limited number of key issues and to obtain agreement that they are important and that something practical can be done. The skills are not unlike those of chairmanship, where analysis and summarising are predominant skills, and many GPs make skilled chairmen.

It is a mistake to ask too much; I rarely suggest that the patient or couple do more than one or two things before the next consultation, and one of these may be to think over some issue.

Style

The GP must watch for co-existent disease and to diagnose it when present. Whatever the doctor's philosophy about psychosomatic disease, it is clear that unhappy and unfulfilled people have more illness and react less favourably to ill health. This role of the doctor may make management easier; it can be useful to carry out an examination and even arrange some blood tests, all the while continuing to explore the relationship. Depression is highly correlated with marital relationship problems and is worth systematic consideration for both partners.

The doctor's style must, as far as possible, be non-judgemental, but more authority can be used in the consulting-room compared with many counsellors, to enforce an equal say for both partners, and to interrupt repetition of statements. It is often helpful for the doctor to adjust the sequence in which problems are dealt with so as to achieve some early successes and thus build up the couple's self-images.

Outcome

About one-third of the marital problems seen in general practice will resolve well, with a happy long-term result, about a third will resolve only partially, with the couples continuing to live together but with recurring tensions, and about one-third will lead to separation or divorce. The GP has special advantages over other agencies in auditing and assessing long-term results, as in many cases the patients will remain on the list for many years, and it is possible to learn at first hand of the progress of the marriage.

Conclusions

Relationship problems are common in general practice and present either directly, or associated with emotional medicine like depression. The family doctor is well placed to understand and manage the majority of these, and they are not as time-consuming as is often thought. Practitioners who do not wish or who do not feel able to handle this work can and should refer to others – counsellors in the practice or organisations such as 'Relate', or to adult or child psychiatrists.

The need is urgent for general practice to evolve techniques of its own, other than long consultations and classic counselling techniques, to exploit its unique set of relationships with several members of families over long periods of time.

For most physical problems and diseases such as asthma, hypertension, hyperlipidaemia, and most infections in most parts of the body, British GPs reckon to deal with about 85% of all problems entirely within the general practice team. The same proportions are true for emotional disorders like depression. There is no reason why 85–90% of relationship problems cannot be well handled within primary care as well.

The consultation approach in psychiatry and general practice is different and complementary. Psychiatrists tend to gather their data in a few long interviews and to document systematically. The advantages of this approach are substantial, and in particular full systematic coverage of all of a list of parameters is usually achieved. However, the specialist in this situation is recording much second-hand (hearsay) data, and often much more than they realise. They learn and write about spouses and parents whom they have never met and homes they have never seen.

General practitioners, in contrast, frequently have professional first-hand knowledge of the way the patient lives, the home, the spouse or partner, access to their medical history and often enough to be useful personal knowledge of parents and grandparents. GPs undervalue and underplay these advantages, largely because they have not often recorded them or codified their information. They often have colleagues in the primary team, such as health visitors or nurses, with whom information and assessments can be checked.

The central failure of general practice is the failure to be systematic and to work through a formal check-list of key questions of parameters needed for assessment. This is reflected in a lack of publications on the ways of working in emotional medicine and the achievements possible in general practice. No branch of medicine is better placed to develop, analyse, and publish the biographical approach to medical care, and the future will be bright as this potential is realised.

References

Balint, M. (1957) *The Doctor, His Patient and the Illness.* London: Pitman.

BERGER, J. & MOHR, J. (1969) *A Fortunate Man*. London: Penguin.
BERNE, E. (1964) *Games People Play*. London: Penguin.
BROWNE, K. & FREELING, P. (1976) *The Doctor–Patient Relationship*. (2nd edn). Edinburgh: Livingstone.
BYRNE, P. S. & LONG, B. E. C. (1976) *Doctors Talking to Patients*. London: HMSO.
COMMITTEE ON CHILD HEALTH SERVICES (1976) *Fit for the Future*, cmnd 6680. London: HMSO.
DEPARTMENT OF HEALTH (1990) *Health and Personal Social Services Statistics for England*. London: HMSO.
DEPARTMENT OF HEALTH STATISTICAL AND INFORMATION DIVISION (1991) *General Medical Practitioners' Workload Survey, 1989–90*. London: DoH.
DRUCKER, P. (1977) *Management*. London: Pan.
FREEMAN, G. & RICHARDS, S. (1990) How much personal care in four group practices? *British Medical Journal*, **301**, 1028–1030.
GENERAL MEDICAL SERVICES COMMITTEE (1992) *Your Choices for the Future: UK Report*. London: Electoral Reform Ballot Services.
HONEY, P. & MUMFORD, A. (1986) *Manual of Learning Styles*. Maidenhead: Honey.
HUYGEN, F. J. A. (1978) *Family Medicine. The Medical Life History of Families*. Nijmegen: Dekker & van de Vegt. (Reprinted (1990) by the Royal College of General Practitioners.)
JOURNAL OF THE ROYAL COLLEGE OF GENERAL PRACTITIONERS (1975) The Nuffield experiment (editorial). *Journal of the Royal College of General Practitioners*, **25**, 547–548.
—— (1978) Looking after children (editorial). *Journal of the Royal College of General Practitioners*, **28**, 519–520.
LANE, K. (1969) *The Longest Art*. London: George Allen and Unwin. (Republished (1992), Royal College of General Practitioners.)
LEWIS, A. P. & BOLDEN, K. J. (1989) General practitioners and their learning styles. *Journal of the Royal College of General Practitioners*, **39**, 187–189.
OFFICE OF POPULATION CENSUSES AND SURVEYS (1991) *General Household Survey 1989*. London: HMSO.
PEREIRA GRAY, D. J. (1978) Feeling at home. James Mackenzie Lecture. *Journal of the Royal College of General Practitioners*, **28**, 6–17.
—— (1979) The key to personal care. *Journal of the Royal College of General Practitioners*, **29**, 666–678.
QURESHI, B. (1989) *Transcultural Medicine*. Lancaster: Kluwer Academic Press.
RITCHIE, J., JACOBY, A. & BONE, M. (1981) *Access to Primary Health Care*. London: HMSO.
ROYAL COLLEGE OF GENERAL PRACTITIONERS (1972) *The Future General Practitioner – Learning and Teaching*. London: British Medical Journal. (Republished by the Royal College of General Practitioners.)
—— (1982) *Healthier Children – Thinking Prevention. Report from General Practice 22*. London: Royal College of General Practitioners.
——, OFFICE OF POPULATION CENSUSES AND SURVEYS & DEPARTMENT OF HEALTH (1990) *Morbidity Statistics from General Practice – 1981–82*. London: HMSO.
WESTCOTT, R. H. (1977) The length of consultations in general practice. *Journal of the Royal College of General Practitioners*, **27**, 552–555.
ZANDER, L. I., BEREFORD, S. A. A. & THOMAS, P. (1978) *Medical Records in General Practice. Occasional Paper 5*. London: Royal College of General Practitioners.

7 Depression

ALASTAIR WRIGHT

Depression is one of Britain's major health problems, not only because of prolonged work absence and poor work performance, but also in terms of human misery. It is a potentially life-threatening clinical illness, as most of the 4000 people committing suicide in the UK each year suffer from depression. Evidently many sufferers do not receive the treatment they desperately need.

Most people who seek medical help for psychological difficulties turn first to their GP. Depression is one of the commonest clinical illnesses found in attending patients, surveys indicating that 1 in 10 attending patients can be diagnosed as suffering from depression, and 1 in 20 would meet criteria for major depressive disorder (Blacker & Clare, 1987).

A significant proportion of this depression goes untreated, and it is clear that there are factors both within the doctor and the patient which make the detection of emotional disturbances less likely. As modern treatment is effective in most cases of depression, it is important to improve case recognition. Recent research (Gask *et al* 1987, 1988) confirms that diagnostic skills can be improved by appropriate training. Over 90% of identified cases of depression are managed exclusively in primary care without referral to a psychiatrist (Goldberg & Huxley, 1980), so GPs bear much of the burden of caring for all mental illness in the community.

What is depression?

In many ways the word 'depression' is an unsatisfactory term. The same word is used to describe an everyday mood, a symptom, or a disease. There is some merit in the use of older terms such as 'melancholia' or 'neurasthenia', as they suggest a clinical picture and add emphasis to our concepts of the disease. What is important is to distinguish individual symptoms of depression from the syndrome, that is when the number and severity of symptoms justifies a clinical diagnosis of depressive illness.

The key feature of all depressive illness is persistent low mood associated with slowed thinking and impaired efficiency. It is accompanied by a range of characteristic physical symptoms. Depressed people are unable to interest themselves in their normal activities or take pleasure in usual pastimes. As depression deepens, a peculiarly negative way of thinking develops with thoughts of personal worthlessness and guilt about past actions. Patients become hopeless, helpless, and intensely pessimistic. Such attitudes on the part of the patient make good compliance with treatment difficult to achieve.

Patients may describe depression as a black cloud, or say they feel that the sun has gone out or that they are living in a green bottle separate from the rest of humanity, unable to love or be loved. Doctors who have suffered from depression as well as physical disease describe the pain of depression as greater than that of myocardial infarction and much less easy to relieve. One doctor has described his ''desperate unhappiness'' and recalls the ''sheer desperation of forcing myself to go to work every day. . . . Depression is very much an illness . . . but it feels different, one feels stigmatised . . .'' (Anonymous, 1989).

Regrettably, depression may be made worse for the patient by the stigma still attached to mental health problems (Sims, 1993), despite a more open attitude to discussing such illnesses. A general public attitude survey, conducted over chosen sites in England in 1991, confirmed the widespread view that psychiatric illness implied weakness, abnormality, and instability (Royal College of Psychiatrists, 1992). Most people considered that physical illness is easier to sympathise with because it is easier to see than mental illness. The commonest perceived 'causes' of depression were life events, such as break-up of a relationship, bereavement, loss of a job, or having a baby. Depression was frequently thought to be linked with the sufferer's ability to cope with life. Depressed patients struggling with thoughts of personal worthlessness and guilt need to be reassured by their doctor that depression is not weakness of character but a well-defined clinical illness.

Psychiatrists have found it constructive to define depression in terms of 'major' depressive disorder (American Psychiatric Association, 1980). Criteria are listed in terms of persistent dysphoric mood and at least four from a list of major symptoms being present for at least two weeks. The term 'major' does not imply that other forms of depression are trivial: milder episodes that do not reach the threshold for major depression are also important in general practice. The concept of a research diagnostic definition is particularly useful in research work, but is of less value in general practice.

Formal specifications emphasise the measuring of symptoms, whereas general practitioners are also guided by sociodemographic or family factors, and social stresses and supports. These non-symptom factors are important in clinical decision-making and management but are difficult to measure or standardise. Attitudes of research psychiatrists have also changed with regard to measuring 'caseness'. Instead of focusing on the number of symptoms complained of, more emphasis is now placed on the type of symptoms, their severity, statistical relationships, and the help-seeking behaviour shown by patients.

It should also be remembered that the demarcation between depression and anxiety disorders is not precise, so that mixed states are common in general practice. The main aim for general practitioners is to recognise and treat depression at an early stage, so it is less suitable to think in terms of exclusive criteria.

It is useful to summarise the clinical features of the depression seen in general practice under three headings:

(a) changed mood
    (i) persistent sadness
    (ii) pathological pessimism
    (iii) abnormal self-reproach
    (iv) lassitude
    (v) inability to feel
    (vi) thoughts of suicide
    (vii) weeping
    (viii) shame
(b) changed drive and thinking
    (i) unable to cope
    (ii) loss of interest and concentration
    (iii) difficulty in making decisions
    (iv) hopeless and helpless
    (v) wish to escape
(c) physical symptoms
    (i) tired all the time
    (ii) aches and pains
    (iii) loss of libido
    (iv) disturbed sleep – early wakening
    (v) loss of weight
    (vi) inability to relax.

Many of the symptoms of depression are non-specific and so common that, on their own, they are of little value for diagnosis or in predicting outcome. Psychomotor retardation is very diagnostic but of little relevance as it is so rare in general practice. Two common and relatively specific symptoms are particularly helpful when the diagnosis is in doubt. These are, firstly, persistent depression of mood with loss of the ability to enjoy normal pleasures (anhedonia), and, secondly, marked impairment of concentration.

Another useful discriminator is the length of time symptoms have been present, especially if they are experienced every day. The longer the symptoms have been present the more likely it is that the patient has a depressive illness rather than simple low spirits. A man who weeps in the consulting-room is almost certainly depressed.

This depression seen by GPs is not a transient or minor illness. It is not weakness of character but a well defined clinical illness. About half of such patients attending their GPs are unable to continue with their normal lives (Johnson & Mellor, 1987).

Subtypes

Depressive illness is sometimes classified in subtypes based on aetiology, symptoms, or other criteria. In general practice this subdivision is not of value in deciding the need for treatment or in predicting outcome. Similarly, subdivision into endogenous or reactive, neurotic or psychotic subtypes is of more value for research and administration than for clinical work. In the community it is more serviceable to think in terms of severity, and to consider whether there are associated problems such as manic features, alcohol abuse, personality disorder, or serious physical illness.

It is also helpful clinically to think of the special features of depressive illness at different ages and in terms of transitions such as childbirth, the menopause, or bereavement. This has the advantage of increasing the doctor's awareness of the possibility of depression, which may not present directly.

Depression becomes more common with increasing age, but it occurs in children as well as the aged. It is commoner in women than men and appears to be more widespread in young men than was recognised formerly. In children, in adolescents, and in the elderly depression may sometimes be recognised in different ways. It may present with different features in ethnic minorities. In all cultures mood disorder is commonly expressed by somatic symptoms.

Depression in childhood and adolescence

Like adults, children can suffer depressed mood, anxiety, and the inability to feel affection, but they rarely complain of this, perhaps because they are less able to verbalise their feelings. The possibility of depression in a disturbed child is often missed because it is not considered.

Typically, a depressed child may develop phobias or hypochondriasis and show obsessional personality features. The child may appear depressed and may show features of anxiety or irritability. School refusal is common, although this may also be a manifestation of maternal depression. As with adults, disturbed sleep is common. School performance quickly deteriorates with the onset of the illness, and unexplained abdominal pain is common. Children who have been sexually abused often develop short-term or delayed depressive reactions, and behaviour disturbances should be a warning to health professionals.

The prevalence of psychiatric illness, including depression, among children and teenagers, is higher than generally realised, so that many sufferers remain unrecognised and untreated (Williams, 1993). This is particularly unfortunate in view of the links between childhood psychiatric disorder and mental illness in later life. Family doctors must also be aware of the interaction within the family when depressive illness is present. There is a clear link between depression in a parent and emotional and cognitive impairment in the children which can have an adverse effect on intellectual attainment, as well as predisposing to adult mental illness.

Adolescent turmoil with low self-esteem is so common that GPs may be reluctant to diagnose depressive illness in this age group. Adolescents look depressed more often than do children. A characteristic sign of depression is an unexpectedly poor performance in examinations due to low levels of interest and concentration. Although GPs may be reluctant to apply the label 'depression' to adolescents, they respond just as well to treatment as do adults.

Depression in older people

Older people may feel that their depressed mood is a normal part of ageing and may not seek help for their depression. Many believe they should consult a doctor for physical complaints only, and are also less likely to accept psychological explanations for their symptoms.

Rather than seeming depressed, older people may appear to be complaining, querulous, difficult, and demanding. They may complain of feeling 'empty' or 'cold inside' rather than saying they are miserable or depressed. Both they and the doctor may attribute symptoms of depression to coexisting physical illness. Chronic somatic disease may precipitate depressive illness just as self-neglect in elderly depressed patients may result in physical illness.

If elderly depressed patients are confused, forgetful or withdrawn, they may be regarded as demented and denied appropriate treatment for their real problem of depression. Depression develops relatively quickly, dementia insidiously. Depressed patients appear more distressed and less blunted than those with dementia. They are guilty, self-reproachful, and often have somatic symptoms which are uncommon in dementia. It is important to distinguish between the two, as response to treatment is much better in depression.

Occasional home visiting is important for these elderly depressed people and the GP should consider having a practice at-risk register. After recognising depression it is important the doctor does something about it (Williamson *et al*, 1964). Older people respond to the same drugs and interventions that are effective in younger patients although special care is needed when prescribing antidepressant drugs in view of the possibility of impaired hepatic or renal function, and the fact that elderly people are more likely to be taking drugs concurrently for chronic physical illness. Electroconvulsive therapy may have a useful place in severe cases and some psychiatrists consider it safer in severe cases than psychotropic drugs.

Bipolar disorder (manic depression)

Most practices will have a number of patients who suffer from depressive symptoms which are associated with dramatic swings in mood. Mania, a state of peculiar excitement in which the patient loses touch with reality, is rarely seen in general practice. The less severe form, hypomania, is an important and not uncommon condition in which patients show pressure of speech, grandiose ideas, and loss of normal social inhibitions. Patients may be so hyperactive that they squander money and may make hasty, irrevocable, and destructive decisions about work or marriage. The introduction of lithium salts in maintenance treatment has much improved the control of this distressing condition. The dose of lithium needs to be adjusted by serial blood sampling, which can be done simply within the practice.

Dysthymia

This condition of chronic low-grade depression is regarded by some as a depressive personality disorder, but it may result from inadequately treated major depression. The essential feature is the chronicity rather than the severity of the depression.

Such patients form an important subgroup of 'frequent attenders' in the consulting-room, tending also to be over-users of medicaments. They form part of the group of "heartsink" patients (O'Dowd, 1988), who can be difficult to help and stressful for the doctor to manage on a long-term basis.

The clinical picture is of a long-lasting disturbance of mood with associated symptoms which are not of sufficient severity and duration to justify a diagnosis of major depressive disorder. Patients show little interest or pleasure in most usual activities or pastimes although they normally function quite well in their social contacts and at work.

Bereavement depression

Most bereaved people pass through recognisable stages of grieving without necessarily suffering frank psychiatric illness. Normal grieving involves:

(a) a short period of emotional blunting, when the individual feels dazed and numb and follows normal activities in a automatic manner; frequently patients have poor subsequent memory of this stage

(b) within weeks or even days patients may become preoccupied with thoughts of the dead loved one, and feel intense yearning and perhaps guilt; most people have some of the symptoms of depressive illness such as disturbed sleep, weeping, and depressed mood without necessarily developing the full-blown illness

(c) within six months most bereaved people come slowly to accept the death of their loved one and readjust to normal life.

A few people will be unable to make this adjustment, and depressive illness supervenes. This type of depression responds better to a behavioural approach than to antidepressants. Benzodiazepine sedatives or hypnotics are best avoided, as patients readily become dependent on them.

Recognising depression in the community

Prevalence of mental illness

As many as one in three patients attending their GP have a demonstrable psychosocial component to the consultation, although not necessarily psychiatric illness (see Chapter 3). Since the early epidemiological research by Shepherd *et al* (1966; Jenkins & Shepherd, 1983), several workers have confirmed frank psychiatric illness in between 20% and 25% of attending patients (Goldberg & Blackwell, 1970; Hoeper *et al*, 1979).

Prevalence of depression

Depression is the commonest psychiatric illness seen by GPs; in fact, it is one of the commonest clinical problems that they have to deal with. Reported prevalence rates for depression based on standardised interviews vary between studies (Neilson & Williams, 1980; Wright *et al*, 1980; Casey *et al*, 1984), but it is likely that at least one depressed patient will be seen at each surgery session.

While GPs efficiently diagnose and manage a large number of depressed patients, there is good evidence that many consulting patients who have depression are not recognised, especially when somatic symptoms are prominent. Patients known to the doctor as having true physical illness are particularly likely to be missed (Wright, 1988).

Reasons for non-recognition

Particular difficulties arise with depressed patients who present with somatic symptoms and act in a less depressed way. The problem is not that the features of depression are absent, but that key symptoms are hidden by a great deal of somatic 'interference'. These patients may prefer to consider themselves as under strain rather than as depressed: the doctor may need to negotiate the diagnosis of depression. Although patient factors are important, better diagnosis depends on the clinical vigilance of the GP. The doctor needs to keep in mind the possibility of depression in disturbed patients presenting mainly somatic symptoms (Wright & Perini, 1987), and also in patients presenting frequently with very varied physical symptoms ('fat file patients').

The reasons for non-diagnosis of depression by GPs have been intensively studied (Marks *et al*, 1979; Davenport *et al*, 1987; Goldberg & Bridges, 1987). There are factors within the doctor, the patient and the consultation process which make the detection of emotional disturbance less likely (Gask *et al*, 1987; Freeling & Tylee, 1992).

Doctor factors

Some doctors are predisposed towards physical explanations for patient symptoms and are uncomfortable dealing with psychological problems. They may behave in ways that make patients less likely to offer clues to their depressive illness. Such doctors tend to use closed questions which can be answered with a simple 'yes' or 'no', allowing patients little chance to explain the problem in their own words. Questions may be asked from a prepared list rather than responding to what the patient has just said.

Patient factors

Depressed patients, who generally suffer low self-esteem as part of their illnesses, may be reluctant to approach a doctor because they are ashamed of their feelings, or fear that the doctor will not have time to listen to them. On the other hand, some patients may not recognise their distress as an illness, so the depression may be masked in various ways when the patient presents. A crucial factor may be the tendency for some patients to somatise their psychological distress, so that they start the consultation by complaining of a physical symptom although their main problem is psychological (Wright, 1990). This somatisation is common but particularly so in some ethnic minorities. Patients may give verbal clues to their depression while about to leave the consulting-room or when the doctor is concentrating on the physical examination.

Organisation of care systems

The pattern of the health care in general practice is radically different from that in specialist practice. Short appointments mean that primary complaints are followed before secondary and tertiary problems can be pursued. High consulting rates leave GPs less time to ask open questions on the emotional and social aspects of the patient's problem.

This explanation cannot, however, be made an excuse, as the decision can be spread over several consultations achieving the same effect. After initial assessment and explanation to the patient, a longer appointment can be arranged at a more suitable time. This extra time is usefully spent in negotiating the acceptance of the diagnosis by the patient and in ensuring compliance with treatment. In times of personal crisis time must occasionally be found even if other patients are kept waiting.

Improving recognition

General practitioners have a challenging responsibility to distinguish, in a comparatively short consultation, a varied assortment of minor problems from covert, potentially life-threatening physical illness. Some doctors are better than others at recognising depression (Freeling & Tylee, 1992). These doctors are generally 'good listeners'. During the consultation they look at the patient rather than the notes and are less likely to interrupt the patient's story. They accept and make use of silence and use the patient's answers in further discussion. Accurate diagnosticians tend to have the directive consulting style that patients prefer, have more factual knowledge about depression, and have a special interest in psychiatry. Gask *et al* (1988), using video feedback techniques, have shown that interviewing skills can be improved, and that these skills can be maintained. It has also been shown that GP trainers can be taught to teach the skills to their own trainees.

The normal 10-minute consultation in general practice can be adequate both for recogniton and management. What is important is not more time, but a better use of the time already available. This time may not necessarily be spent in detection but in negotiating what is to be done about the illness. It is also important to organise the practice so that there is continuity of contact between the patient and a specific GP.

Screening for depression using questionnaires or computer-administered interviews has been shown to improve recognition under research conditions (Johnstone & Goldberg, 1976). Instruments can be used to identify probable psychiatric cases but these tests cannot make a clinical diagnosis. Screening can be useful clinically in raising the doctor's awareness of the possibility of depression, and it is known that recognition improves outcome even when the patient does not comply with treatment (Freeling *et al*, 1985). Screening may be useful in high-risk groups, especially when the doctor is skilled and prepared to discuss social and psychological problems with the patient.

Managing depression in the community

General practitioners are well placed to treat their depressed patients, who may also have physical and social problems. Most people regard the GP as the best person to treat depression initially, with the psychiatrist as the best option for severe depression and family or friends for milder, everyday symptoms (Royal College of Psychiatrists, 1992). Most depressed patients can be fully and effectively managed in general practice without referral, providing that the GP is interested, and prepared to be systematic and to follow-up the patient carefully.

Treating depression in general practice should be seen against the background of continuing medical care of all kinds to the same few thousand people over time – often three generations. GPs, who often see and can treat the early stages of depressive illness, deal with a different population of psychiatrically ill people, who have different needs, from hospital in-patients or day patients. There are therefore some differences of approach to managing depression from that appropriate to patients who are referred to a psychiatrist.

Before deciding on management for an individual patient, an individual assessment is needed. The type of patient who has the illness is as important as the illness itself, so the personality and circumstances of the patient should be carefully considered when deciding appropriate treatment. The doctor must also evaluate how well the patient is coping with everyday life, what are the main psychosocial stresses, and what is the effectiveness of support from family and friends.

Assessment of suicide risk

Assessment of suicide risk is essential in all patients in whom suicide is a reasonable possibility. Most severely distressed patients are grateful to have the subject explored tactfully, and should be referred promptly if a serious risk is identified. It is best to work up from relatively gentle questions, otherwise denial may be too ready. It is not unusual for depressed patients to have occasional thoughts about suicide, but special care is needed when the patient becomes preoccupied with thoughts of suicide, has active plans, or fears that the urge might prove irresistible. Factors predisposing patients to suicide risk are:

(a) intense feelings of hopelessness and worthlessness
(b) depression with marked sleep disturbance
(c) poor physical health or much pain
(d) living alone
(e) recent stress, or loss
(f) being male, especially if over 45 years

(g) alcoholism or heavy drinking
(h) previous psychiatric illness or suicide attempt
(i) family history of mental illness or suicide
(j) family history of alcoholism.

Much of the patient's background and some of these risk factors will already be known to the GP, who must remember to use this information.

Special risk factors in women have been identified in a large survey by Brown & Harris (1978). These are:

(a) loss of mother by death or separation before the age of 12 years
(b) three or more children under five years
(c) lack of either a close caring relationship or a job.

General management

The basis of effective menagement in general practice is to offer the patient a series of short appointments, first weekly and then at longer intervals, depending on progress. This is not only supportive for patients, but regular attendance helps ensure compliance with treatment. It also allows the history and symptoms to be explored in a systematic way without being too disruptive of ordinary consulting sessions. This approach is appropriate to the realities of general practice and is derived from clinical experience. It is as sophisticated and effective in general practice populations as the more comprehensive, traditional approach is in out-patient clinics. A good understanding of the patient's view of problems and life events can sometimes permit the primary care team to prevent more serious psychiatric illness as well as treat established depression.

Initially, the patient should be seen briefly at least weekly to assess progress, check compliance, and offer simple counselling and support. The patient can be encouraged to talk about symptoms and perceived contributing problems. The doctor can suggest ways of dealing with problems, emphasising practical solutions or the need to come to terms with what cannot be changed.

Treatment possibilities

Reassurance, support, and the offer of further appointments are important for all patients, but this is not enough. Management possibilities include medication, supportive psychotherapy, or behaviour therapy (e.g. relaxation techniques, tapes). Cognitive therapy may be useful where there is prominent negative thinking, and social intervention where an unrewarding lifestyle seems remediable. Associated physical illness also requires treatment. Referral to a consultant psychiatrist should be considered where appropriate.

Depressed patients are an important group because of their numbers and because they are less likely to be helped by social measures. More could probably be achieved within the existing system by making greater use of psychological therapies, but these treatments may not be available to every practice. A significant component in improving outcome is simply recognition of the disease by the doctor and acceptance by the patient that he/she is suffering from an illness and that the prospects for cure are good.

Antidepressant medication

While not the doctor's only response to depressive illness, antidepressant drugs have a key role in relieving the misery of a great many patients suffering from this painful illness. Successful treatment depends on adequate dosage and duration of therapy. Antidepressants are used to relieve suffering, to shorten an episode of depression, and sometimes to prevent relapse.

Antidepressant therapy should not be withheld solely because the depression is apparently a reaction to stressful life events or whether or not the depression is understandable to the doctor. It is recommended that antidepressants are used where, irrespective of cause, there is a persistent picture of depressive syndrome, that is, symptoms additional to the depressed mood such as pessimistic thought, suicidal feelings, sleep and appetite disturbance, severe impairment of energy, interest or concentration, so that the patient's capacity to cope with normal living is impaired (Paykel & Priest, 1992).

Most available antidepressants have been shown to be superior to placebo, but no convincing difference in efficacy between individual drugs has been demonstrated. A wide range of effective drugs is now available for use in general practice. The standard tricyclic antidepressants have the advantage that doctors are familiar with their efficacy, side-effects, and the consequences of long-term use. They are also much cheaper than the newer compounds which, nevertheless, are less toxic in overdose and have fewer side-effects in normal use. Their improved side-effect profile may make these drugs more acceptable to patients, thus improving compliance.

Although there is a wide choice of antidepressants, it is not yet possible to define which patients will respond to one group of drugs rather than another. Apparent failure of treatment may be the result of inadequate dosage or poor compliance, which in turn may be due to side-effects. Change to another type of antidepressant drug will not necessarily eliminate adverse effects, but the changed pattern of drug effects may be more acceptable to the patient.

Tricyclic antidepressants

There is good evidence (Blashki *et al*, 1971; Paykel *et al*, 1988) from general practice populations that tricyclic antidepressants are efficacious in moderate to severe depression using doses customary in psychiatric practice

(125–150 mg daily). It is less clear whether they are effective in doses of 75 mg daily or lower, although there are patients who seem to stay well on such doses and to relapse on withdrawal.

The older tricyclics, such as amitriptyline, trimipramine, and their direct derivatives, are probably still the first choice of most GPs, although care is required with the elderly, and with patients with heart disease, hypertension, epilepsy, diabetes, glaucoma, prostatism, or suicidal tendencies. They are contraindicated in recent myocardial infarction and in heart block, in pregnancy, or where there is severe liver disease.

Normally, if prescribing a tricyclic, the doctor would start with a relatively small dose, especially in elderly patients, and increase the dose in stages until the full therapeutic level has been reached (e.g. 150 mg per day for a tricyclic antidepressant). The patient should be reassured that the treatment is not addictive but should be warned of both the expected delay in response and the common side-effects. The antidepressant effect from drugs should not be expected earlier than two to three weeks on full therapeutic dose. In the meantime, side-effects can be more acceptable to the patient as 'a sign that the medicine is working'.

Selective serotonin reuptake inhibitors

The place of the newer antidepressant drugs, including the selective serotonin reuptake inhibitors (SSRIs, also called 5-HT antagonists), is still controversial (Matthews & Eagles, 1991; see also correspondence in the *British Journal of General Practice* (1991), vol. 41, pp. 260, 302–303, 346). They have fewer side-effects, which helps compliance, and they are significantly less toxic in overdose. It is too early to be confident of their long-term safety, and as yet there have been few trials in elderly people. It would seem that this group of drugs has a place in patients with heart disease, glaucoma, or marked obesity, in those who are unable to tolerate tricyclics, or where there is a risk of deliberate overdose. They have been summed up by Edwards (1992) as "A modest though welcome advance in the treatment of depression".

Side effects are commonly gastrointestinal, such as nausea, vomiting and diarrhoea, although dizziness and tremor do occur and headache can be troublesome. Rare serious problems such as spontaneous bleeding, paranoid reactions and extrapyramidal effects have been reported from the USA, where drugs of this group have been extensively prescribed. In a meta-analysis of 63 randomised clinical trials, drop-out rates for patients taking SSRI antidepressants were not significantly different from those on tricyclic drugs (Song *et al*, 1993).

Preventing relapse

After successful treatment of the acute episode of the illness, the question of preventing relapse should be considered and discussed with the patient.

Following successful treatment with relief of the patient's symptoms, management can be considered in two phases, the first, or maintenance stage, lasting for six months, and the second, or prophylactic stage, extending beyond six months. Further episodes of illness during the first phase can be thought of as relapses, and any during the second phase as recurrences.

First stage

Studies show that inadequate therapy in the first six months results in relapse rates as high as 50% compared with 20% where treatment is continued. To prevent relapse, a further four to six months of treatment is recommended after symptoms have been relieved, at the dose at which a clinical response was achieved (Royal College of Psychiatrists & Royal College of General Practitioners, 1992). It is often difficult to convince a well patient to continue prophylactic drug therapy for this length of time, and compliance with such prophylaxis is often poor.

Second stage

Long-term prophylactic drug therapy is still a matter for clinical judgement. As yet there is neither consensus on appropriate dosage of antidepressants for long-term use nor on recommended total duration of prophylaxis. It would appear necessary to continue relatively high doses to ensure effective prophylaxis. Long-term antidepressant drug treatment should be carefully considered for recurring severe depression and for manic–depressive illness, for which lithium is specific.

The decision regarding long-term prophylaxis should be a joint one with the patient, with the risks and advantages being balanced against the benefit.

Non-drug prophylaxis

When available, non-drug methods of prophylaxis (e.g. cognitive therapy) should be offered to the patient in order to provide a choice of options. Patients should be made aware of facilities for group support and of self-help schemes in their locality.

The role of psychosocial management

Some patients do not respond to drugs alone, and others do not wish to take drugs for their depression. Most are helped by appropriate psychosocial management.

General practitioners should identify the problems that the patient is facing and the patient's personal priorities. It is often worthwhile to seek the support of family and friends, self-help groups, or support groups run by community psychiatric nurses or other health professionals. Discussing chronic social difficulties or relationship problems often brings relief to patients, even though they may feel powerless to change them.

Special therapies

Specific psychological therapies (Tyrer, 1988; Andrews, 1991) based on a recognised theoretical model can be useful in the type of depression found in general practice. In particular cognitive techniques with depressed patients can be effective and cost efficient in general practice (Ross & Scott, 1985). The gain from treatment has been shown to be maintained after 12 months, and patients likely to respond can be identified on the basis of chronicity and social stresses. The place of these therapies is dealt with in greater detail in Chapters 17 and 18.

Cognitive therapy

Cognitive therapy may be useful where there is prominent negative thinking. Major disadvantages of cognitive therapy are that it is not readily available to all GPs and that a course of treatment usually takes a total of 15 hours. When formal cognitive therapy is not available, the GP can adopt a general problem-solving approach with the patient. The doctor's management plan should be shared with the patient, who may be given written material. The patient may be set simple self-help tasks and asked to keep a diary of daily activities recording thoughts and feelings.

Counselling

Studies of brief counselling conducted by GPs have tended to be concerned with anxiety-reduction techniques rather than the management of depressive illness. Depressed people with marital problems do well when treated by counsellors attached to general practices. Women with postnatal depression have been shown to benefit from simple counselling by health visitors.

Appropriate referral to secondary care

In the community at large, one in 20 persons is depressed. Only one in 400 is referred to a psychiatrist for depression, and only one in 1000 is admitted to hospital for depression (Blacker & Clare, 1987). The traditional view that the more severely depressed patients are all likely to be referred and managed by a consultant is probably true only of patients suffering from psychotic illness.

Referral to a consultant psychiatrist is appropriate whenever the GP feels that guidance or help is required with diagnosis or management. It is usually necessary when there is a high risk of suicide or progress is unsatisfactory in spite of adequate treatment. When patients show markedly disturbed behaviour, particularly psychomotor retardation or agitation, or exhibit psychotic features, they should be referred to a psychiatrist without delay.

While many severely depressed patients are rightly referred for specialist help, referral of depressed patients is often made on the basis of additional complicating factors such as personality disorder, alcohol abuse, or family pressure for admission. In some areas the only access to care by community psychiatric nurses or clinical psychologists is by referral to a consultant psychiatrist.

Depression and physical illness

Physical and psychological disorder frequently coexist, and some individuals seem to be especially susceptible to both types of illness. Patients who are dependent on others for care seem more likely to become depressed. Working in the community with responsibility for a defined population of patients, the GP is well placed to identify and manage concurrent physical and mental illness. In practice this can be difficult to do, particularly as the doctor may become accustomed to see the patient fairly frequently for follow-up of a chronic physical illness.

It is easy to understand how long-term painful or incapacitating illness can lead to low spirits and depressed mood. Some illnesses are particularly associated with depressive disorder, for example, cancer, Crohn's disease, diabetes, and other endocrine and metabolic diseases. Cataclysmic physical events such as myocardial infarct, coronary artery bypass surgery, or stroke can be followed by a severe depressive reaction, perhaps due to the psychological trauma of facing death. Vigorous treatment of the depressive reaction can take precedence over the management of the physical disease, for example, a patient with advanced cancer of the lung who becomes severely depressed.

Viral illnesses such as influenza have long been associated with depression. The so-called post-viral syndrome, or ME, has recently been prominent in the columns of the medical journals. The nature of the syndrome is hotly disputed, but the clinical picture would seem to show more similarities to depressive illness than infection (Kendell, 1991).

The depression suffered by patients with physical illness is often concealed: it may present as an exacerbation of the existing physical disorder or by producing new physical symptoms. Unless the depression is recognised and treated, full recovery from the organic disease may be delayed or prevented.

Auditing management

Primary care teams are progressively developing protocols for the management of common chronic diseases in their practices and monitoring their compliance with these protocols through clinical audit. Teams now expect to know what they are trying to do, where they are, and whether they are reaching their standards of clinical care. Such management protocols are common in the management of diabetes, asthma, and hypertension, but are not yet commonly accepted for the care of mental illness. The care of depressive illness in general practice is a worthwhile area for audit of both process and outcome. Management could be improved by prescribing adequate doses of antidepressant for an adequate length of time. Systematic performance review of patient follow-up would provide valuable information, especially on how successfully patients are being convinced to comply with treatment.

Burton & Freeling (1982) have proposed a practical method for performance review of primary care management of depression. They recommend that a standardised record is kept at each consultation, so that both the patient's progress and the process of care can be reviewed reliably. Such audit has the potential for substantial benefits to the patient.

Conclusions

Depression is a common condition worldwide, causing much misery and underachievement, yet it is likely to be underdiagnosed to a significant degree. Improved recognition requires vigilance at each consulting session. Depression should be carefully sought and diligently treated, as it can now be effectively managed with a high probability of cure and improvement in the quality of our patients' lives.

References

AMERICAN PSYCHIATRIC ASSOCIATION (1980) *Diagnostic and Statistical Manual of Mental Disorders* (3rd edn) (DSM–III). Washington, DC: APA.

ANDREWS, G. (1991) The evaluation of psychotherapy. *Current Opinion in Psychiatry*, **4**, 379–383.

ANONYMOUS (1989) *RCGP Connection*. London: Royal College of General Practitioners.

BLACKER, C. V. R. & CLARE, A. W. (1987) Depressive disorder in primary care. *British Journal of Psychiatry*, **150**, 737–751.

BLASHKI, T. G., MOWBRAY, R. & DAVIES, B. (1971) Controlled trial of amitriptyline in general practice. *British Medical Journal*, i, 133–138.

BROWN, G. W. & HARRIS, T. (1978) *Social Origins of Depression: A Study of Psychiatric Disorder in Women*. London: Tavistock.

BURTON, R. H. & FREELING, P. (1982) How general practitioners manage depressive illness: developing a method of audit. *Journal of the Royal College of General Practitioners*, **33**, 558–561.

CASEY, P. R., DILLON, S. & TYRER, P. J. (1984) The diagnostic status of patients with conspicuous psychiatric morbidity in primary care. *Psychological Medicine*, **14**, 673–683.

DAVENPORT, S., GOLDBERG, D. & MILLAR, T. (1987) How psychiatric disorders are missed during medical consultations. *Lancet*, *i*, 439–441.

EDWARDS, J. G. (1992) Selective serotonin reuptake inhibitors. *British Medical Journal*, **304**, 1644–1645.

FREELING, P., RAO, B. M., PAYKEL, E. S., *et al* (1985) Unrecognised depression in general practice. *British Medical Journal*, **290**, 1880–1883.

—— & TYLEE, A. (1992) Depression in general practice. In *Handbook of Affective Disorders* (ed. E. S. Paykel) (2nd edn). Edinburgh: Churchill Livingstone.

GASK, L., MCGRATH, G. & GOLDBERG, D. (1987) Improving the psychiatric skills of established general practitioners: evaluation of group teaching. *Medical Education*, **21**, 362–368.

——, GOLDBERG, D., LESSER, A. L. *et al* (1988) Improving the psychiatric skills of the general practice trainee: an evaluation of a group training course. *Medical Education*, **22**, 132–138.

GOLDBERG, D. P. & BLACKWELL, B. (1970) Psychiatric illness in general practice. A detailed study using a new method of case identification. *British Medical Journal*, *ii*, 439–443.

—— & HUXLEY, P. (1980) *Mental Illness in the Community: The Pathway to Psychiatric Care*. London: Tavistock.

—— & BRIDGES, K. (1987) Screening for psychiatric illness in general practice: the general practitioner versus the screening questionnaire. *Journal of the Royal College of General Practitioners*, **37**, 15–18.

HOEPER, E. W., NYCE, G. R., CLEARY, P. D., *et al* (1979) Estimated prevalence of RDC mental disorder in primary care. *International Journal of Mental Health*, **8**, 6–15.

JENKINS, R. & SHEPHERD, M. (1983) Mental illness in general practice. In *Mental Illness: Changes and Trends* (ed. P. Bean). Chichester: Wiley.

JOHNSON, D. A. W. & MELLOR, V. (1987) The severity of depression in patients treated in general practice. *Journal of the Royal College of General Practitioners*, **27**, 419–422.

JOHNSTONE, A. & GOLDBERG, D. (1976) Psychiatric screening in general practice. *Lancet*, *i*, 605–608.

KENDELL, R. E. (1991) Chronic fatigue, viruses and depression. *Lancet*, **337**, 160–161.

MARKS, J., GOLDBERG, D. P. & HILLIER, V. E. (1979) Determinants of the ability of general practitioners to detect psychiatric illness. *Psychological Medicine*, **9**, 337–353.

MATTHEWS, K. & EAGLES, J. M. (1991) Which antidepressant? *British Journal of General Practice*, **41**, 123–125.

NEILSON, A. C. & WILLIAMS, T. A. (1980) Depression in ambulatory medical patients. *Archives of General Psychiatry*, **37**, 999–1004.

O'DOWD, T. C. (1988) Five years of "heartsink" patients in general practice. *British Medical Journal*, *ii*, 528–530.

PAYKEL, E. S., HOLLYMAN, J. A., FREELING, P., *et al* (1988) Predicters of therapeutic benefit from amitriptyline in mild depression: a general practice placebo-controlled trial. *Journal of Affective Disorders*, **14**, 83–95.

——, PRIEST, R. G., on behalf of Conference Participants (1992) Recognition and management of depression in general practice: consensus statement. *British Medical Journal*, **305**, 198–202.

ROSS, M. & SCOTT, M. (1985) An evaluation of the effectiveness of individual and group cognitive therapy in the treatment of depressed patients in an inner city health centre. *Journal of the Royal College of General Practitioners*, **35**, 239–242.

ROYAL COLLEGE OF PSYCHIATRISTS (1992) *Attitudes Towards Depression. Research Study Conducted for the "Defeat Depression" Campaign*. London: Royal College of Psychiatrists.

SHEPHERD, M., COOPER, M., BROWN, A. C., *et al* (1966) *Psychiatric Illness in General Practice* (2nd edn, 1981). London: Oxford University Press.

SIMS, A. (1993) The scar that is more than skin deep: the stigma of depression. *British Journal of General Practice*, **43**, 30–31.

SONG, F., FREEMANTLE, N., SHELDON, T. A., *et al* (1993) Selective serotonin reuptake inhibitors: efficacy, acceptability and effectiveness: a meta-analysis. *British Medical Journal*, **306**, 683–687.

TYRER, P. (1988) The Nottingham study of neurotic disorder: comparison of drug and psychological treatments. *Lancet, ii,* 235–240.

WILLIAMS, R. (1993) Psychiatric morbidity in children and adolescents: a suitable cause for concern. *British Journal of General Practice,* 43, 3–4.

WILLIAMSON, J., STOKOE, I. H. & GRAY, S. (1964) Old people at home: the unreported needs. *Lancet, i,* 1117–1120.

WRIGHT, A. F. (1988) Psychological distress in a general practice: outcome and consultation rates in one general practice. *Journal of the Royal College of General Practitioners,* 38, 542–545.

—— (1990) A study of the presentation of somatic symptoms in general practice by patients with psychiatric disturbance. *British Journal of General Practice,* 40, 459–463.

—— (1993) *Depression. Recognition and Management in General Practice.* London: Royal College of General Practitioners.

—— & PERINI, A. F. (1987) Hidden psychiatric illness: use of the General Health Questionnaire in general practice. *Journal of the Royal College of General Practitioners,* 37, 164–167.

WRIGHT, J. H., BELL, R. A., KHUN, C. C., *et al* (1980) Depression in family practice patients. *Southern Medical Journal,* 73, 1031–1034.

8 Anxiety

LYNNE M. DRUMMOND

Anxiety is a universal experience. The amount of anxiety experienced by an individual depends on a number of factors, including genetic constitution, life experiences, and current situation. There are two main forms of anxiety, which have been defined as *trait* and *state* (Lader, 1975).

Firstly, trait anxiety refers to the baseline levels of anxiety which vary from person to person. For example, Mr A is a man who is rarely anxious and indulges in hang-gliding and rock-climbing. He is sociable, loves an audience, and is always confident in his work. Mr B, in contrast, describes himself as always having been a worrying and anxious person. His hobbies are stamp-collecting and reading. He avoids sport as he fears making a fool of himself and also fears bodily injury. His family are always being cautioned to be careful whenever they leave the house. He works in the same office as Mr A but is always quiet and withdrawn at office social gatherings, worries for weeks in advance of his having to present reports to an audience, and constantly is concerned about his work performance. Both these men are useful and valued employees, and both have normal levels of anxiety.

State anxiety refers to anxiety which occurs in response to specific situations, and these situations also vary from person to person. Mr A rarely experiences much anxiety but is always more anxious when a wasp is in his vicinity. This fear does not lead him to avoid any situations where there are wasps but does mean that he prefers other people to remove them. Mr B, however, has no fear of wasps and frequently will dispose of any which come into the office when Mr A is there.

With the wide range of degree of anxiety experienced by different people, there is no clear dividing line between normal and abnormal anxiety. Abnormal anxiety can therefore only be truly defined by the sufferer as being more severe, frequent, persistent or restricting than he/she can tolerate or is used to. Thus most patients who present to a GP complaining of anxiety symptoms have usually had a recent change in the severity of these symptoms or the life-restricting side-effects of excessive anxiety has become clear to them.

The symptoms of anxiety can be divided into the emotional and the physical. Common emotional symptoms include the feeling of dread, impending doom, out of control, difficulty in concentrating, and difficulty in thinking of other things. The physical symptoms can affect any system of the body and are mostly caused by an increase in sympathetic activity, an imbalance between sympathetic and parasympathetic systems, or an increase in muscular tension. Common symptoms include heart racing, difficulty breathing, 'butterflies in the stomach', and headache.

The function of anxiety

Anxiety can be viewed as having three main roles in shaping a person's behaviour. Firstly, it can act as a conditioned response to a particular situation. For example, a young child shows no fear of fire. However, if the child puts out a hand to the candles on the birthday cake and gets burnt, it experiences pain and fear. In future it is likely to react to fire with caution and apprehension. Thus anxiety has become the conditioned response to the stimulus of the sight of a burning flame. Fortunately we do not have to learn to be justifiably fearful of all situations, but can learn vicariously by being told of danger by others and by observing others in different situations, as well as having phylogenetic tendencies to respond to certain situations with fear.

Secondly, anxiety acts as a negative reinforcer. For example, Ms A has spider phobia. The presence of a spider makes her feel extremely anxious. She escapes from the situation by running from the room. This escape behaviour reduces her anxiety. Her escape has thus been reinforced by the reduction in her anxiety and this increases the likelihood that she will try and escape again, which will lead eventually to total avoidance of any situations where there may be spiders.

Lastly, anxiety can also be viewed as a secondary drive state. In other words, very high or very low levels of anxiety impede, whereas moderate levels of anxiety improve performance of tasks. An extremely anxious driver is likely to drive badly and may cause an accident. An overconfident driver is similarly dangerous. The safest drivers are ones who are appropriately apprehensive, vigilant, and aware of any potential dangers.

It can be seen that anxiety has been an important factor in evolutionary terms in ensuring the survival of our species. Without it the human race would have been attacked, been preyed upon, and fallen down mountain ravines into extinction. Experiments have demonstrated that it is much easier for people to learn to be fearful of certain situations which have particular evolutionary significance rather than those with little or no evolutionary significance (Ohman & Dimberg, 1984; Ohman *et al*, 1984).

Classification of anxiety disorders

Excessive anxiety may present as a symptom of almost any psychiatric diagnosis. However, excessive anxiety is often more prevalent in the neurotic disorders than in the psychotic, personality, and habit disorders. Patients with neurotic disorders are common in general practice, and these patients who present with anxiety are described in detail.

In recent years there has been the tendency, particularly in the North American literature, to separate those patients with panic into a separate category (American Psychiatric Association, 1987). Panic refers to extreme levels of anxiety and also episodes of this extreme anxiety occurring in an apparently unprovoked manner when the sufferer is not in the presence of any fear-provoking situation. Whereas many clinicians choose to separate those anxiety disorders with panic from those without, in practice it may be easier to view panic as an extreme level of anxiety and to treat the underlying disorder with or without additional help for any unprovoked anxiety episodes.

Patients with neurotic disorders who frequently present to the GP with excessive anxiety may be suffering from one of the following (classification from ICD-9, World Health Organization, 1978):

anxiety states
phobic state
obsessive–compulsive disorders
neurotic depression
hypochondriasis

In addition, patients suffering from post-traumatic stress disorder or abnormal grief reactions (see Chapter 7) may frequently present with anxiety which may mimic any of the above diagnoses.

Depression and abnormal grief reactions are discussed in Chapters 5 and 7, and are not covered here.

Differential diagnosis

Any of the anxiety disorders can be confused with each other, but a careful history will normally reveal which is the correct diagnosis. There are, however, a number of physical illnesses which can present with symptoms which are difficult to distinguish from anxiety disorders. Inquiry about physical health, physical examination, and even investigations should not be overlooked in a patient who presents with apparent anxiety symptoms.

Examples of physical conditions which can mimic an anxiety disorder include:

thyrotoxicosis
temporal lobe epilepsy
asthma
migraine
pheochromocytoma
adrenal insufficiency
carcinoid syndrome
Zollinger–Ellison syndrome (hypoglycaemia leads to increased sympathetic outflow)
poorly controlled diabetes
paroxysmal atrial tachycardia

As well as recognised medical syndromes, other physical factors may cause symptoms indistinguishable from anxiety. Examples of these include:

excessive intake of caffeine, nicotine, or alcohol (withdrawal in the form of a 'hangover' is partially characterised by increased sympathetic outflow)
drug abuse (cannabis excess generally leads to increased vagal output; amphetamines to increased sympathetic output)
withdrawal from benzodiazepine medication
irregular meals leading to hypoglycaemia
reactive hypoglycaemia
insufficient regular exercise
excessive tiredness

Anxiety state (generalised anxiety; anxiety neurosis)

This diagnosis refers to the presentation of a patient with an increase in anxiety. Patients may have predominantly physical or emotional symptoms, and the symptoms may either be persistent or episodic. The anxiety is not provoked by any particular object, situation, or thought, nor is it precipitated by any obvious life event. Although the patient is disturbed by the symptoms, there are no symptoms suggestive of a depressive disorder.

The differential diagnosis of this condition includes the physical disorders mentioned previously. Psychological conditions which are frequently misdiagnosed as generalised anxiety include depression; grief (not only provoked by loss of relatives and friends, but also loss of a pet, material possessions, job, etc.); social phobia; agoraphobia (phobias which include a wide range of anxiety-provoking stimuli can often be misdiagnosed unless care is taken to ask exactly what thoughts run through the patient's mind at the time of the anxiety episodes); and obsessive–compulsive disorder (patients with obsessions may be secretive about the basis of their worries as they often fear being thought 'mad').

Practical management

Lifestyle management

The first step to helping these patients can be for the GP to examine their lifestyle to see if this has any changeable factors which are implicated in the disorder. This can be done by asking the patient to keep a diary for a week. In this diary should be recorded the frequency and severity of anxiety episodes. It is often easier to record severity of anxiety using a scale. A nine-point scale is favoured by Marks (1986) and many other clinicians. On this scale 0 = no anxiety; 2 = mild anxiety; 4 = moderate anxiety; 6 = severe anxiety; and 8 = panic.

In addition patients should be asked to record: their meals, with details of food consumed; cigarette consumption; alcohol consumption; coffee, tea and cola-type drinks; drugs; details of working hours; and sleep. To avoid being presented with a heavy tome of notes at the end of the week it is often useful to provide a sample diary sheet to the patient which can then be completed with minimum words (Fig. 8.1).

Name   Date

	Anxiety (0-8)	Food	Drink	Cigarettes or drugs	What I was doing
6.00 a.m.					
7.00 a.m.					
8.00 a.m.					
9.00 a.m.					
10.00 a.m.					
11.00 a.m.					
12.00 m.d.					
1.00 p.m.					
2.00 p.m.					
3.00 p.m.					
4.00 p.m.					
5.00 p.m.					
6.00 p.m.					
7.00 p.m.					
8.00 p.m.					
9.00 p.m.					
10.00 p.m.					
11.00 p.m.					
12.00 m.n.					
1.00 a.m.					

Fig. 8.1. A sample diary sheet for lifestyle management of patients with anxiety disorders

After a week of recording information in this way it is possible precipitants for the problem may be seen. Advice can then be given to the patient about improving lifestyle. Once this has been given, the patient should continue to record anxiety and lifestyle on the diary sheets to see if these simple measures do help. Anyone who is making a major change in their lifestyle is likely to require to see a professional on a weekly basis for several weeks or even months to receive encouragement and praise for maintaining the changes. Changes of this type can initially produce a temporary worsening of symptoms; for example, many patients who are used to a high caffeine intake will complain of headache, palpitation, and feeling unwell for several days after it is withdrawn.

Prolonged regular exercise has also been shown to reduce anxiety symptoms. This needs to be tailored to the patient's age and physical health. Some people may enjoy running and jogging, whereas to others it is their idea of hell on earth. If any activity is to be regularly incorporated into a patient's life, the benefits have to be clearly seen by them to outweigh the disadvantages. It is often useful to ask if they had any sport which they enjoyed at school to see if they could build up to taking part in this again. Even brisk walking and using the stairs rather than lifts can be a useful life change. The patient should be warned to start with gradual exercise and not expect rapid changes in their general fitness.

Avoiding avoidance

This may seem to be a contradiction as, by definition, there is no real avoidance in anxiety neurosis. However, there may be subtle avoidance of activities which might bring on symptoms.

Case 1

A 54-year-old man had made a good recovery from a heart attack but avoided intercourse with his wife. The onset of his anxiety symptoms had started shortly after this myocardial infarction. They began during intercourse. Treatment involved him facing up to the feared activity and when he had done so he made a rapid recovery.

Prediction testing

Many patients with anxiety believe that frightening or humiliating things are likely to happen in everyday situations. It can be helpful for these patients to plan situations in which they can test out their prediction of impending disaster. In these patients there is no avoidance, however subtle, and the GP has to work out with the patient a purely artificial situation to carry out a behavioural experiment.

Case 2

John was a young man with general anxiety symptoms which were especially bad if he thought people were looking at him. He never avoided social situations, but he was asked to devise an imagined situation that would bring on the most symptoms, and he pointed out that if he was to walk past a group of school-children he would feel very bad indeed, because this would make him very self-conscious. He would fear that the children might laugh at him, and then he would become awkward and make a fool of himself. He had no children of his own and in the normal way would never come into contact with children. After some discussion he agreed that it would be useful to walk past a school just as the children were coming out and force himself to do this difficult task on a number of occasions. Prediction testing in this way served to prove to him that the worst feared consequences would not happen, and was a useful part of the therapeutic strategy in his case.

Voluntary hyperventilation and controlled breathing

Many patients who complain of anxiety symptoms overbreathe when they feel anxious. This serves to worsen their symptoms, and particularly can produce sensations of dyspnoea, flushing paraesthesia, and dizziness. Some patients become so fearful of these sensations that they use many techniques to avoid provoking the symptoms. Voluntary hyperventilation can be used in these patients to help them to realise how overbreathing causes these symptoms and also to allow them to experience the symptoms, recognise they are not life-threatening, and become less anxious about them.

This is done by asking the patient to breathe rapidly in and out. After about two minutes of hard overbreathing the patient is asked to report what actual symptoms were experienced, and then asked whether these feelings are similar to those experienced in a panic attack. Most patients have difficulty in performing overbreathing to a sufficient extent to reproduce symptoms if just asked to do so. For this reason it is better to perform the exercise along with the patient. The resultant symptoms and signs produced in the therapist can be an additional useful learning experience for the patient. This technique does produce a number of unpleasant symptoms and it is advisable not to drive for at least 30 minutes after performing this exercise.

There are some medical conditions where hard hyperventilation may be contraindicated, for example, recent myocardial infarction, and some forms of obstructive airways disease.

Voluntary hyperventilation may be useful in many patients with panic attacks, but there may be some difficulty enabling the technique to be practised outside the clinic. Clark *et al* (1985) have devised a way round this by using audio-tape recordings of a voice saying 'in' for two seconds, then 'out' for the same period; after a short period, 'in' again, and so on. The therapist chooses the rate most suitable for the patient and patients are asked to follow the pacing on the tape. Next the patient is asked to turn the tape off and carry on breathing at the same pace for progressively longer periods.

In addition to teaching the patient how to produce symptoms of hyperventilation, it is necessary to teach controlled breathing to reduce symptoms and prevent a recurrence. This can be done by asking the patient to place his/her hand on the abdomen. They should feel their abdomen going out on inspiration and in on expiration. If this is not the case then diaphragmatic breathing is not being used and practice is needed to achieve it. Once this is achieved then the patient can be asked to breathe in to the slow count of five seconds, hold their breath for five seconds, and then breathe out for five seconds. This technique is useful as patients can put a hand on their abdomen any time they feel they may experience symptoms and prevent or abort an episode.

Relaxation training

Relaxation can be seen as a coping skill, that once acquired can be used by the patient to reduce symptoms in anxiety disorders. It is something positive a patient can do in an anxiety attack and serves to reduce the sense of helplessness. In some oriental cultures relaxation is part of the lifestyle, but this is not so in most Western cultures. Therefore relaxation has to be taught, and it is worth emphasising to patients that, as with other things that have to be taught, a number of practice sessions will be needed. Various methods are available (e.g. Bernstein & Borkovec, 1973; Stern & Drummond, 1991).

It is wise to remember that relaxation has only a limited role in helping anxiety and should rarely, if ever, be used alone. For example, most people can be taught to relax at home. However, if after being taught relaxation, the person is taken for the first time into a light aircraft and told to jump with a parachute, they are likely to experience anxiety. Anyone who suggests that they do their relaxation to cope with this is likely to be subjected to a very rude reply. Thus although relaxation may be helpful for general stress and tension, it is not helpful for situational anxiety.

Cognitive treatments

These include anxiety management training and Beck's cognitive therapy. Further details of cognitive therapy are given elsewhere in Chapter 18, as well as being described in detail in practical guides on the subject (e.g. Beck & Emery, 1985; Stern & Drummond, 1991). In patients who require detailed cognitive treatments it is advisable to refer the patient to a specialised cognitive–behavioural therapist.

Drug treatments

Many drugs are used in the primary care of patients with anxiety disorders, and more are being developed. However, there are two main problems with any kind of pharmacological treatment of anxiety. Firstly, anxiety neurosis tends to be a chronic condition, and thus treatment may need to be continued for many years. When the cost of the drugs and the time of the doctor seeing the patient is considered over several years, it becomes clear that any psychological treatment which produces lasting results is more cost-effective. Secondly, no drug is perfect, and all have the potential to produce side-effects and psychological dependence.

In the past, benzodiazepine drugs (see Chapter 16) were the most commonly prescribed for anxiety. The tendency for these drugs to produce tolerance and psychological and physical dependence has meant that they are not recommended for anything that is likely to be a chronic condition.

Low doses of phenothiazine drugs, such as chlorpromazine and trifluoperazine, can be used. However, they do produce autonomic side-effects, including dry mouth and dizziness. Extrapyramidal effects have also been noted even at these low doses.

Tricyclic antidepressants with sedative properties, such as amitriptyline and doxepin, have not been widely accepted in the treatment of pure anxiety states, although some workers have shown that they can reduce anxiety symptoms (Kahn *et al*, 1987).

Monoamine oxidase inhibitors have been used for atypical depression and phobic disorders. They have many side-effects and require dietary restrictions, and thus are rarely suitable for chronic anxiety states.

Beta-adrenoceptor agonists, such as propranolol, do appear to reduce the somatic symptoms of anxiety which are mediated by beta neurons (Tyrer, 1980). Thus a patient with palpitations and tremor may find that these improve without improvement of psychological symptoms.

Newer drugs, such as buspirone, which act on the serotonin system, have now been developed. Their efficacy in generalised anxiety is still being assessed (*Lancet*, 1988).

Prognosis

Whereas acute anxiety state following a traumatic life event will generally reduce and abate after a few weeks or months, many patients have chronic problems. Drug treatment may alleviate at least some of the symptoms, but there is a real danger of the patient becoming a long-term regular anti-anxiety drug user (Mellinger *et al*, 1984).

Many of the psychological treatments are in their infancy, and thus have been subject to relatively few controlled trials. However, a study by Butler *et al* (1987) showed that most patients with chronic severe anxiety symptoms were helped by an anxiety management package. There are no studies on the less severe cases.

Phobic disorder

A phobia is a morbid fear which is out of proportion to the threat of the stimulus, is involuntary, cannot be explained away, and leads to avoidance of the feared object or situation (Marks, 1969). Although this definition appears straightforward, there are frequent difficulties which can lead to misdiagnosis. Firstly, nearly all of us have some irrational fears which do not, however, amount to a phobia. For example, Ms B had a strong dislike of earwigs. If an earwig came into the room she would ask her husband to remove it. If she was alone, she could just about steel herself to pick it up in a paper tissue and flush it down the toilet. She did not avoid any situation because of her dislike of earwigs. Ms B suffers from a minor fear of earwigs but does not meet the criteria listed above for the diagnosis of phobic disorder. However, as it can be seen that these fears are on a spectrum with more severe phobias, epidemiological research has been variable owing to different criteria being used by researchers.

A second diagnostic confusion is with obsessive–compulsive disorders. In this condition there is marked fear of certain objects or situations which also leads to avoidance. The fear in obsessive–compulsive disorder is not, however, of the object itself but of the consequences of the object or situation. For example, Julie had a fear of dogs. This fear was an example of a specific animal phobia, as the fear was purely related to the presence of dogs in her vicinity. Bert had a 10-year history of fear of contamination by dirt from dog faeces as he was concerned that he might catch a variety of diseases which could then be passed on to others and which would result in him feeling responsible for this plague. This problem caused him to avoid any situations where he had seen dogs in the past. Even if he saw a dog through his window he would feel anxious and resort to cleaning rituals. His anxiety-reducing rituals consisted of stripping off all his clothes which were then considered contaminated and washing these: he would bathe in a set pattern and would repeat this ritual washing in multiples of four, which he considered a good number.

In Julie's case she had a classic dog phobia which led to avoidance of dogs or any situations which reminded her of dogs. Bert's problem is different. His fear is not of dogs, but of the consequences which he worries may result from contact with dogs. Unlike Julie, whose anxiety is relieved by escaping from the dog, Bert would still remain anxious after the dog had left until he had performed his washing rituals. The development of elaborate belief systems in people with obsessive–compulsive disorders is also demonstrated by Bert performing his stereotyped washing rituals in multiples of four.

These belief systems are only part of the story, however, as people with obsessive–compulsive disorders generally realise that their fears are irrational and that their ritualistic patterns are unrealistic.

Treatment in both Julie and Bert's cases was similar. Both received graduated prolonged exposure to their feared situation. There was an additional component in Bert's treatment because of the rituals. This is called self-imposed response prevention, in other words, explaining to the patient the effect of rituals on anxiety and then asking him not to ritualise.

It should also be remembered that a phobia is an irrational fear. In other words, one cannot have a phobia of man-eating tigers but can have a cat phobia, the difference being the actual amount of threat presented by each stimulus.

Phobias can also be confused with general anxiety states; the differential diagnoses of these are discussed below.

Common types of phobias

The tendency of humans to develop fears of situations of particular evolutionary significance has been discussed above. The most frequent phobic syndromes are listed in Table 8.1.

Treatment

Prolonged graduated exposure

A full description of the behavioural treatment of phobic disorder using prolonged, graduated exposure in real life to the feared situation, is given in Chapter 18, and is not described in detail here.

In the past, exposure treatments in which the therapist was expected to spend many hours helping the patient in the programme were clearly impractical for the general practice surgery. However, recent developments in the field have demonstrated that many patients with mild to moderately severe phobias and obsessive–compulsive disorder require only minimal therapist intervention. Indeed, a study by Ghosh *et al* (1988) demonstrated that self-exposure methods were as effective as therapist-aided exposure.

For a GP to help a patient successfully complete an exposure programme, the following steps may be helpful. Firstly, it is useful to educate the patient about anxiety and its symptoms and how prolonged exposure works by allowing anxiety to reduce. It is then useful to draw up a hierarchy of feared situations with the patient, together with an anxiety rating (using a scale like the 0–8 scale mentioned previously). The patient's spouse or other relatives can often be incorporated to help the patient perform the exposure tasks.

Once this has been done, patients are asked to decide which exposure task they would feel able to tackle first. The task should be something which

TABLE 8.1
The most frequent phobic syndromes

Type of phobia	Percentage of patients with phobic disorder (Marks, 1969)	Sex ratio	Usual age at onset: years	Other comments
Agoraphobia	60%	F > M	15–35 years	Fear of shopping, crowds, travelling, enclosed spaces
Social phobia	8%	F = M	10–20 years	May have general social anxiety or fear of specific activities, e.g. eating, drinking, blushing, shaking
Specific animal phobia	3%	F > M	<7 years	Specificity to a particular animal
Miscellaneous specific phobias	14%	Varies, but overall F = M	Variable	Fear of thunder, heights, air travel, etc.
Blood and injury phobia	c.3% of adults (often do not seek medical help)	F = M	2–15 years	Fear of medical and dental procedures. Unlike other phobias exposure results in a bradycardia with a risk of fainting

causes them some anxiety but which they feel able to do for at least one to two hours until their anxiety reduces, and to repeat daily or at least four times a week. They should be asked to record their exposure and the anxiety level before, during, and after the exposure, in a diary. Once a substantial reduction in fear has occurred in performing the task, the patient should move on to more difficult tasks. The therapist should aim to see the patient weekly initially to monitor progress, give praise and encouragement, and to trouble-shoot any difficulties.

Many patients find that a self-help book can be an additional help when performing a self-exposure programme. There are several such books available and some are more helpful than others. Marks's (1978) book *Living with Fear* is an excellent self-help manual, which has advice and help for the whole range of phobias and obsessive–compulsive disorders. However, few patients are able to follow this advice without some additional input from a professional, as described here.

The major pitfall to exposure treatment is that patients often do not expose themselves to the feared situation for long enough. Often they try it out for half an hour and forget that more than twice this time is usually needed for anxiety to reduce substantially. Also, it is sometimes difficult for the therapist to advise a patient when the therapist has never had the experience of being in exposure with a phobic patient. Books which give detailed case histories of problems and pitfalls can help to alleviate this problem (e.g. Stern & Drummond, 1991) but clearly some experience of conducting exposure *in vivo* is preferable.

Despite the success of self-exposure, there are a few patients who cannot be helped in this way and who need referral to a specialist behavioural–cognitive psychotherapist.

Self-help organisations

There has been a burgeoning of self-help organisations for patients with phobias in recent years. Some have been no more than social groups where patients are not helped to overcome their problems. Some offer a telephone help-line, and produce leaflets for sufferers and their families. Some provide local support groups.

Drugs

The drugs used for most phobic disorders are the same as those listed for anxiety states, and have the same problems for this chronically disabled group of patients.

Agoraphobia, however, deserves a separate discussion, as it has been the phobia most often studied in drug trials. Imipramine has been shown to be superior to placebo in the treatment of agoraphobia (e.g. Klein, 1967;

Michelson & Mavissakalian, 1985). Phenelzine has also been shown to be superior to placebo in a group of patients with agoraphobia or social phobia (Tyrer & Steinberg, 1975). In all of these studies relapse was common on stopping the drug.

The combination of drugs with exposure therapy has also been studied. Imipramine and phenelzine were found to have no additional advantage when combined with exposure treatment (Solyman *et al*, 1981; Marks *et al*, 1983).

Prognosis

Most phobias have a chronic course without treatment. Fortunately graduated exposure treatment is successful for most patients with phobic disorder.

The efficacy of exposure treatment for the treatment of agoraphobia has been repeatedly demonstrated in studies over the past 25 years (see Mathews *et al*, 1981). Significant improvements in symptoms have been reported in two-thirds of agoraphobic patients which persist for as long as nine years (Munby & Johnston, 1981). The outcome with exposure treatment for the other phobias demonstrate an even higher success and lower relapse rate (see Marks, 1986).

Post-traumatic phobias (post-traumatic stress disorder)

Recently attention has focused on the prevalence and severity of psychological sequelae following a traumatic life event or disaster. These patients may often present with a phobia which dates to the time of the disaster or shortly afterwards. In addition, they often suffer from irritability, tension, depression, insomnia, nightmares, and flashbacks, as well as fear and avoidance of objects or situations which remind them of the disaster (see Marks, 1987).

Treatment involves graduated exposure to the avoided fear-provoking cues. This often involves fanstasy exposure – thinking about the traumatic event itself. This exposure must be sufficiently prolonged to allow anxiety to reduce. As this may well be too time-consuming for the primary care team, severe cases might best be referred to a specialist cognitive–behavioural psychotherapist.

Although case studies suggest a good outcome after treatment for many of these patients, controlled trials have not yet been reported.

Obsessive–compulsive disorder

Although this condition has been thought to be rare, recent studies suggest that as many as 3% of the population may suffer from it during their lifetime (Karno *et al*, 1988). This staggeringly high figure means that a GP would be expected to have several patients with this disorder. It is however likely that few of these patients ever seek medical help for their problems and also it may be that these prevalence figures have been inflated by including everyone who has any obsessional symptoms.

The definition of obsessive–compulsive disorder is best tackled by defining the two main symptoms of obsessions and compulsions, as done in DSM–III–R (American Psychiatric Association, 1987). Obsessions are intrusive and unwanted thoughts, images or impulses, which the patient tries, at least in the early stages of the illness, to resist. These thoughts are recognised as being a product of the patient's own mind but are seen as contrary to his/her wishes or personality, for example, a parent thinking of harming a loved child, or a religious person having blasphemous thoughts.

Compulsions may be either overt actions or covert 'neutralising' thoughts. These are activities which are designed to reduce the anxiety caused by the obsessional thought or to 'put the thought right' in some way; for example, a person with an obsessional thought that they may have been contaminated by a dreaded disease may compulsively wash to 'undo' the contamination; the minister plagued by blasphemous obsessions may have the covert compulsion of thinking a stereotyped prayer to 'undo' or neutralise the obsessional thought. These activities, however, may not in reality be linked with the fear. For example, a spinster with thoughts of having sex with strangers in a shop may have the compulsion to wash her hands repeatedly. Alternatively, such activities may be clearly excessive. For example, a man with the obsessional thought that his home may be burgled, may check that he has locked the front door 25 times.

In addition, many patients with obsessive–compulsive disorder seek reassurance from others. They may repeatedly ask a relative or friend if the front door was locked. This reassurance acts in a similar way to compulsions or rituals. Although it temporarily reduces anxiety, which reinforces the behaviour, the effect is short-lived; more reassurance is then required.

The differential diagnosis of obsessive–compulsive disorder includes phobias, depression, anorexia nervosa and Gilles de la Tourette syndrome.

Practical management

Prolonged graduated exposure plus self-imposed response prevention

The principles of exposure treatment for obsessive–compulsive disorder are identical to those previously discussed for phobic disorder. In these cases, however, the exposure is to situations and objects which induce the anxiety-provoking thoughts.

Compulsions or rituals serve to maintain anxiety. Although they initially reduce anxiety, they do this by a small amount and for a limited time (Fig. 8.2).

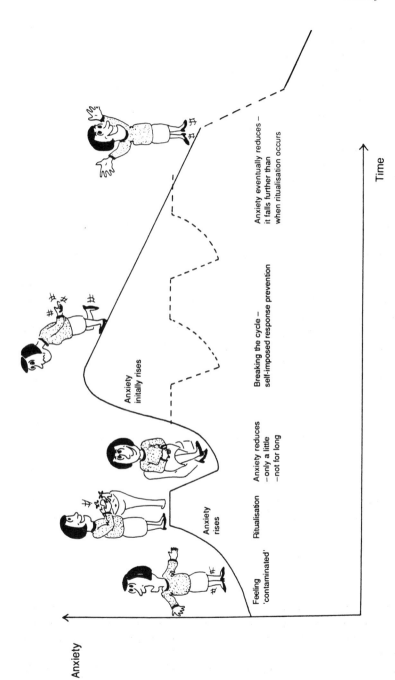

Anxiety

Feeling 'contaminated'

Ritualisation

Anxiety rises

Anxiety reduces
– only a little
– not for long

Anxiety initally rises

Breaking the cycle –
self-imposed response prevention

Anxiety eventually reduces –
it falls further than
when ritualisation occurs

Time

Fig. 8.2. Breaking the cycle of anxiety and ritualisation (from Stern & Drummond, 1991, reproduced with permission of Cambridge University Press)

This limited efficacy of the rituals leads to them being repeated many times. Overall, they serve, therefore, to prolong anxiety and do not allow the anxiety to reduce naturally.

It is, therefore, necessary to ask the patient not to perform their rituals. This can be achieved by educating the patient about the effect of rituals, and grading exposure tasks so that they start with tasks which will cause *tolerable* anxiety, such that the patient will not need to perform the ritual. Even with the best-motivated patients, slips will occur and they will find themselves performing the rituals on the odd occasion. It is therefore advisable to tell them that this is to be expected on the rare occasion and will not interfere with the efficacy of therapy as long as they repeat the exposure task immediately.

An identical approach is taken with reassurance-seeking, although in this case it may be necessary for the doctor also to educate relatives, friends or professionals who are providing the reassurance as to what is an appropriate response from them. It is often difficult for relatives to withhold reassurance, and it is often useful to role-play situations where reassurance is requested with them and suggest they reply by saying, "Dr X has asked me not to answer questions like that".

Self-exposure and self-imposed response prevention has been shown to be effective in patients with obsessive–compulsive disorder (Marks *et al*, 1988). The self-help book *Living with Fear* (Marks, 1978) covers this area. In a similar way to the treatment of phobias, family members can often be usefully incorporated in the treatment programme with the patient. The role of the GP in seeing the patient regularly for support, encouragement, and advice is vital for most of these patients.

Patients with complex problems or who fail to respond rapidly to self-treatment methods are best referred to a specialist cognitive–behavioural therapist.

Self-help groups

The charitable organisation Phobic Action provides telephone helplines, informative leaflets and local support groups for sufferers of obsessive–compulsive disorder and their families.

Drugs

The first drug to be found to be useful in obsessive–compulsive disorder was clomipramine. Although this drug reduced symptoms in many patients, it does have serious side-effects. Indeed, as well as the commonly reported anticholinergic side-effects, Monteiro *et al* (1987) found that 70% of previously sexually active patients became anorgasmic on therapeutic doses of clomipramine.

More selective 5-hydroxytryptophan reuptake inhibitors have been introduced in the past few years. These include fluvoxamine, fluoxetine, and sertraline. The advantage of these drugs are that they have a lower incidence of side-effects. They have been found to be useful in reducing symptoms in many patients.

There are, however, two main problems with drug therapy for obsessive–compulsive disorder. Firstly, relapse is common on stopping the drug, and thus treatment is usually necessary for many years (see review by Marks, 1987). Secondly, 40–60% of patients fail to derive any benefit from drug treatment (McDougle & Goodman, 1991). This has led to the investigation of combination therapies. Many of these investigations have taken the form of open studies and are therefore difficult to evaluate fully. Examples include combinations of fluoxetine with buspirone (Markovitz *et al*, 1990), and fluvoxamine with a neuroleptic (McDougle & Goodman, 1990).

Some clinicians have tried combining drug treatment with exposure therapy. However, there is evidence that the drug treatment has no additional benefit to the effect of exposure therapy (Marks *et al*, 1988).

Prognosis

Without treatment, obsessive–compulsive disorder is a chronic condition which often persists for several decades and causes considerable suffering and social handicap.

Exposure therapy has been shown by controlled trials to be effective in most patients who undergo treatment. Success rates have ranged from 75% (Marks *et al*, 1975) to 85% of patients (Foa & Goldstein, 1978). A number of studies have also shown that these gains are maintained for at least four years after stopping treatment (see Marks, 1981).

Drug treatment has been shown to improve symptoms in 40–60% of obsessive–compulsive patients (McDougle & Goodman, 1991). Relapse is common after stopping the drug.

Hypochondriasis

The term 'hypochondriasis' is commonly misused among lay people and health-care workers alike. Indeed, it has only recently been included in the various classifications of diseases, having previously been included under phobic disorders, obsessive–compulsive disorder, hysteria, and atypical depression.

According to DSM–III–R (American Psychiatric Association, 1987), for the diagnosis of hypochondriasis to be made, the following criteria should be met:

(a) preoccupation with the fear of having, or the belief that one has a serious disease; this is based on interpretations of physical signs or sensations
(b) physical evaluation does not show evidence of serious disease
(c) medical reassurance does not reduce the belief about having a serious disease
(d) the duration of the disturbance is more than six months
(e) the patient is not frankly psychotic.

Closer examination of these patients has led to the development of cognitive–behavioural models of hypochondriasis (Salkovskis & Warwick, 1986; Barsky *et al*, 1988; Barsky & Wyshak, 1990). According to this model, the patient begins to interpret normal bodily symptoms as evidence of disease. This is normally precipitated by a life event or even being given information about a particular pathology (a familiar example being medical students' hypochondriasis). The increased awareness of bodily symptoms leads to worry and often checking. Checking and worry increase physiological arousal and increase bodily symptoms. The increase in bodily symptoms is interpreted as further evidence of physical illness (Fig. 8.3).

An important factor which often perpetuates the anxiety in hypochondriacal patients is medical reassurance.

Case 3

Joy was a 25-year-old secretary who was worried that she might have cervical cancer. The concern had started when she had seen a television programme about screening for this disease. Her worry was increased as she noticed she had a clear, non-purulent vaginal discharge. She visited her GP, who reassured her. This reassurance initially reduced her anxiety but rapidly Joy remembered that the programme had said that cervical cancer was difficult to diagnose without a smear. She returned to her GP, who performed a cervical smear examination. Again this initially reduced her anxiety until she remembered that some smears gave false-negative results. Over the next year, Joy attended all the GPs in her area, had five cervical smear examinations, attended a well-woman clinic monthly, and eventually was seen at a specialist oncology unit at her local hospital. Despite all this reassurance, she remained convinced that she had cervical cancer.

It can be seen that medical reassurance in these patients works in a similar way to reassurance in obsessive–compulsive disorder. In other words, the reassurance initially reduces anxiety, which reinforces the reassurance-seeking, but this reduction is short-lived, and soon more reassurance is sought.

Indeed, many hypochondriacal patients have symptoms identical to those of obsessive–compulsive disorder. They have the worrying thought or obsession about illness which leads to checking rituals, reassurance-seeking, and often avoidance of cues which precipitate the thoughts.

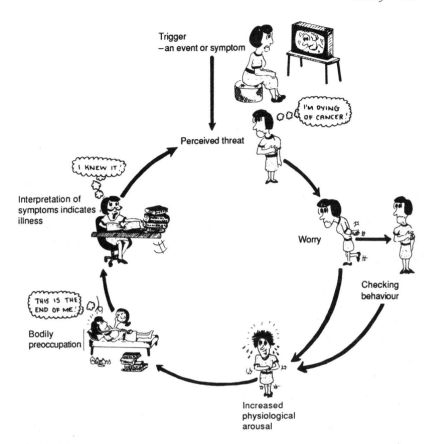

Fig. 8.3. The cognitive–behavioural model of hypochondriasis (from Stern & Drummond, 1991, reproduced with permission of Cambridge University Press)

Practical management

The management of these patients is similar to that of obsessive–compulsive disorder, and consists of the following stages.

Education

Educating the patient about how anxiety can worsen real symptoms until they get out of hand can be difficult to achieve, as patients may feel the doctor is doubting the validity of their symptoms and suffering. It can be useful to suggest that although the patient believes the symptoms are due to serious disease, the GP believes that the symptoms are caused by stress and worry. Therefore as the constant attendance at doctors' surgeries and hospitals has not helped, it might be useful to test out the theory that the symptoms are stress-induced for the next two months.

Ban on reassurance and checking

This may require liaison with other medical agencies, with the patient's permission.

Cognitive restructuring

This is needed for some patients to help them see alternative explanations for their symptoms.

Prognosis

The behavioural–cognitive treatment of hypochondriasis has only recently been developed, and controlled trials are currently being performed which appear to be producing good results. Uncontrolled work suggests that most patients who agree to receive this type of therapy, even in groups, can benefit significantly (Stern & Fernandez, 1991).

Conclusions

Patients with anxiety disorders are often discussed in terms of being the 'worried well'. This can often be viewed in a pejorative way and can lead health planners to consider anxious patients as a drain on precious resources. Not only is this untrue – Marks (1986) has shown that the handicap of obsessive–compulsive disorder can be at least as great as that of chronic schizophrenia – but it also leads to these patients being overlooked in the planning of health-care facilities.

Patients with severe anxiety disorders will generally require referral to specialist clinics. The patient with a mild or moderately severe condition often needs considerable input from the GP. Medication has been the chief weapon which the GP has used to conquer anxiety symptoms in the past. We now know that prolonged use of benzodiazepine drugs is unsafe. The general public are increasingly wary about taking medication for psychological distress.

Fortunately, developments in psychiatric and psychological research have shown that psychological treatments do not need to be time consuming, and need not require years of training to be effectively applied to most anxious patients. Indeed, the judicious use of a simple technique, such as self-exposure instructions for an agoraphobic lady, can reduce the time a GP needs to spend with the patient. Prescribing for this lady means that she needs to be seen, albeit intermittently, for many years. With self-exposure guidance, she might need to be seen weekly for eight weeks and then be sufficiently recovered to require little or no input thereafter.

Overall, as our knowledge of the possible causes and maintaining factors in anxiety disorders increase, so does the potential to abort, prevent and treat these distressing conditions.

References

AMERICAN PSYCHIATRIC ASSOCIATION (1987) *Diagnostic and Statistical Manual for Psychiatric Disorders* (3rd edn, revised) (DSM–III–R). Washington, DC: APA.

BARSKY, A. J., GERINGER, E. & WOOD, C. A. (1988) A cognitive–educational treatment for hypochondriasis. *General Hospital Psychiatry*, **10**, 322–327.

—— & WYSHAK, G. (1990) Hypochondriasis and somatosensory amplification. *British Journal of Psychiatry*, **157**, 404–409.

BECK, A. T. & EMERY, G. (1985) *Anxiety Disorders and Phobias: A Cognitive Perspective.* New York: Basic Books.

BERNSTEIN, D. A. & BORKOVEC, T. D. (1973) *Progressive Relaxation Training: A Manual for the Helping Professions.* Champaign, Illinois: Research Press.

BUTLER, G., CULLINGTON, A., HIBBERT, G. *et al* (1987) Anxiety management for persistent generalised anxiety. *British Journal of Psychiatry*, **151**, 535–542.

CLARK, D. M., SALKOVSKIS, P. M. & CHALKLEY, A. J. (1985) Respiratory control as a treatment for panic attacks. *Journal of Behavior Therapy and Experimental Psychiatry*, **16**, 23–30.

FOA, E. B. & GOLDSTEIN, A. (1978) Continuous exposure and complete response prevention in the treatment of obsessive–compulsive neurosis. *Behavior Therapy*, **9**, 821–829.

GHOSH, A., MARKS, I. M. & CARR, A. C. (1988) Therapist contact and outcome of self-exposure treatment for phobias: a controlled study. *British Journal of Psychiatry*, **152**, 234–238.

KAHN, R. J., MCNAIR, D. M. & FRANKENTHALER, L. M. (1987) Tricyclic treatment of generalized anxiety disorder. *Journal of Affective Disorders*, **13**, 145–151.

KARNO, M., GOLDING, J. M., SORENSON, S. B., *et al* (1988) The epidemiology of obsessive-compulsive disorder in five U.S. communities. *Archives of General Psychiatry*, **45**, 1095–1099.

KLEIN, D. F. (1967) Importance of psychiatric diagnosis in prediction of clinical drug effects. *Archives of General Psychiatry*, **16**, 118–126.

LADER, M. H. (1975) *The Psychophysiology of Mental Illness.* London: Routledge & Kegan Paul.

LANCET (1988) Buspirone – a radical advance in the treatment of anxiety? *Lancet*, *i*, 804–806.

MARKOVITZ, P. J., STAGNO, S. J. & CALABRESE, J. R. (1990) Buspirone augmentation of fluoxetine in obsessive–compulsive disorder. *American Journal of Psychiatry*, **147**, 798–800.

MARKS, I. M. (1969) *Fears and Phobias.* New York: Academic.

—— (1978) *Living with Fear.* New York: McGraw-Hill.

—— (1986) *Behavioural Psychotherapy: Maudsley Pocket Book of Clinical Management.* Bristol: Wright.

—— (1981) *Cure and Care of Neurosis: Theory and Practice of Behavioural Psychotherapy.* New York: Wiley.

——, GRAY, S., COHEN, D., *et al* (1983) Imipramine and brief therapist-aided exposure in agoraphobics having self-exposure homework. *Archives of General Psychiatry*, **40**, 153–162.

——, HODGSON, R. & RACHMAN, S. (1975) Treatment of chronic obsessive–compulsive disorder by *in vivo* exposure. *British Journal of Psychiatry*, **12**, 349–364.

——, LELLIOT, P., BASOGLU, M., *et al*, (1988) Clomipramine, self-exposure and therapist-aided exposure for obsessive–compulsive rituals. *British Journal of Psychiatry*, **152**, 522–534.

MATHEWS, A. M., GELDER, M. G. & JOHNSTON, D. W. (1981) *Agoraphobia: Nature and Treatment.* New York: Guilford Press.

MCDOUGLE, C. J. & GOODMAN, W. K. (1990) Obsessive–compulsive disorder: recent neurobiological developments. *Current Opinion in Psychiatry*, **3**, 239–244.

—— & —— (1991) Obsessive–compulsive disorder: pharmacotherapy and pathophysiology. *Current Opinion in Psychiatry*, **4**, 267–272.

MELLINGER, G. D., BALTER, M. B. & UHLENHUTH, E. H. (1984) Prevalence and correlates of the long term regular use of anxiolytics. *Journal of the American Psychiatric Association*, **251**, 375–379.

MICHELSON, L. & MAVISSAKALIAN, M. (1985) Psychophysiological outcome of behavioural and drug treatments of agoraphobia. *Journal of Consulting and Clinical Psychology*, **53**, 229–236.

MONTEIRO, W. O., NOSHIRVANI, H. F., MARKS, I. M., *et al* (1987) Anorgasmia from clomipramine in obsessive–compulsive disorder: a controlled trial. *British Journal of Psychiatry*, **151**, 107–112.

MUNBY, M. & JOHNSTON, D. W. (1980) Agoraphobia: the long-term follow-up of behavioural treatment. *British Journal of Psychiatry*, **137**, 418–427.

OHMAN, A. & DIMBERG, U. (1984) An evolutionary perspective on human social behaviour. In *Sociopsychology* (ed. W. M. Waid). New York: Springer.

—— , —— & OST, L-G. (1984) Animal and social phobias: biological constraints on learned fear responses. In *Theoretical Issues in Behavior Therapy* (eds. S. Reiss & R. R. Bootzin). New York: Academic.

SALKOVSKIS, P. M. & WARWICK, H. M. C. (1986) Morbid preoccupations, health anxiety, and reassurance: a cognitive–behavioural approach to hypochondriasis. *Behaviour Research and Therapy*, **24**, 597–609.

SOLYMAN, L., SOLYMAN, C., LaPIERRE, Y., *et al* (1981) Phenelzine and exposure in the treatment of phobias. *Biological Psychiatry*, **16**, 239–247.

STERN, R. S. & FERNANDEZ, M. (1991) Group cognitive and behavioural treatment for hypochondriasis. *British Medical Journal*, **303**, 1229–1231.

—— & DRUMMOND, L. M. (1991) *The Practice of Behavioural and Cognitive Psychotherapy*. Cambridge: Cambridge University Press.

TYRER, P. (1980) Use of beta-blocking drugs in psychiatry and neurology. *Drugs*, **20**, 300–308.

—— & STEINBERG, D. (1975) Symptomatic treatment of agoraphobias and social phobias: a follow-up. *British Journal of Psychiatry*, **127**, 163–168.

WORLD HEALTH ORGANIZATION (1978) *Glossary of and Guide to the Classification of Mental Disorders in Accordance with the Ninth Revision of the International Classification of Diseases* (ICD–9). Geneva: WHO.

9 Alcohol problems

JAMES DUNBAR

Alcohol consumption is a major cause of premature death and avoidable ill health throughout the whole population (Anderson, 1991). One-fifth of the adult patients in any general practice are consuming harmful amounts of alcohol. The total cost of this public health problem in the UK is difficult to estimate, but may be £2 billion annually (Robinson *et al*, 1989), and 5000 to 40 000 deaths in England and Wales could be attributed to alcohol each year (Anderson, 1988). The main instruments for controlling consumption and therefore damage are in the hands of government: taxation, licensing laws, and setting national consumption targets. But the role of primary care is far from insignificant. Screening programmes and early intervention by primary care teams are effective and necessary. Each year, intervention by GPs could reduce the alcohol consumption of 250 000 men and 67 500 women to moderate levels.

General practitioners think alcoholics incurable

Many GPs dislike dealing with 'alcoholic' patients. The GP sees alcoholics as sliding downhill with few, if any, recovering. This stereotype is based on the small number who continually relapse and turn up in surgery (Babor *et al*, 1986). However, a more complete picture of the process indicates that prospects for full recovery are rather more hopeful.

Few GPs have the knowledge or skills to diagnose, intervene, and adequately treat their patients with alcohol problems, since undergraduate teaching concentrates on the 'skid-row' alcoholic, or the patient with advanced physical problems, and gives a false picture of alcohol problems in the community. Furthermore, lack of success with such patients reinforces the view that intervention is futile. Conversely, the more GPs have been trained and educated to manage early alcohol problems in primary care, the more effectively and enthusiastically they do it (Anderson, 1984, 1985).

General practitioners may find their own ambivalence to alcohol is a bar to helping patients with alcohol problems. Until recently GPs ran a high risk of dying from the results of excessive consumption. This has changed recently, but one in five GPs still drinks too much (Plant, 1987).

The patient's well kept drinking secret

Patients may be secretive or sensitive about their drinking; indeed, the patient may deny there is any problem. Consequently, doctors should ask about it in a matter-of-fact way.

The sooner affected drinkers are helped, the better the results. In the Malmo study, which involved screening the adult male population for gamma-glutamyl transpeptidase (GGT) levels, advice and feedback of blood results resulted in the treatment group's hospital admission rate being 39% of the control rate, and the mortality rate was halved (Kristensen & Hood, 1984). In a study of in-patients on medical wards in Edinburgh, a half-hour intervention reduced alcohol problems when compared with controls one year later (Chick *et al*, 1985).

General Practitioners are well placed to intervene early, and can therefore expect good results. Over 98% of the population are registered with a GP. Two-thirds of the practice population consult their doctor within one year and nine-tenths within a five year period (Cartwright & Anderson, 1977). This presents unique opportunities for prevention and early intervention. Three British studies have demonstrated that 10–15 minutes of GP advice results in a 15% reduction of alcohol consumption and a 20% reduction in the proportion of excessive drinkers (Heather *et al*, 1987; Wallace *et al*, 1988; Anderson & Scott, 1992).

Programmes to persuade patients to give up smoking, have their high blood pressure controlled, and be screened routinely for cervical carcinoma all met with initial resistance. It was hardly surprising, as patients who felt perfectly well were being advised to accept a change. Asking about smoking is now routine, and, in time, asking about alcohol consumption will be carried out routinely and evoke no surprise from a patient. There is even some evidence that patients expect this advice from their GPs (Wallace & Haines, 1984).

Who has the alcohol problem?

Patients can be categorised by defining their alcohol consumption in standard units, where one unit is equivalent to half a pint of beer, or a measure of spirits, sherry or wine (Table 9.1).

TABLE 9.1
The alcohol content of various drinks (Royal College of Physicians, 1987)

Beverage	Grams of alcohol	Units of alcohol
Beers and lagers		
Ordinary strength	8 g per ½ pint	1
Beer or lager	12 g per can	1.5
(3% alcohol)	16 g per pint	2
Export beer	16 g per can	2
(4% alcohol)	20 g per pint	2.5
Strong beer	16 g per ½ pint	2
or lager	24 g per can	3
(5.5% alcohol)	32 g per pint	4
Extra-strength	20 g per ½ pint	2.5
beer or lager	32 g per can	4
(7% alcohol)	40 g per pint	5
Ciders		
Average cider	12 g per ½ pint	1.5
(4% alcohol)	24 g per pint	3
Strong cider	16 g per ½ pint	2
(6% alcohol)	32 g per pint	4
	64 g per quart bottle	8
Spirits		
Whisky 70° proof	8 g per single measure	1
(40% alcohol)	in England and Wales	
Brandy 70° proof	12 g per single measure	1.5
(40% alcohol)	in Scotland and N. Ireland	
Whisky, gin, vodka	240 g per bottle	30
(40% alcohol)		
Wines		
Table wines	8 g per standard glass	1
(10% alcohol)	56 g per bottle	7
	100 g per litre bottle	12.5
Fortified wine, sherry, port	8 g per standard measure	1
Vermouth (20% alcohol)	120 g per bottle	15
Liqueurs (20% alcohol)	8 g per small measure	1
	100–240 g per bottle	12.5–30

Recently the categorisation into 'alcoholics' and 'social drinkers' has been replaced by the concept of drinking spread along a continuum (Royal College of General Practitioners, 1986). At one end there are low consumers, who are free of harm, and at the other end are the highly dependent drinkers, with multiple medical and social consequences. An individual's position on the continuum can be seen as the result of a behaviour learned and modified by experience. At any stage in a person's life the position on the continuum may change favourably or adversely, depending on circumstances. There is good evidence that many drinkers 'treat themselves', and move out of harmful drinking without any professional contact or help. Vaillant (1983),

TABLE 9.2
The spectrum of alcohol abuse in the average general practice

	Low risk	Moderate risk	High risk/dependent
Intake: units per week			
men	less than 21	21–50	more than 50
women	less than 15	15–35	more than 35
Number of patients			
men	487	140	40
women	679	77	15
Action	review in 3 years	advise to reduce consumption, review annually, including GGT and MCV	advise to reduce consumption, monitor closely, including GGT and MCV

in his longitudinal study of drinking careers in Boston, reported that one-third of those experiencing problems became abstinent without professional help. Significantly, many of them had a medical problem which deteriorated immediately with drinking.

Most alcohol problems seen in general practice are among moderate drinkers – that is, men who drink between 21 and 50 units per week, and women who drink between 15 and 35 units per week. The spectrum of alcohol abuse in the average general practice is shown in Table 9.2.

Environment and culture play a part in developing drinking behaviour. Heavy-drinking husbands are more likely to have heavy-drinking wives. The Irish and Scots are more likely to have alcohol problems than the English, and working in a brewery or pub is more hazardous to the liver than working in an office.

Sex differences

Men drink much more than women, but the difference between the drinking habits of the sexes is changing steadily (Plant, 1987). During the past two decades there has been a steady increase in alcohol problems among women. Female problem drinkers are:

(a) more socially isolated
(b) more often divorced
(c) have experienced more childhood disruption
(d) are in poorer general health than male problem drinkers.

Husbands are probably less willing or able to tolerate and support a heavily-drinking wife than wives who are expected to help or accept a heavily drinking husband.

Women appear to be:

(a) more vulnerable to liver disease than men; this may be attributable to lower average body weight and a higher proportion of body fat – alcohol is dispersed in body water only, so the same volume of alcohol leads to a higher blood level in women than in men
(b) less likely than men to become problem drinkers for purely casual social reasons, but especially likely to develop alcohol problems in reaction to specific events such as bereavement or divorce
(c) more likely to feel guilty about their drinking
(d) changing their drinking habits, although there is still greater stigma attached to misuse by women than men.

What constitutes abuse?

Although drinking behaviour should be seen as a continuum, it is useful to be able to describe the many different types of alcohol abuse, and a whole range of physical, psychological and social problems associated with excessive drinking. (The hazards of alcohol abuse are listed in Appendix 1.) The spectrum of alcohol abuse includes the 'social drinkers' at one end and 'skid-row' alcoholics at the other. Between the two are moderate drinkers, problem drinkers, and dependent drinkers.

Social drinkers drink usually not more than two to three units of alcohol a day and do not become intoxicated; they are not likely to harm themselves or their families through drinking. The amount that can be drunk without harm varies widely, but greater amounts than this are associated with increasing risk of harm.

Moderate drinkers regularly drink more than five units of alcohol a day but without apparent immediate harm. Moderate drinkers are at risk in the long term.

Problem drinkers are those who experience physical, psychological, social, family, occupation, financial, or legal problems attributable to drinking, regardless of the amount.

Dependent drinkers have a compulsion to drink, take roughly the same amount each day, have increased tolerance to alcohol in the early stages and reduced tolerance later, and suffer withdrawal symptoms, which are relieved by consuming more. Drinking takes precedence over all other activities, and the dependent drinker tends to resume drinking after a period of abstinence.

General practitioners have a contractual obligation to advise their patients about sensible drinking, and to recognise alcohol-related problems at an early stage (Department of Health, 1989). Remember:

(a) advice is more readily accepted if it is given in the spirit of concern for health

(b) dire warnings are rarely heeded

(c) simple advice from the GP about changing habits is often surprisingly effective

(d) relapse is not inevitable

(e) habits are often hard to change because of the patient's ambivalent attitude to his/her drinking pattern. This can be harnessed by asking the patient to draw up a balance sheet of good and bad consequences of continuous drinking. Such evidence allows GP and patient to discuss goals for changing a drinking pattern.

(f) initially aim at specific, short-term goals.

Identifying 'at risk' patients

Patients with alcohol problems may be identified in one of three ways:

(a) during a consultation when alcohol is found to be the cause of the problem – the 'hidden diagnosis' (Wilkins, 1974)

(b) at a 'well-person' check, blood pressure, diabetic clinic or other screening programme

(c) self-referral or referred by a relative.

The 'hidden diagnosis'

Alcohol is the great mimic, a common cause of medical problems, and should be considered for the following presentations and indications (Department of Health, 1989):

(a) frequent consultations with the GP

(b) dyspepsia

(c) diarrhoea

(d) hypertension

(e) tranquilliser prescription

(f) anxiety

(g) depression

(h) marital disorder

(i) liver disease.

(j) occupational risk group

(k) alcohol noted on casualty slip.

The screening programme

Alcohol intake should form part of the routine questioning in the 'well-person' check. The GP or nurse should know how to ask about intake, and how to convert the answer to units per week; patients may then be classified according to risk (Table 9.2, above). Patients attending for blood pressure or diabetic control should be asked about alcohol consumption and have GGT and mean corpuscular volume (MCV) measured annually, as alcohol often plays an aetiological role in the problem.

Low risk

Reinforce knowledge about safe limits and review at next 'well-person' check. Remember that even a low-risk drinker may increase the risk within the three years and present with an alcohol-related problem (Anderson, 1987).

Moderate risk

This group is particularly important as it is the most numerous 'at-risk' group, and with whom GPs expect most success in preventing more risky drinking (Kreitman, 1986). Measuring GGT and MCV with feedback on progress towards normalisation, along with a pack such as *So You Want to Cut Down on Your Drinking?*, will usually be sufficient for this group. The key elements of the packs are:

(a) information about safe limits and alcohol-induced harm
(b) drinking diary
(c) a medical questionnaire to elicit alcohol-induced symptoms
(d) tips on avoiding drinking situations and on drinking more slowly
(e) a balance sheet to encourage the drinker to weigh up the pros and cons of harmful drinking.

High risk

The aim with this group is to bring their drinking into the safe range by either control or abstinence. The drinker will go through three phases before achieving this aim (Prochaska & Di Clemente, 1984).

(a) Pre-understanding. A drinking diary provides a record of drinks consumed, the time, the quantity, and the occasion. This is a useful form of self-audit. Show the patient how to keep the diary and how to convert the amount of alcohol consumed into standard units. The diary should be completed each day, kept for a few weeks, and discussed at each consultation. It may help identify occasions when the patient has drunk more than intended by identifying times of the day or days of the week, people with whom drinking occurs, particular emotional state, or conflicts with other people. Anticipating these circumstances and finding ways of avoiding them may reduce drinking. Many people are surprised at how much alcohol they have actually

consumed in a week when they have been made to write it down. Listing alcohol-related problems that the person might experience is also useful. Some will already be apparent from the medical notes. Relating the cause of any medical problems to alcohol may bring understanding. Insomnia, for instance, may be given as a reason for drinking and not seen as its cause. Understanding the problem may break the vicious cycle.

(b) Understanding. At this stage alcohol is understood to be the cause of the problem but no decision to act on it has been made. Drawing up a balance sheet of advantages and disadvantages of drinking may tip the balance.

(c) Action. At this stage the patient needs guidance towards the most realistic goal-controlled drinking or abstinence.

Self-referral or referred by a third party

It is becoming commoner for patients to refer themselves because they are concerned about their drinking. Relatives and employers too are more likely to express concern to the GP. Perhaps advertising alcohol clinics as part of health-promotion activity and mentioning an interest in alcohol problems in the practice leaflet makes it easier for people to report the adverse consequences of drinking.

The protocol for managing these patients is the same as for those found in a screening clinic, but the following guidelines are given to provide a more comprehensive approach.

Taking a complete history

The clues to alcohol abuse are listed above (p. 140). Questions about alcohol should not stand alone but be part of a general inquiry, even at routine visits, for instance for cervical cytology, blood pressure clinics, and other screening programmes. Ask about alcohol consumption over the last week and then relate the result to safe limits. Elicit whether drinking started following some unpleasant life event, and determine whether heavy drinking persisted after the original provocation, perhaps because of additional problems, such as difficulties at work. Ask about previous attempts to reduce drinking and any reason for the attempt, and about attitudes towards relapses. Ask whether the patient has: indigestion, nausea, diarrhoea, insomnia, lassitude, depression, arguments at home, difficulties at work, money problems, problems with the police, accidents, a tendency to drink in the morning, or trembling the following day.

Some of the other clues to alcohol abuse include a history of frequent consultations and tranquilliser prescriptions.

Physical signs

Look out for:

(a) bloated plethoric face with puffiness around the parotid
(b) telangiectasia
(c) blood-shot eyes
(d) acne rosacea
(e) smell of alcohol
(f) poor oral hygiene
(g) tremor
(h) palmar erythema
(i) Dupuytren's contracture
(j) beer belly, gynaecomastia
(k) bruising from falls
(l) hypertension.

Further laboratory investigations

No single laboratory test is an unequivocal indicator of alcohol abuse, as tests may be affected by other diseases or drugs (Baxter *et al*, 1980; Chick *et al*, 1981; Rosalki, 1984; Kristensen, 1989).

The most sensitive markers are serum enzyme GGT and red-cell MCV. Together these identify 9 out of 10 chronic excessive consumers of alcohol in general practice when used with another indicator such as admitted high consumption or an alcohol-related problem (e.g. indigestion). Both tests have limitations when used alone as screening instruments, and are best used to monitor successful drinking control. Levels of GGT (normal values: male 0–50 IU/l, female 0–35 IU/l) is the best screening test available and values above 50 IU/l are found in 80% of problem drinkers. This is not a measure of liver damage but of enzyme induction. An MCV of greater than 92 is found in 60% of problem drinkers, more commonly in women than men. With abstinence, MCV returns to normal more slowly than GGT, but both revert to abnormal fairly rapidly after any relapse.

Supporting evidence of alcohol abuse can come from:

(a) raised serum urate (normal 170–520 mmol/l)
(b) raised fasting triglycerides (normal < 1.8 mmol/l)
(c) raised aspartate aminotransferase (normal 5–40 IU/l).

Other diseases which may raise GGT are: obstructive liver disease, hepatic malignancy, hepatitis, cirrhosis, pancreatic disease, and infectious mononucleosis. Drugs which may raise GGT levels include: salicylate, barbiturates, carbamazepine, chlorpromazine, rifampicin, azathioprine, cocaine, and warfarin.

Blood alcohol concentration

This test is not used often enough. An alcometer of the type used by the police gives an accurate reading. Alternatively, a blood sample may be taken into a fluoride/oxalate container. Raised concentrations can provide incontrovertible evidence of excessive drinking and break down the denial mechanism.

Because alcohol is eliminated relatively slowly from the blood, appreciable amounts may be found even 24 hours after a drinking session.

Alcohol levels above 150 mg/100 ml are fairly diagnostic of chronic excessive drinking, particularly where the patient shows no obvious signs of intoxication.

Questionnaires

These are useful for epidemiological research but have little value in identifying individual patients, since honesty and personality influence the response. Their role in primary care has never been validated but some specific uses have been found (Wallace & Haines, 1985; Cutler *et al*, 1988; Anderson, 1992).

Management and outcome

The predictors of a good outcome are:

(a) youth
(b) stable job
(c) stable marriage
(d) higher occupational status
(e) sound underlying personality.

Impediments to progress are:

(a) alcohol available at work
(b) family or financial stress
(c) neurosis or depression
(d) withdrawal symptoms
(e) leisure-time activities where alcohol is available.

The following advice should be given to patients:

(a) aim for activities that do not involve drinking
(b) take up relaxation training for anxiety
(c) involve your spouse.

The role of the spouse

Frequently, it is worth interviewing the spouse since he/she may experience physical, social, or psychological harm. Furthermore, he/she may have a positive or negative effect on successful outcome for the drinking partner – for instance, having a row about drinking behaviour when the spouse is sober. It is important for the spouse to understand that sobriety should be rewarded and drinking punished. Partners need to learn to increase their involvement with non-drinking activities.

The DRAMS kit

The DRAMS kit (Drinking Reasonably and Moderately with Self-Control) consists of: (a) a DRAMS medical record card for the doctor's use, with questionnaire, space for blood test results, and a record of alcohol consumption; (b) an initial two-week drinking diary for the patient and a self-help booklet with a further drinking diary.

Other self-help manuals are available (see Appendix 2). *Let's Drink to Your Health* is particularly suitable for better-educated patients. Many GPs would gain useful knowledge and skills from reading it.

Abstinence or controlled drinking?

If drinking is excessive but with no signs of harm, then safe drinking limits can be attempted once the biological markers have returned to normal. Most seriously affected patients – for example older, physically addicted, physically damaged patients, or those who fail on controlled drinking – should aim for abstinence.

Relapse

Do not regard relapse as failure, but as an opportunity to learn more about the nature of the drinking problem in the individual patient. It can be analysed for how and why it happened.

Follow-up

Review progress regularly. Progress in the first six months gives a fairly good indication of the likely outcome.

Indications and reasons for referral to specialist services

It seems that in the majority of cases seen, patients do not actually need referring to specialist services, and on most occasions can be adequately helped by their own GP (Lock, 1982). There may be times when there are indications that require a referral to a psychiatrist at an alcohol treatment centre. Some of these symptoms are:

(a) severe withdrawal symptoms
(b) fits or delirium tremens
(c) lack of supportive environment
(d) neurosis or psychosis
(e) need for help in restructuring social activities
(f) requirement for intensive counselling.

These units have detoxification facilities and many now run on a behaviourist approach, with great emphasis placed on group work.

On the other hand, there are some signs that a patient may need a referral to a local counsellor:

(a) lack of supportive environment
(b) need for help in restructuring social activities
(c) requirement for intensive counselling in the absence of other psychiatric indications.

Local counsellors who are dealing with the problems of alcohol are highly trained and, as a result, the patient has the pleasing benefit of being able to remain in the community.

Patients should be referred to a physician if they have:

(a) major physical disease
(b) cirrhosis
(c) peripheral neuropathy.

Detoxification

A few patients with a history of severe withdrawal symptoms will require formal detoxification. This can take place at home but, in my view, is probably better undertaken in hospital, as such patients will require intensive support. For the same reasons, initiation of disulfiram therapy should be confined to in-patients.

Alcohol and its effects in the workplace

Some occupations have particularly high rates of alcohol problems. Until recently medical practice was one, but now there is some evidence that the cirrhosis rate is down to just above the average risk.

Employees in the alcohol trades are particularly likely to have heavy intakes and develop alcohol problems (Plant, 1987). It is difficult to identify common factors which might link occupations at risk, but some explanations are:

(a) availability of alcohol at work
(b) social pressure to drink at work (e.g. servicemen, seamen)
(c) separation from normal social or sexual relationships (e.g. servicemen, seamen, commercial travellers)
(d) freedom from supervision (e.g. executives, doctors, lawyers)
(e) very high or very low income levels (e.g. professionals, the unemployed, unskilled workers)
(f) collusion by colleagues (e.g. fear of dismissal or exploiting a colleague's incapacity)
(g) strains and stresses, danger (e.g. seamen, servicemen), responsibility (e.g. doctors, lawyers, executives), job insecurity (e.g. actors), boredom
(h) recruitment of 'unusual people' predisposed to drink heavily (e.g. merchant navy).

Alcohol problems at work lead to absenteeism, accidents, poor performance, and poor leadership (Royal College of Physicians, 1987; McNeill, 1989).

Alcohol may potentiate some cerebral depressants used in industry such as trichlorethylene.

The vast majority of people with drinking problems are men in full-time employment. It is not only problem drinkers who are likely to have difficulty at work. Lunchtime drinking increases the likelihood of an accident, and impairs judgement and decision making.

The workplace provides an ideal setting for early identification and treatment. GPs working as occupational physicians are in a position to make employees aware of the dangers of alcohol abuse and to assist employers in formulating alcohol policies. GPs advising in occupational medicine should take a stand against: the practice of allowing employees to consume alcohol before reporting for work or during rest periods; a bar being provided where alcohol is available at subsidised rates and whose profits are ploughed back into sports or social activities; alcohol provided free for executive hospitality; alcohol consumed at in-house meetings or when entertaining clients. They should lead by example, and have an alcohol policy for the practice.

Alcohol policies at work

Until comparatively recently, problem drinking at work has been dealt with by either collusion or dismissal (McNeill, 1989). Now an increasing number of employers have adopted policies aimed at early identification, treatment, and rehabilitation of employees who abuse alcohol. The Post Office is a good example. Managers are trained to identify problem drinkers on the basis of absenteeism, poor work performance, and unacceptable behaviour, and these are referred to a specialist. This may be the GP occupational physician.

Provision should be made for employees who believe they have an alcohol problem to consult an occupational health service, and to be regarded as on sick leave while undergoing a recovery programme within general practice. Help needs to be given in strict confidence and job security guaranteed. It is important that employees are aware that an occupational alcohol policy exists and are encouraged to report early, and that managers realise they should recognise alcohol problems at the earliest stage to increase the effectiveness of treatment.

The relevance of drinking and driving to primary care

Drinking and driving has increased fourfold in the last 20 years. A mass of evidence has now accumulated to demonstrate the relationship between drinking and driving and accidents.

(a) It is associated with one-quarter of all fatal road traffic accidents
(b) It is a major cause of death in 18–24-year-olds
(c) The higher the level of alcohol, the greater is the accident risk. At 150 mg/100 ml, the average for arrested drivers, the accident risk is increased 25-fold.

Drivers are generally unaware of how long it takes to eliminate alcohol from the body. In one experiment, two out of three drivers who were drinking socially between 7.30 p.m. and midnight still exceeded the legal limit at 9 a.m. the next day (Dunbar *et al*, 1983*a*). Perhaps less well known is that one in four drinking and driving offenders is a problem drinker (Dunbar *et al*, 1983*b*). These problem drinkers are particularly likely to be involved in road accidents and to drive while under the influence of alcohol, including during the day when children are about (Dunbar *et al*, 1985).

The first indication that a patient is a problem drinker may be a conviction for drinking and driving. There is a good case for the courts notifying GPs when their patients are convicted, but at present this does not happen. In the meantime receptionists frequently glean this information from reports in the local newspapers. Any driver over the age of 30 who has been convicted should be screened for alcohol problems.

A large proportion of professional drivers are problem drinkers and therefore should be screened for alcohol problems when being examined for licensing for load-carrying and passenger-carrying vehicles.

Conclusions

Early identification of alcohol problems is a challenge to the skill of any GP, but the success of early detection and treatment is rewarding. The role of the practice team is expanding to include health promotion, and the importance of providing advice, counselling, and treatment for alcohol is increasing.

Appendix 1. The hazards of alcohol abuse

The following list is derived from the Royal College of Physicians (1987).

Centre nervous system

Acute intoxication – 'blackouts'

Neuropsychiatric

Insomnia
Anxiety
Depression, suicide
Amnesia
Other substance abuses
Persistent brain damage:
   Wernicke's encephalopathy
   Korsakoff's syndrome
Cerebellar degeneration
   Dementia
Cerebrovascular disease
   strokes, especially in young people
   subarachnoid haemorrhage
   subdural haematoma after head injury
Withdrawal symptoms
   tremor
   hallucinations
   fits
Nerve
   weakness
   paralysis
   paraesthesiae of hands and feet

Liver

Fatty infiltration of liver
Alcoholic hepatitis
Cirrhosis and eventual liver failure
Hepatoma

Gastrointestinal system

Reflux oesophagitis
Tearing and occasionally rupture of the oesophagus
Cancer of the oesophagus
Gastritis
Aggravation and impaired healing of peptic ulcers
Diarrhoea and impaired absorption of food
Chronic pancreatitis leading to diabetes and malabsorption
Malnutrition from reduced intake of food, toxic effects of alcohol on intestine, and
    impaired metabolism leading to weight loss
Obesity, particularly in early stages of heavy drinking

Heart and circulatory system

Palpitations
Abnormal rhythms and sudden death
High blood pressure
Chronic heart muscle damage leading to heart failure

Respiratory system

Bronchitis
Pneumonia from inhalation of vomit

Muscular/skeletal

Fractured ribs
Myopathy
Low back pain due to muscle weakness
Gout
Repeated injuries

Endocrine system

Overproduction of cortisol leading to obesity, acne, increased facial hair, and high
    blood pressure
Condition mimicking overactivity of the thyroid with loss of weight, anxiety,
    palpitations, sweating and tremor
Severe hypoglycaemia, sometimes leading to coma
Intense facial flushing in many diabetics taking the antidiabetic drug chlorpropamide

Reproductive system

Loss of libido
Reduced potency
Shrinkage in size of testes and penis
Reduced or absent sperm formation and infertility
Loss of sexual hair
Breast swelling
In women
    sexual difficulties
    menstrual problems
    shrinkage of breasts and external genitalia

Social problems

Domestic violence
Absenteeism
Arguments
Aggression
Inefficiency
Divorce
Legal problems
Accidents and reduced chance of survival
    at leisure
    at work
    at home
    at sea
    on the roads
Drunkenness
Breach of peace
Vagrancy
Drinking and driving
Assault
Manslaughter
Homicide

Appendix 2. Useful self-help materials

DRAMS Pack. Edinburgh: Scottish Health Education Group.
Let's Drink to Your Health: A Self Help Guide to Sensible Drinking, by I. Robertson &
    N. Heather. British Psychological Society, Blackhorse Road, Letchworth,
    Herts SG6 1HN.
That's the Limit, and *So You Want to Cut Down on Your Drinking Pack*. Health Education
    Authority, London.

References

ANDERSON, P. (1984) Early intervention in general practice. In *Helping the Problem Drinker* (eds
    T. Stockwell & S. Clement). London: Croom Helm.
——— (1985) Managing alcohol problems in general practice. *British Medical Journal*, **290**,
    1873–1875.
——— (1987) A strategy for helping people who are drinking excessively. *Practitioner*, **231**,
    297–306.
——— (1988) Excess mortality associated with alcohol consumption. *British Medical Journal*,
    297, 824–826.
——— (1991) Alcohol as a key area. *British Medical Journal*, **303**, 766–769.
——— (1992) Self administered questionnaires for diagnosis of alcohol abuse. In *Diagnosis of
    Alcohol Abuse* (ed. R. R. Watson). Baton Rouge: CRC Press (in press).
——— & SCOTT, E. (1992) The effect of general practitioners' advice to heavy drinking men.
    British Journal of Addiction, **87**, 891–900.
BABOR, T. F., RITSON, B. & HODGSON, R. (1986) Alcohol related problems in a health care
    setting: a review of early intervention strategies. *British Journal of Addiction*, **81**, 23–46.

BAXTER, S., FINK, R., LEADER, R., *et al* (1980) Laboratory tests for excessive alcohol consumption evaluated in general practice. *British Journal on Alcohol and Alcoholism*, **15**, 164–166.

CARTWRIGHT, A. & ANDERSON, R. (1979) *Patients and Their Doctors, 1977*, Occasional Paper No. 8. London: Royal College of General Practitioners.

CHICK, J., KREITMAN, N. & PLANT, M. (1981) Mean cell volume and gamma glutamyl transpeptidase as markers of drinking in working men. *Lancet*, *i*, 1249–1251.

——, LLOYD, G. & CROMBIE, E. (1985) Counselling problem drinkers in medical wards: a controlled study. *British Medical Journal*, **290**, 965–967.

CUTLER, S. F., WALLACE, P. G. & HAINES, A. P. (1988) Assessing alcohol consumption in general practice patients – a comparison between questionnaire and interview (findings of the Medical Research Council's general practice research framework study on lifestyle and health). *Alcohol and Alcoholism*, **23**, 441–450.

DEPARTMENT OF HEALTH (1990) *General Practice in the National Health Service. The 1990 Contract*. London: Department of Health.

DUNBAR, J. A., HAGART, J., MARTIN, B. T., *et al* (1983*a*) Drivers, binge drinking and gamma glutamyl transpeptidase. *British Medical Journal*, **285**, 183.

——, MARTIN, B. T., DEVGUN, M. S., *et al* (1983*b*) Problem drinking among drunk drivers. *British Medical Journal*, **286**, 1319–1322.

——, OGSTON, S. A., RITCHIE, A., *et al* (1985) Are problem drinkers dangerous drivers? An investigation of arrest for drinking and driving, serum gamma glutamyl transpeptidase activities, blood alcohol concentrations and road traffic accidents: the Tayside safe driving project. *British Medical Journal*, **290**, 827–830.

HEATHER, N, CAMPION, P. D., NEVILLE, R. G., *et al* (1987) Evaluation of a controlled drinking minimal intervention for problem drinkers in general practice (the DRAMS scheme). *Journal of the Royal College of General Practitioners*, **37**, 358–363.

KREITMAN, N. (1986) Alcohol consumption and the preventive paradox. *British Journal of Addiction*, **81**, 353–363.

KRISTENSEN, H. (1989) Biological markers and traffic safety. *Journal of Traffic Medicine*, **17**, 3–5.

—— & HOOD, B. (1984) The impact of alcohol on health in the general population: a review with special reference to experience in Malmo. *British Journal of Addiction*, **79**, 139–145.

LOCK, S. (ed.) (1982) *Alcohol Problems. An ABC of Alcohol and Alcoholism*. London: British Medical Journal.

MCNEILL, A. (1989) *The Industrial Alcohol Pack*. London: Institute for Alcohol Studies.

PLANT, M. A. (1987) *Drugs in Perspective*. London: Hodder and Stoughton.

PROCHASKA, J. O. & DI CLEMENTE, C. C. (1984) *The Transtheoretical Approach*. Illinois: Dow Jones-Irwin.

ROBINSON, D., MAYNARD, A. & CHESTER, R. (1989) *Controlling Legal Addictions*. London: Macmillan.

ROSALKI, S. B. (1984) Identifying the alcoholic. In *Clinical Biochemistry of Alcoholism* (ed. S. B. Rosalki), pp. 65–92. London: Churchill Livingstone.

ROYAL COLLEGE OF GENERAL PRACTITIONERS (1986) *Alcohol – A Balanced View*, Report from General Practice, no. 24. London: Royal College of General Practitioners.

ROYAL COLLEGE OF PHYSICIANS (1987) *A Great and Growing Evil*. London: Tavistock.

VAILLANT, G. E. (1983) *The Natural History of Alcoholism*. Cambridge, Mass: Harvard University Press.

WALLACE, P. G. & HAINES, A. P. (1984) General practitioner and health promotion: what patients think. *British Medical Journal*, **289**, 534–536.

—— & —— (1985) Use of a questionnaire in general practice to increase the recognition of patients with excessive alcohol consumption. *British Medical Journal*, **290**, 1949–1953.

——, CUTLER, S. & HAINES, A. (1988) Randomised controlled trial of general practitioner intervention in patients with excessive alcohol consumption. *British Medical Journal*, **297**, 663–668.

WILKINS, R. H. (1974) *The Hidden Alcoholic in General Practice*. London: Elek Science.

10 Older people

IDRIS WILLIAMS

Mental health is an important factor in achieving successful ageing and maintaining a good quality of life as the years pass. Most old people live in the community in their own homes, and GPs have responsibility for their health care, both physical and mental. Demographic changes have had a significant effect on the volume and type of work which family doctors do with their old patients. The average number of consultations per person per year in the 75 and over age group is 6.1 (Office of Population Censuses and Surveys, 1984). However, the proportion of psychiatric problems presented at consultation decline slightly in this age group (Wilkin & Williams, 1986).

The last 20 years has seen a steep rise in the number of elderly people, and the number of patients aged over 65 years has increased both in total and as a proportion of the general population (Fig. 10.1). The overall increase in numbers has probably now reached its peak, and numbers will not increase again until the effect of the post-war 'baby-boom' becomes apparent around 2010. But within the over-65-year age group, there will be an increase in the most elderly group, that is those aged 74–84, and particularly in the over-85-year age group. This means a relative increase in the number of frail old people. This age group has been shown to have the highest level of disability (Martin *et al*, 1988) (Fig. 10.2). It can be expected therefore that the prevalence of disability – and this includes mental disability – among the elderly will increase. Thus, although the incidence of senile dementia or depression will remain the same, the actual numbers of people who will need treatment and care for these conditions will increase.

The psychology of ageing

The normal biological ageing process, for instance hair turning grey and losing weight, is clear for all to see. Inherent in this process is the increasing

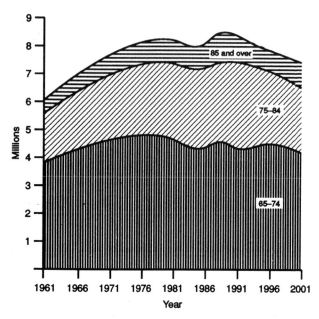

Fig. 10.1. Populations and population predictions for the over-65s to 2001 (from Department of Health and Social Security, 1981, reproduced with permission)

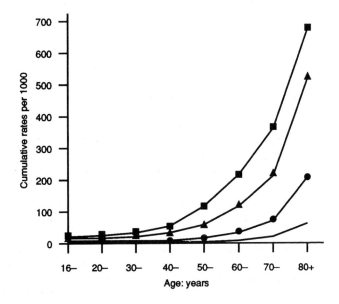

Fig. 10.2. The prevalence of disability in Britain (private households) (——— most severe, ——●— very severe, ——▲— intermediate, ——■— all severities) (from Martin et al, 1988) reproduced with permission)

likelihood of death. Ageing also brings decline in social function, and people gradually cease to undertake various activities of daily living as the years go by. This usually starts with declining sociability and progresses to inability to cope with domestic and personal tasks (Williams, 1986). Side by side with these changes, psychological ageing diminishes the capacity of an old person to adapt to emotional and external changes. These three age-related processes – biological, social, and psychological – are linked, and all need to be understood when considering what is normal. A basic feature, however, of old age is heterogeneity – people vary in the rate of ageing, and biological age does not necessarily equate with chronological age. Similarly, physical, social and psychological ageing can occur at different rates in the same person. Distinctions need to be made between normal changes which occur in every person and, for instance, pathological changes such as senile dementia, which is found in older people but is not typical of all old people. An understanding of the wide spectrum of psychological ageing is therefore necessary when dealing with undesirable deviations from the norm.

The wide variety of normal human experience means that everyone has to make different psychological adjustments along the pathway from early adulthood through middle age to the pre-retirement phase. The adaptations needed are often complex, but if achieved successfully can help enormously when coping with the next stage.

It is normal for people as they get older to review their lives, and this is often constructive. Most accept that some ambitions will not be fulfilled, and they become more realistic about what can be achieved. This minimises feelings of frustration later and a sense of failure once retirement has started. Some, however, despair of their physical and mental decline as age advances, or deny its existence. Men and women can respond differently in this respect, but probably less so than previously, with more women having careers. Women do, however, tend to live longer than men, and psychological adaptions may occur at different times and in different ways. A common happening is for women to become concerned about their husbands' health and consider the possibility of widowhood, even to the extent of forward planning. Sometimes these plans are sensible, and are put into effect long before widowhood. Examples would be moving into a smaller house, restructuring the family's finances, and developing independent interests.

There is a risk as age advances of disengagement, with withdrawal from the mainstream of life. Ideally an old person should assess what is practical, always however with the aim of achieving integration into a new stage of life and so gaining additional fulfilment. These changes are influenced by such things as culture, economic difficulties, stress, family responsibilities, and indeed latent marital strife. Successful adaptations may be hindered by subtle factors such as pride, attitudes towards friends, or previously held prejudices. Nevertheless there is evidence (Clarke, 1984) that most people react positively to old age. The provision of a good pension has allowed many to use their freedom to enable late development and the opportunity to fulfil ambitions previously denied by the demands of working life. The period between 65 and 75 is often the best part of people's lives. An old person in good mental health is likely to be able to maximise his/her potential and adapt to changing circumstances and abilities. Birren & Renner (1981) list some features which mark good mental health in old age. These are: self-acceptance; integration into a harmonious unit; relative personal autonomy; an accurate perception of abilities; adaption to environmental demands; and an ability to overcome the limitations of function.

A stage is however sometimes reached when an old person, because of the demands of daily living, becomes unable to cope. This may be due to physical disability, but social circumstances, for instance the loss of a spouse, can also be the cause. Psychological momentum is lost and dependency results. Previous personality traits may affect this, for instance lack of confidence, impatience, high expectations. Dependency may result in role reversal, with children adopting a parental role. Conflicts may ensue and lead to neglect and isolation of the old person.

There is a fine line between normal psychological responses to circumstance and mental ill health, for instance associated with depression or dementia. Depression in old age is often put down to ageing itself and goes unreported to, or not identified by, professional health workers, and as a result therapy is denied with sometimes tragic results. An understanding of psychological ageing is therefore important, and much can be learned by observing old people day-to-day in practice.

Assessment in the community of elderly patients with disordered thinking

In the community, mental state is assessed in two situations. With the introduction of the new contract for GPs, each person aged 75 years and over has to be offered a health check every year. This is part of a health-promotion programme and has the aim of identifying problems at an early stage in the hope of preventing or reducing disability. An assessment of mental function is included in the health check. The procedure has to be short and is usually carried out by a nurse. The format of this check is discussed below.

The second situation is where a patient presents to a doctor with problems which indicate mental disorder. Because the presentation of mental illness in old age may be subtle and complex, a reliable framework of assessment of a patient's mental state is needed. The aim of such assessment is to identify and clarify the problem, and will entail history-taking, physical examination, mental examination, and perhaps some investigation.

History-taking

History-taking is all important, and with old people it is often necessary to corroborate the story with a relative or carer. Often it is not the patient who is the complainant, and a clear understanding of the reason for the consultation must be gained. Timing of symptoms or changes in behaviour, collateral life events, presence of physical symptoms, previous medical problems, and especially previous psychiatric episodes are all relevant pieces of information. A family history of psychiatric disorder, for instance depressive illness, is also significant. An indication of the patient's psychological adaption to old age and previous personality is helpful when separating mental illness from behavioural idiosyncrasy. The GP is often in an extremely good position to judge these events, having probably known the patient for some years. Inquiry about work experience, marriage relationships, sociability, interests, smoking and alcohol intake give information about the patient's lifestyle and experience.

Physical examination

A full physical examination is necessary, including special attention to the neurological system, and this follows the normal lines.

Mental state examination

An examination of the mental state should also be structured, taking into account general appearance including demeanour, what is said and how it is said, mood, thought processes, and cognitive functions such as memory, intelligence, ability to think abstractly, and orientation.

Gradually developing mental illness can reduce ability to undertake basic activities of daily living; a person can cease to go out shopping, get behind with housework, and fail to attend to personal cleanliness and clothes (Williams, 1986). These are important signs to note. Patients may look sad or happy, anxious or confused, and indeed a sense of disorientation can be observed by just watching a patient's reaction to his/her surroundings. What patients say and how they say it are also relevant. Speech may be fast or slow, jumbled and obscure, or clear and precise. There may be slowing of speech or dysarthria. Ideas experienced may be paranoid, obsessional, fanciful, or doom laden. An assessment of mood involves looking at emotional or affect changes. These may be too much depression, irritability, hostility, fear, worthlessness, and guilt – or incongruous happiness. All these may be apparent in the major mood disorders. Inappropriateness of affect may be the result of chronic schizophrenia. Organic dementias also impair mood. Differentiating between dementia and depression may be difficult (see below).

Looking for abnormal thought processes means detecting for instance paranoia (not uncommon in the elderly), delusions, false perceptions, and irrational obsessions. Cognitive function is assessed by simple memory tests, determination of orientation and testing concentration by, for instance, remembering the months of the year. Abstract thinking can be tested by asking the patient the meaning of proverbs.

Further investigation

Investigations such as urinalysis, blood count, and chest X-ray are often routine. Associated physical illness may be responsible for the mental state and may require specific tests to be undertaken. Schedules are available to test for depression and dementia (see below).

It is important to link these tests with the findings of clinical history-taking and examination.

Clinical disorders

There are complex classifications for psychogenic disorder, but there are for those practising in the community three commonly recognised main themes in old age. These are *mood disorders*, consisting of depression/mania and paranoia/schizophrenia; *organic disorders*, consisting of acute confusional state and dementia; and a mixed group of *personality disorders, behavioural problems*, and *neurosis*, for instance anxiety states, obsessional states, hypochondriasis, hoarding, sexual aberrations. For the GP, the three important conditions practically are acute confusional state, the dementia syndrome, and depression.

Acute confusional state

The sudden onset of confusion in an old person presents an emergency in general practice which needs considerable skill and patience to manage effectively. Dementia can predispose an individual to confusion, but there are many other possible causes; it is necessary when confronted with a confused old patient to search for underlying conditions, and there can be several of these present at the same time. A summary of possible causes is provided by Williams (1988):

(a) intracranial
   (i) space-occupying lesion
   (ii) low-pressure encephalitis
   (iii) infection
   (iv) vascular episode
   (v) trauma
(b) toxic
   (i) systemic infection
   (ii) gangrene
   (iii) alcohol

(c) endocrine
    (i) thyroid disease
    (ii) diabetes mellitus
(d) organ failure
    (i) renal
    (ii) hepatic
    (iii) respiratory
    (iv) anaemia
(e) vitamin deficiency
    B group
(f) medication
    (i) altered response in old age
    (ii) withdrawal symptoms
    (iii) polypharmacy
(g) mental
    (i) presence of Alzheimer's disease or multi-infarct dementia, especially when associated with chronic constipation, pain and discomfort
    (ii) depression
(h) social stress
    (i) acute worries regarding family ⎫
    (ii) harassment   ⎬ especially when dementia
    (iii) unfamiliar surroundings   ⎪ is present
    (iv) change in residence   ⎭

Mental disorder in the form of dementia and depression are frequently associated, but the trigger to the confusion may be infection, over-medication, and social stress. The latter is normally associated with basic care provision and can include change in environment, temporary absence of a carer, and family tensions. The development, and particularly the presentation, of confusion in an old person often occurs at awkward hours and is frequently accompanied by strong demands by neighbours and relatives that the doctor or social worker 'do something', urgently.

Acute confusional states usually have a rapid onset. Consciousness is clouded and disorientation is a marked feature. The mood is one of fear and anxiety, but occasionally the patient can be incongruously jocular and oblivious to reality. Speech is often incoherent, and agitated restlessness is prominent. The mental state can fluctuate over time although the confusion is usually fairly short lived. Eventual recovery is the rule, although death is a possible outcome.

Faced with such an old patient the GP has very quickly to decide whether hospital admission is indicated or whether the situation can be managed at home. This means determining if possible the cause of the confusion and will involve a careful history from carers and a physical examination. Further investigations may be necessary. If care is not available at home, the decision to admit is inevitable; however, when the episode is clearly associated with dementia, management at home has advantages because a move to hospital can deepen the confusion.

If it is decided that it is possible to manage the patient at home it is nevertheless useful to seek the help of a psychiatrist or geriatrician. This allows confirmation of the diagnosis and discussion of possible investigations. A plan of management can be formulated which the hospital understands, so that if deterioration occurs admission can be effectively arranged.

Management of an acute confusional state at home therefore depends on a clear knowledge of the diagnosis, adequate nursing care, and full social support. A nurse and social worker must be involved in the decision taken at the case conference, which should occur between the GP and consultant, so also must be the relatives and carers on whom most of the burden will fall. As important as the history and physical examination of the patient is the assessment to determine the needs of the patient and the resources which are available to satisfy them.

A nursing assessment will include note of other conditions, such as infections and ulcers, problems that may occur with diet, medication, and dealing with a bedridden patient.

A social assessment should include noting any difficulties that will occur in feeding, dressing, toileting, bathing the patient, and with food preparation, laundry, and cleaning of the house. Ensuring adequate heating will also be necessary. A suitable room for nursing the patient will be required and when assessing this the needs of other people, especially children in the household, should be considered. Safety is important and account must be taken of the risks of fires, electricity and gas, and the opportunities available for the patient to wander. The carers will need careful support and it is necessary to assess how much help they can realistically give in providing 24-hour cover. Financial assistance such as attendance allowance should be considered. Often voluntary services, for example Age Concern and the Alzheimer's Disease Society, are useful.

Drugs should be used sparingly, as they can make the situation worse. In a restless patient sedation may be used, but the dosage should be small and careful watch kept for reactions. Long-term supervision is usually necessary once the initial crisis has passed. Established nursing and social-worker services need to be reassessed and placed on a maintenance basis. Short-term respite may be needed for carers.

The dementia syndrome

Dementia is a syndrome that has been defined as "acquired global impairment of memory and personality, but without impairment of consciousness"

(Lishman, 1978). The incidence increases as age advances, so that it affects 4% of 65–69-year-olds, 26% of 75–79-year-olds, and 60% of those over 85 years old (Nielson, 1962). It is an important disorder in general practice; 5% of old people over 65 living at home will be severely demented and a further 5% less severely demented (Hodgson & Jolley, 1985). The most important causes of the syndrome are senile dementia of the Alzheimer type (SDAT) and arteriosclerotic dementia, sometimes called multi-infarct dementia. The two have different courses; SDAT patients show a slow, steady decline in mental ability, whereas arteriosclerotic dementia deterioration takes place in a series of steps. SDAT is more common in women and arteriosclerotic dementia more common in men. The forms can exist together.

Dementia usually results in the complete disruption of thinking. In the early stages there are minor changes of intellectual ability, commonly with forgetfulness. The loss of memory becomes, however, much more severe than is associated with normal ageing. The memory loss is most evident for recent events, and happenings that occurred many years previously are sometimes remembered with astonishing accuracy, although objective tests show that these are also unreliable. There is a gradual reduction in the ability to learn new skills and adapt to changing environments. The emotions are often disorganised, with inappropriate outbursts of crying and laughing.

Sometimes other factors contribute to the dementing syndrome, such as physical illness, sensory impairment, emotional disturbance, or changes in environment. Depression, anxiety, and paranoia can coexist with dementia. The differentiation between depression and dementia is particularly important, as the former is susceptible to treatment. Dementia is most likely if impairment of memory and thinking is reported before the depression. When tested, dementia patients tend to try to respond, but give the wrong answers, whereas depressed patients fail to try, or say 'I don't know'. Early dementia can of course cause depression. Sometimes both can lead to excess alcohol consumption, which in itself can complicate the diagnosis. Self-neglect and social isolation can be a feature of all these conditions and lead eventually to malnutrition.

Management at home, particularly in the early stages, is feasible, but is entirely dependent upon family support, social services input and, very importantly, help from voluntary organisations. At the present time there is nothing in the way of therapy, although occasionally some mild sedation is required. Attention to the patient's physical condition, keeping an eye on weight, blood pressure, diet, alcohol intake, exercise, cleanliness, and other diseases which may also be present is important.

Safety needs to be considered, especially environmental hazard and heating arrangements. As mentioned earlier, financial assistance through attendance allowances should be considered. Maintaining a patient's interest by orientation and awareness devices appears to help and at least counteract the feelings of helplessness and nihilism which sometimes overwhelm the carers.

It cannot be emphasised too strongly that carers need all the support possible: occasional visits from doctor, health visitor, and practice nurses are greatly valued, as also are some respite periods organised through the local hospital. Often when wandering becomes a feature and incontinence develops, carers cannot provide the 24-hour watch that is necessary, and admission to a nursing home or hospital is required. Nursing homes now have a high proportion of patients who are at various stage of the dementia syndrome (Williams *et al*, 1992).

Long-term continuing care for demented patients has become part of the community responsibility through nursing and rest homes, and the GP will continue the management in these institutions. Whereas some dementing patients settle easily into a nursing home, others are more vulnerable and become confused or develop what sometimes turn out to be terminal chest infections.

Depression and the affective disorders

These consist of the manic–depressive illnesses and are associated with dysfunction in the patient's emotional state. Depression is the commonest feature and is important because there is a tendency for the depressed patient not to seek medical help and for the doctor not to recognise it at consultation (Freeling *et al*, 1983). It is difficult to get an accurate idea of the prevalence of depression among the elderly, but the 1977 Age Concern study (Abrams, 1987) of a large sample of men and women of 75 years or more living in their homes showed that 14% had long spells of depression. The scores for men and women were similar, but the proportion of high depression scores among those living alone greatly exceeded those of people not living alone.

Clinically, depression in the elderly may present in many different ways. Classically a patient has a weary air of overall depression, and there is a marked degree of apathy. The mood change may not, however, be apparent, and the patient may present principally with physical problems – headache, chest pains, fatigue, and poor appetite. The word 'depression' is rarely used, and phrases like 'emptiness'; 'nothing to live for'; 'life's getting on top of me' are frequently used. Sometimes these feelings are attributed to old age itself, which results in a resigned acceptance that nothing can be done. Relatives and professional workers sometimes collude with these sentiments. The stigma of mental illness is still felt among old people, and they prefer to have physical explanations for their symptoms.

Clues to the presence of depression include a recent deterioration in abilities to undertake the various activities of daily living (Williams, 1986), recent bereavement (see Chapter 7), or a change in environment. Other physical illness may be contributing and, as indicated earlier, depression and dementia may sometimes be present together. A possibility of depression must always be there if a patient complains of guilt, worthlessness, or despair – especially in an old person ruminating about events in the past. These feelings can sometimes be dismissed with an air of false jocularity which belies the true feelings. It is also important to realise that anxiety is commonly associated with depression. A past history or family history of depression, including a suicidal attempt, may be present. Suicides are not uncommon among old people, and the threat of such action must be taken seriously.

Hypochondriasis is a common feature of depressive illness in old age. Old people also have genuine multiple pathology.

The general spectrum of depressive disease seen in the community ranges from the mild to the very severe, and this is also true in old age. Most mild to moderate depressions respond to the usual antidepressant drugs, with care about the dosage. Most severe depression may need electroconvulsive therapy and psychiatric help.

The manic phase of the illness occurs less commonly, but when it does the patients are difficult to help. They are hyperexcited and agitated, often impressed by their own importance, and undertake outrageous and expensive activities. Compulsory admission to hospital may be necesary in these situations.

Behavioural disorders, personality disorders, and psychoneurosis

The GP sees a wide variety of non-psychotic mental illness. This is true of all age groups, but is particularly so when working with old people. Some are unique to old age, and some are exaggerations of earlier personality trends which become abnormal. Some are bizarre and poorly understood and are likely to have underlying mental pathology. An example of this is an interesting condition sometimes referred to as *paraphrenia*.

Patients with paraphrenia, usually women, present in old age with symptoms which are predominantly paranoid. This exhibits itself most commonly as a feeling of being watched or persecuted in some way. The patient is usually unmarried and suffering also from problems with hearing or vision. The patient might have had a degree of paranoia throughout life, but in old age develops delusions, particularly about neighbours, whom they see as a threat. Others develop fantasies about sex and imagine that they are being watched while undressing and also have worries about being molested.

Anxiety is common in old age. The patients present with agitation and the usual physical symptoms (see Chapter 6). There are often predisposing circumstances such as financial or family worries. Harassment may be a problem, and old people living alone may be easily upset by the uncalled for attention of certain neighbours. Particularly unpleasant cases occur where old women are attacked and raped.

Personality problems and eccentricities are common in old age and may be developments of earlier tendencies: awkwardness, miserliness, bad temper, and stubborness are all common among old people. Dislike of a person or relative may take on a more sinister aspect as age advances. Hidden jealousies or resentments come to the surface. The effect is that the old person loses friends and with them support systems. At the extreme, the old person becomes a hermit – quite unapproachable and difficult to help.

Institutional neurosis is thought mainly to apply to patients in hospital, but it can equally well apply to people confined to their own home. Apathy and loss of initiative ensues.

Old people rarely consult about *sexual problems*, although this is changing as many old people now expect to remain active sexually. The family might, however, consult about aberrant sexual behaviour. This usually involves an old man suddenly developing a preoccupation with sex, and this may produce difficulties for female relatives and helpers. Sometimes indecent exposure is a problem, and occasionally indecent assaults on children occur. A sexual problem may manifest itself in quite unrealistic jealousies and can result in physical violence.

Alcoholism is seen in old age, and this may be a feature of anxiety state or depression. There is often tell-tale evidence of large numbers of empty bottles around the house and in dustbins.

Obsessive neurosis is not uncommon in old age; cleanliness, position of furniture, timing of meals, the amount of sleep taken, regular bowel habits, needing to sit in a particular armchair, can dominate out of all proportion. Obsessive collecting (of objects or magazines, etc.) can result in chaos.

Hypochondriasis occurs, as does denial. The hypochondriac pays frequent visits to the doctor with a variety of symptoms, and usually has an underlying fear of cancer; little can be done to convince that there is no serious illness. More commonly perhaps is denial, where patients refuse to accept the real nature of symptoms which they attribute to 'old age' and therefore do not consult.

Preventive aspects

The contract for general practice introduced in April 1990 includes provision for health checks for patients aged 75 and over. These checks are mandatory and are to be undertaken yearly. Their purpose is early recognition of problems, with the aim of improving or preserving functional ability. Included in these checks is mental assessment. As they have evolved in practice, the checks have turned out to have three stages: problem identification; further assessment and management in primary care; and full assessment, which usually means using secondary-care facilities. At stage 1, problem identification is undertaken, often in the patient's home, by either a GP or more usually a practice nurse. The mental assessment is largely concerned with identifying early dementia and depression. To decide on the instruments which will do this effectively and not take too long to administer has needed careful thought. The contract offered no guidelines, and the profession was left to construct the protocols.

Each general practice team at the end of the day has needed to make its own arrangements. The Royal College of General Practitioners has, however, offered guidelines, and these are published as an Occasional Paper (Williams & Wallace, 1993). The initial mental assessment can be limited to a few questions which alert the interviewer to the possibility of mental problems (see Appendix) and these questions can be followed up by more detailed tests. Those recommended are the Abbreviated Mental Test (for identifying dementia) and the Geriatric Depression Scale (for identifying depression) (see Appendix). Both are standardised, relatively easy to administer, and validated. Ideally they should be used on all patients who receive a health check. These schedules should, however, always be used with common sense and alongside clinical findings.

Preliminary studies show that about 8% of new problems identified at health check are concerned with mental health (Brown *et al*, 1992). Most of these problems are dealt with by primary care workers. The health checks of the elderly have turned out to be controversial, although they have been better accepted than other forms of health promotion. The health benefit of such activities has not been fully demonstrated. Early research was concerned largely with assessing the effect of screening on the prevention and cure of disease, and not with improvement in ability to undertake activities of daily living and in the quality of life.

It would be wrong however to consider that yearly health checks were the limit of a preventive approach. The opportunity provided by the regular contact a GP has with old patients (Williams, 1983) and within the consultation itself (Stott & Davis, 1979) allow for an eye to be kept on developments or deteriorations of known illness. Good acute care is good preventive care. Early detection of a decline in mental health can be observed in diminishing ability to undertake activities of daily living. If the problem is depression, prompt treatment can be effective; if dementia, early knowledge of the condition can at least alert the carers and health team to future difficulties. Stroke and Parkinson's disease are common in the elderly, and depression is associated with both conditions; its presence can diminish the chances of successful rehabilitation. Early treatment of physical conditions may reduce the possibility of depression.

In old age there is a close link between physical disability and depression. This needs to be identified and both need treating. Patients' perceptions of a disability are in some cases more important to note than objective ratings. Pain from arthritis leading to poor mobility and isolation can often lead to depression. Dealing with each may prevent or ameliorate that depression. A confiding relationship in old age is important in avoiding depression.

Finally, activity seems to be good for both physical and mental health, and should be encouraged.

The law and vulnerable old people

Mental incapacity in old age brings with it the need for both legal protection and representation. Recently legislation has helped to make arrangements for these easier. Power of attorney (see also Chapter 4) enables a person to give authority to another, or others, to act on his/her behalf. It is needed particularly when the infirmity is physical and where the person has full mental capacity. The Enduring Powers of Attorney Act 1985 provides that a power of attorney does not expire when the donor of the power becomes mentally incapable. This is the form which is now most usually used and is reasonably simple to execute. The attorney appointed can be either an individual or two persons jointly. They are chosen by the donor and can be given full authority, or authority limited to certain things. If the donor becomes mentally incapacitated, the power is registered at that point with the Court of Protection (Chapter 4). When an enduring power of attorney is not in existence when an old person becomes mentally incapable of managing his/her affairs, it is necessary to go to the Court of Protection which exists to safeguard the elderly person's interests. The Court's responsibility is for financial matters. Evidence is needed from the appropriate medical practitioner before the person is registered and thereafter all the affairs of that person are placed under the supervision of the Court, usually through a person known as the receiver, who may be a close relative or professional adviser of the old person. Normally an order is made for regular payments to be made to the donor, but disposal of assets such as a house or investments will need the specific sanction of the Court.

Caring in the community

There have in recent times been many changes in the way that care has been offered to psychiatrically ill old persons, although nationally the developments have been patchy. Important has been the growth of old-age psychiatry, the development of a community psychiatric nurse service, the increased importance of shared care owing to the closure of mental hospitals and long-stay beds, and the changes resulting from new NHS legislation.

There are some causes for concern, both organisational and clinical. The transfer of psychiatrically ill old patients needing continuing care from the hospital to the community has not been properly planned. The rapid growth in the number of nursing homes has meant that long-term medical care for mentally disturbed old people has been shifted from the consultant to the GP – without necessarily ensuring that skills and resources exist. The rapidly changing scene in the community – with contract setting, budget-holding practices, trust-status community units – has changed the balance of responsibility between hospital and primary care. Lines of responsibility and accountability need defining. Communication channels need to be clarified and decisions taken about, for instance, prescribing and clinical responsibility. Contracts will need to address: day-to-day management, pathways for consultation, management of emergencies, access to community psychiatric nurses, considerations of best place of management, joint assessments, discharge procedures, and protocols for shared care. The principle of shared care is important, and a team approach is vital.

The community has a wide network of help available. This starts with the patient's carers, who themselves require support, and includes a large number of professional workers. Old people with psychiatric problems often also have physical problems, and so the help of community nurses, physiotherapists, speech therapists, and occupational therapists is invaluable. More attention is being paid now to environmental and financial aspects. The new arrangements in the community following the '*Caring of People*' legislation (The National Health Service and Community Care Act 1990), which comes into effect in 1993, will involve the social service departments of local authorities more closely with the care of the mentally ill. Health services will need to liaise with providers of social care in planning support for both the clients and carers. Acute social crises are common among mentally ill old persons, and there will need to be close cooperation between the services when providing acute care to deal with these aspects. Joint education and evaluation of services will be essential if these new arrangements are to succeed.

Appendix

Test of mental function

From Williams & Wallace (1992):

1. Do you feel sad, depressed or miserable?	Yes*
2. Do you have problems with your everyday memory?	Yes*
Does the elderly person's attitude or behaviour suggest agitation, depression or mental impairment?	Yes*

*Further mental assessment indicated.

Abbreviated Mental Test Scale (AMTS)

From Hodkinson (1972).

May I ask you some routine questions to gauge your memory?

What is your age?
What is the time (to nearest hour)?
  Please remember this address (for example): '42 West Street'
What year is it?
What is your home address?
Who are these two people? (Photographs of Pope and Queen)
What is the date of your birth?
What year did the First World War start?
What is the name of the present monarch?
Please count backwards from 20 to 1.
Please repeat the address I asked you to remember.

Score 1 *only* for each correct answer.
Score 0–3 severe impairment
      4–6 moderate impairment
      >6 normal.

Geriatric Depression Scale (15 questions)

Sheik & Yesavage (1986).

Are you basically satisfied with your life?	yes/NO
Have you dropped many of your activities and interests?	YES/no
Do you feel that your life is empty?	YES/no
Do you often get bored?	YES/no
Are you in good spirits most of the time?	yes/NO
Are you afraid that something bad is going to happen to you?	YES/no
Do you feel happy most of the time?	yes/NO
Do you often feel helpless?	YES/no
Do you prefer to stay at home, rather than going out and doing new things?	YES/no
Do you feel you have more problems with memory than most?	YES/no
Do you think it is wonderful to be alive now?	yes/NO
Do you feel pretty worthless the way you are now?	YES/no
Do you feel full of energy?	yes/NO
Do you feel that your situation is hopeless?	YES/no
Do you think that most people are better off than you are?	YES/no

For each answer in capitals, score 1.
Score: >5 indicates probable depression.

References

ABRAMS, M. (1987) *Beyond Three-Score and Ten*. Research Unit, Age Concern Publications, Mitcham, Surrey.

BIRREN, J. E. & RENNER, V. J. (1981) Concepts and criteria of mental health and ageing. *Orthopsychiatry*, **51**, 242–254.

BROWN, K. P. H., WILLIAMS, E. I. & GROOM, L. (1992) Health checks on patients 75 years and over in Nottinghamshire after the new GP contract. *British Medical Journal*, **305**, 619–621.

CLARKE, M. E. (1984) Problems of the elderly: an epidemiological perspective. *Journal of the Royal College of General Practitioners*, **18**, 128.

DEPARTMENT OF HEALTH AND SOCIAL SECURITY (1981) *Growing Older*, cmnd 8173. London: HMSO.

FREELING, P., RAO, B. M., PAYKEL, E. S., *et al* (1983) Unrecognised depression in general practice. *British Medical Journal*, **290**, 1880–1883.

HODGSON, S. P. & JOLLEY, D. J. (1985) Psychiatry of the elderly. In *Principles and Practice of Geriatric Medicine* (ed. M. S. J. Pathy). Chichester: Wiley.

HODKINSON, H. M. (1972) Evaluation of a mental test score for assessment of mental impairment in the elderly. *Age and Ageing*, **1**, 233–238.

LISHMAN, W. A. (1978) *Organic Psychiatry*. Oxford: Blackwell Scientific.

MARTIN, J., MELTZER, H. & ELLIOT, D. (1988) *The Prevalence of Disability Among Adults. OPCS Surveys of Disability in Great Britain, Report 1*. London: HMSO.

NIELSON, J. (1962) Geronto-psychiatric period prevalence investigation in a geographically delimited population. *Acta Psychiatrica Scandinavica*, **38**, 307.

OFFICE OF POPULATION CENSUSES AND SURVEYS (1984) *General Household Survey 1982*. London: HMSO.

SHEIK, J. I. & YESAVAGE, J. A. (1986) Geriatric Depression Scale (GDS): Recent evidence and development of a shorter version. In *Clinical Gerontology. A guide to Assessment and Intervention* (ed. T. L. Brink). New York: Haworth Press.

STOTT, N. & DAVIS, R. H. (1978) The exceptional potential in each primary care consultation. *Journal of the Royal College of General Practitioners*, **29**, 201–205.

WILKIN, D. & WILLIAMS, E. I. (1986) Patterns of care for the elderly in general practice. *Journal of the Royal College of General Practitioners*, **36**, 567–570.

WILLIAMS, E. I. (1983) The general practitioner and the disabled. *Journal of the Royal College of General Practitioners*, **33**, 296–299.

—— (1986) A model to describe social performance levels in elderly people. *Journal of the Royal College of General Practitioners*, **36**, 422–423.

—— (1988) Crisis managment of acute confusions. *MIMS Magazine – The Journal of Prescribing and Therapeutics* (1 March), 87–93.

—— & WALLACE, P. (1992) *Health Checks for People Aged 75 and Over*, Occasional Paper 59. London: Royal College of General Practictioners.

——, SAVAGE, S. McDONALD, P. S. *et al* (1992) Residents of private nursing homes and their care. *British Journal of General Practice*, **42**, 477–481.

11 Emergencies, crises and violence

RICHARD WESTCOTT

Psychiatric emergencies defined

What is a psychiatric emergency? A medical definition – a situation "in which, on account of his or her abnormal mental state or behaviour, the life of a patient, or someone else, is in jeopardy" (Berrios, 1982) – which excludes lesser, non-life-threatening crises is obviously inadequate. But the working GP, influenced by daily exposure to the word 'emergency' which is regularly used to gain immediate attention, bypassing appointment systems, receptionists, and other barriers to the doctor – and who may even have contributed to the further erosion of the word him/herself by, for example, designating Saturday morning surgeries as 'Emergency Only' – might have and transmit a quite different concept of 'emergency'. As for the patient – the word can mean anything from 'the acute which cannot be put off to the next day' through 'a matter of urgency' to the 'critically overwhelming', via the 'increasingly intolerable': a wide spectrum indeed, but one which we might well adopt, since emergencies and crises are (at least initially) defined by patients.

Perhaps therefore a good definition of a psychiatric crisis is that it represents a situation in which the demands exceed a person's ability to cope (Markus *et al*, 1989). At its worst then, it is pandemonium – the wild, unrestrained uproar of a tumultuous assembly – frightening to all concerned, especially the summoned. But a crisis can be a turning point in the progress of anything, a state of affairs in which a definitive change for better or worse is imminent: it can represent a point at which some action, property, or condition passes over into another. Hippocrates interpreted these ebbs and flows as tidal, with the crisis – the point of decision and judgement – the moment when the physician could determine which way the disorder was going.

Such archaic remarks are not deliberately wayward. This chapter has something to say about time and tide; the inadequacy of present definitions and classifications; teaching, growth and development and support – we may yet learn about psychiatric emergencies by bearing in mind some Hippocratic concepts. Specifically, having considered some definitions of psychiatric emergencies, I shall deal with their classification and their management – in both the immediate and longer terms – including problems associated with compulsory admission. The use of the whole primary care team is described, with an emphasis on the GP's approach – a responsible and deliberate use of time, an encouragement of development, growth and autonomy, and an awareness of the importance of feelings (not least in the helpers) – factors which have been, for most of us, only minimally addressed in our medical education.

The classification of psychiatric emergencies

While psychological disorders are one of the most common reasons for consultation in general practice, their classification in general, and that of psychological emergencies in particular, remains a problem for all concerned, with psychiatric diagnosis remaining at the descriptive or syndromal level.

A study using 27 experienced GPs showed that even with specific instruction in the use of the World Health Organization's *International Classification of Diseases* and the *International Classification of Health Problems* (adapted for primary care physicians), the GPs tended to use an idiosyncratic, multidimensional framework, finding the existing schemes inadequate or unsuitable (Shepherd, 1991).

Of the four ways in which GPs classify, the use of the traditional diagnosis is probably the least common. The problems which constitute the majority of mental problems in primary care – psychosomatic conditions, organic disorder with associated emotional distress, and psychosocial problems – are indeed poorly served by traditional diagnostic systems (Sharp & King, 1989). The other three possibilities are to classify on the basis of loose aggregates of symptoms, to use a problem-orientated approach to rationalise management decisions, or to proceed directly from symptoms to treatment and then if necessary place a diagnostic label on afterwards.

With such a background it is not surprising that conventional classifications are of only limited help. Another scheme, Frank's (summarised by McGrath & Bowker, 1987) looks more promising, with its four main categories: patients with psychotic illness, those with neurotic illness, those who are 'psychologically shaken', and those who are 'unruly'. But there are curiosities, such as the placing of severe depression, delirium, dementia and even severe anorexia in the first group, so perhaps understandably this system too has not been widely adopted.

The GP therefore takes a pragmatic approach to psychiatric emergencies. Rather than considering whether the emergency is, for example, organic, functional, or social, the GP will more likely take a personalised, practical management approach. The questions are immediate and action-orientated (befitting an emergency), as follows:

> What is the simplest and easiest way I can cope with this crisis so that it stops being an emergency?
>
> Will listening on the telephone now to the patient (or to someone else) be enough to calm the anxieties?
>
> Can a talk on the telephone now, followed by contact later, settle the crisis?
>
> Do I know this person well enough to be able to make some recommendations about starting, stopping or altering treatment which might allay the present problem?
>
> Should I offer an appointment? At an early opportunity? Or right away?
>
> Is a visit required?
>
> If so, can it wait until the present task is completed or must it be done immediately?
>
> Can some other member of the primary care team help me with this emergency?
>
> Might the patient need admission?
>
> If so, might it be compulsory?
>
> Does a social worker need to be involved?
>
> Is it an overdose?
>
> If so, is it substantial, potentially serious, gestural only – or unclear?
>
> Would it be best to get on and arrange the urgent admission to hospital here and now, with the appropriate telephone calls?
>
> Can I call on any other person (e.g. neighbours, relatives, community psychiatric nurse) or organisation (police, psychiatric day hospital, etc.) to help with this emergency?

Such is, in reality, the 'classification' of the GP.

It is important to be honest: neither the inadequacy of our inherited classification systems – which are not owned by primary care – nor our preference for a management-orientated rather than a quasi-scientific approach need be a cause for embarrassment. Perhaps a clear description of what actually happens in practice can enable the construction of better frameworks, as well as encouraging more openness in other areas, where there may be discrepancies between theory and reality, teaching and practice. Once again, the GP can feel let down by his/her medical education.

The management of psychiatric emergencies

The immediate crisis

This is best addressed by continuing to pursue the pragmatic classification, using the acute management approach as described above, with some reflections later on the chronic, ongoing, and more preventive-orientated aspects of management.

Collecting information – 'taking a history' as we are taught – remains the first task. A fuller description helps the first questions to be answered, whether the informer is the patient or not, as well as enabling the doctor to enter the scene, if only figuratively. We all well know how reassuring it can be to be able to describe and explain what is going on (or has happened) when we or others are upset, to an attentive listener – the more so if that person is respected, authoritative, or in a position to do something. Even speaking on the telephone can satisfy this need. I continue to be surprised at the number of times such a simple service succeeds in defusing an apparent crisis, whether it be pandemonium or a family tiff.

Sometimes a visit seems necessary anyway, but the knowledge that help is on its way, or the actual presence rather than the ear of the doctor, can help. Most GPs will have had the experience of rushing to an apparently desperate patient only to find him sleeping soundly in bed (Holmes, 1990).

Having assessed the information, the GP has to make a decision about appointments, visits – and urgency. Urgency is above all the pressure of time: time is crucial when considering emergencies and crises. "Have I got time to finish what I am doing, how much time should I give now, can I take my time, how many times has this happened before or is it the first time, above all how can I make the time? . . ." It is in the use of time that the doctor's skill in managing the crisis emerges.

A critical decision is whether admission is a possibility. There are certain categories of patients who will probably need admission: those with a first psychotic episode, those in whom an organic psychosis is suspected, patients who are dangerous (either to themselves or others), and unstable patients who are poorly supported or likely to show poor compliance (Holmes, 1990). Suicidal and most parasuicidal patients are covered in these categories, but there may be some parasuicidal patients who do not need admission.

Although one study showed a fourfold increase in parasuicide between 1962 and 1972, it has now levelled out (Markus *et al*, 1989). The associated factors are well documented – poor social conditions (including high unemployment locally, a large family, early parental death, and a criminal or antisocial record) with a disturbed relationship with a key individual (a recent quarrel perhaps) – producing an impulsive act in two-thirds of cases. As this proportion will have recently visited their GP and one-third will be receiving treatment from him/her for a physical disease, many if not most will be known to them. Depending therefore on the seriousness of the gesture (in terms of the amount of agent taken and the possibility of repetition), against the background of supportive influence the GP can bring to bear, the GP may or may not admit the patient. As ever, good assessment is the key to management. This helps to define those at risk of further attempts and those needing formal psychiatric treatment, and determines the strategy for further management (Markus, 1989).

On the other hand, sometimes the GP will need to request admission when it may be hard for the receiving team, separated from the patient's situation, to understand the reason. Admissions and referrals were ever thus – fortunately our hospital colleagues recognise this: "To psychiatrists used to dealing with acute distress a problem might not seem urgent, but urgent referrals indicate anxiety in those trying to help the patient. It is best to respond rapidly to such anxiety" (McGrath & Bowker, 1987).

Admission raises the question of compulsory admission. If the GP suffers in an emergency from decisions about and the pressures of time, then how much more he/she will feel anxious concerning this decision – possibly quite stressful, not least in terms of the time required. If compulsory admission seems probable, time will be well spent making preparations before the visit is made – with the GP's own receptionist helping track down the approved social worker, duty section 12 psychiatrist, on-call senior house officer and the ambulance, as well as perhaps the police. Such an agenda is more easily accomplished in the relative peace of one's own territory than in the additionally difficult environment of the emergency itself.

If there is time to make the right arrangements, the GP can enter the house with the others nearby but out of sight, introduce the appropriate colleagues, and matters can then proceed relatively smoothly, with the GP feeling supported. However, there are times when such emergencies become crises for more than just the patient, the family and neighbours: unsupportive, unavailable or just unpunctual colleagues can leave the GP dangerously isolated, undermine his/her confidence, and create a situation where demands threaten to exceed a person's ability to cope.

Guidelines for compulsory admission are summarised in Fig. 11.1. In short, patients can be admitted to hospital under a section of the Mental Health Act if they are a danger to themselves or others, or if their health is likely to deteriorate if left untreated (see Chapter 4).

The management of potentially violent patients may be mentioned here. Although only relatively few incidents of dangerous behaviour are likely to be caused by mental illness, it is important to know how to cope with dangerous behaviour, not least since this ability will increase confidence and reduce the doctor's stress. Violence can come from those seeking drugs, the intoxicated, the angry, or the mentally ill, or a combination of all or some of these categories (Bradley, 1989). Anticipation of dangerous behaviour and appropriate preventive action can reduce the risk of harm. Youth, male sex, alcohol and drugs are classic predictors. Of mental illnesses schizophrenia is a relatively uncommon cause of violence, although hallucinations and delusions can provoke a motiveless attack. In the affective disorders, mania can lead to brawls, and the organic psychoses can cause violence too.

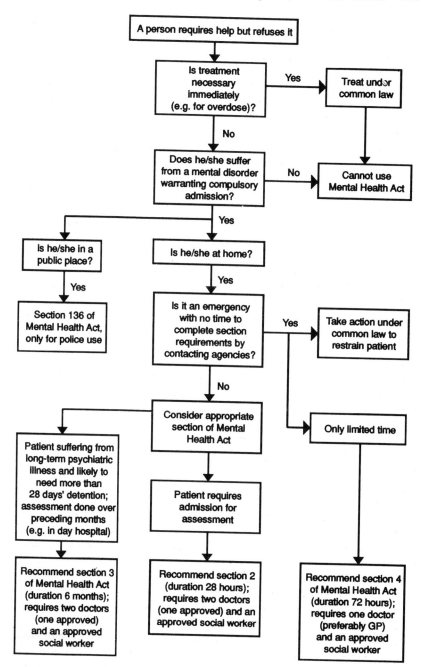

Fig. 11.1. Guidelines for compulsory admission (adapted from Holmes, 1990)

A courteous, quiet, friendly approach is recommended, with attentiveness and common-sense care concerning position: the doctor should be able to leave the room easily and summon help. In the presence of weapons, we are advised to make no attempt to restrain or disarm but to talk calmly, to maintain only intermittent eye contact, and to make no sudden movements (Bradley, 1989). Another suggestion is for the doctor to sit on a chair with the back facing the patient, so that on the rare occasions a paranoid or psychotic patient attacks, the chair can be used as a shield (Holmes, 1990). It is permissible under common law to restrain and administer sedation: haloperidol (5–10 mg) or chlorpromazine (100–150 mg) intramuscularly would be suitable (Bradley, 1989). Happily, such measures are rarely needed. The great majority of psychiatric emergencies being psychosocial problems, emotional distress associated with an organic disorder, or psychosomatic conditions, the GP can proceed with his/her practical approach based as it is on essential GP skills.

Patients present as emergencies because of acute, distressing and destabilising changes, and the initial response must be towards stabilisation of the patient and the situation (McGrath & Bowker, 1987). Assessment – already taking place, as described – enables clarification, as well as being therapeutic in its own right by encouraging patients to express their feelings. This leads naturally to discussion, negotiation, and agreement on further action, along the well-known lines of the various models of the consultation (Pendleton *et al*, 1984). For although this occasion may be a crisis, the contribution of the GP is no more and no less than the bringing to bear of his/her traditional skills, never more needed and never more appreciated than in a psychiatric emergency.

A crisis-intervention technique can be useful when dealing with parasuicide, other abnormal behavioural responses to social crises, severe or inappropriate responses to acute stress such as bereavement, and other socially disrupted patients (McGrath & Bowker, 1987). It also represents an aspiration of GPs: to help patients define and take control of the crisis, working with their strengths to renew their feelings of competence and mastery. The GP brings a structured, empathic, problem-solving approach which enables the patient to identify the problem, propose alternative solutions, consider the implications of the alternatives, make a choice, define the steps required, implement the decision, and check its result.

Of course, some patients can be especially difficult. Every GP has some multiproblem families who go from crisis to crisis with perhaps intractable mental illness, personality disorders, or life circumstances that are apparently irremediable, leaving them vulnerable to life events that most people would take in their stride (Markus, 1989). But even – especially – here, these principles hold good – their crisis is an acute failure of normal coping which needs to be understood, and they above all need to be helped to choose and develop better solutions.

Longer-term management

The paradox of longer-term management of psychiatric emergencies is resolved by looking at crisis-intervention techniques: while they represent a suitable acute approach, they also produce an ongoing agenda. It may well be that the first, vital stage of trying to understand what it feels like to be that person at that moment will take a lot of time – much more than the initial crisis meeting. Such a task is hard enough in the best of circumstances (which a psychiatric crisis certainly is not): how much more difficult then when coping mechanisms have broken down and powerful emotions are released. But a start will have been made and further plans will follow.

At this stage the GP may call upon other members of the team. The health visitor is in contact with many of the more vulnerable people whose psychosocial problems make up a large part of the workload: 'mental health care' was discussed in nearly 20% and 'social care' in another 25% of their visits (Clark, 1973). Significant psychosocial factors are present in about half the consultations concerning children (Royal College of General Practitioners, 1981). With their attachment to primary care teams and their acceptance by their communities, they represent an important source of help for people with emotional and psychological problems, who may find it difficult to ask for help. The routine care they offer not just to mothers and children, but also to the disadvantaged, provides an ongoing relationship which the GP can use for the longer-term management of breakdown in coping ability.

The same applies to the practice nurse, the midwife, and the district nurse, to whom the GP may appropriately turn for help. If the team incorporates a community psychiatric nurse the GP will undoubtedly call upon him/her. The team may even be fortunate enough to include a counsellor or the services of a clinical psychologist, well equipped to promote adaptive coping skills (Milne & Souter, 1988). These team members have special skills and understanding of problems – be they physical, psychosomatic, or psychological – associated with times of life change. And attention to these sensitive periods can help prevent crises.

The well functioning primary care team will, if unable to predict psychiatric emergencies, at least be able to place the many that are psychosocial transitional crises in a context of education, anticipation, crisis intervention, and therapy; to work within a logical framework with its own structure – its own time and tide (Fig. 11.2).

Education can inform people about the nature of the changes that may be expected and how they can be coped with – patients who enter any critical transition with knowledge of what it might involve are naturally better able to cope; anticipation can give guidance to those approaching a crisis. The crisis itself passes with whatever help the GP and team can give (Markus *et al*, 1989). It is at these sensitive periods that the behaviour of individuals

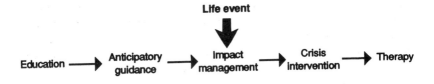

Fig. 11.2. The long-term management of psychiatric emergencies

and families can take on a new form (Royal College of General Practitioners, 1981) – ''The GP has a role in ensuring that changes that do occur during these sensitive periods allow as far as possible for subsequent healthy development and adaptation.''

Another resource available within the practice is the skills and goodwill of patients themselves. Groups – mutual support, educational or therapeutic – can be set up or, more simply, the experiences of individuals ('veterans' who have survived) can be used.

In summary, the GP will try to structure continuing care so that developments can take place at the right time, growing naturally in their own time. He/she will work with the grain of events, sensitive to the natural currents, and using the tide.

Conclusions

The management of psychiatric emergencies is the re-creation of security: the unbalancing of the patient's homeostasis has to be restored, and the doctor's confidence, which, starting in him/herself, is extended to include the patient. This begins the process of re-establishment of significance and order. From this re-alignment arise opportunities for improvement and greater self-reliance in coping with challenges. This statement applies to both doctor and patient.

As always, when dealing with the printed word rather than the action, it can all sound so simple. But the responsibility is great if indeed ''the GP now plays a vital role in providing the psychological containment and expertise that was formerly the provenance of the mental hospital'' (Holmes, 1990). Carrying such a potentially heavy emotional burden means that there is a longer-term management need for the GP – and the team – as well as for the patient. After the crisis, ''the GP should not feel ashamed or embarrassed by a need to 'offload' or debrief himself with the help of a spouse, partner or support group'' (Holmes, 1990). Here there may well be a special role for the team to help itself and thereby the others it purports to help.

There is fortunately a greater awareness now of such needs, which has of itself happily contributed to better patient care: if we can begin to talk about our own emotions, thus recognising them and attributing importance to them, learn how each other feels and thus improve our listening skills and give support and understanding to each other – then we shall be practising on ourselves the prevention which we are increasingly expected to preach (Holmes, 1990). And in such mutual caring we can all find growth and development.

"A well-handled psychiatric crisis can be very rewarding, creating the special bond between patient, family and GP that comes from adversity overcome, and providing an opportunity for learning and change" (Holmes, 1990). Such an experience reminds us of the paradoxical synchrony of continuity and change – Hippocrates' tide perhaps – and underlines the centrality of relationships, with their understanding, communicating and sharing (Button, 1988), so crucial to the management of psychiatric emergencies in particular, and to general practice in general.

References

BERRIOS, G. E. (1982) Psychiatric emergencies. *Hospital Update* (March), 303–313.

BRADLEY, J. J. (1989) Coping with dangerous patients. *Update* (1 March), 520–526.

BUTTON, E. (1988) *Psychological Problems in Primary Health Care*. London: Croom Helm.

CLARK, J. (1973) *A Family Visitor: A Descriptive Analysis of Health Visiting in Berkshire*. London: Royal College of Nursing and National Council of Nurses of the United Kingdom.

HOLMES, J. (1990) Psychiatric night calls. *Practitioner*, **234**, 772–775.

MARKUS, A. C., MURRAY PARKES, C., TOMSON, P., *et al* (1989) *Psychological Problems in General Practice*. Oxford: Oxford University Press.

McGRATH, G. & BOWKER, M. (1987) *Common Psychiatric Emergencies*. Bristol: Wright.

MILNE, D. & SOUTER, K. (1988) A re-evaluation of the clinical psychologist in general practice. *Journal of the Royal College of General Practitioners*, **38** 457–460.

ROYAL COLLEGE OF GENERAL PRACTITIONERS (1981) *Report from General Practice 20: Prevention of Psychiatric Disorders in General Practice*. London: Royal College of General Practitioners.

SHARP, D. J. & KING, M. B. (1989) Classification of psychosocial disturbance in general practice. *Journal of the Royal College of General Practitioners*, **39**, 356–358.

SHEPHERD, M. (1991) Primary care psychiatry: the case for action. *British Journal of General Practice*, **41**, 252–255.

PENDLETON, D., SCHOFIELD, T., TATE, P., *et al* (1984) *The Consultation: An Approach to Learning & Teaching*. Oxford: Oxford University Press.

12 Personality problems

PETER TYRER

In all clinical practice, the most worrying personality disorders are those that present with hostility, both verbal and physical. However, it would be wrong to assume that those psychiatric patients who manifest violent propensities are necessarily personality disordered, or, conversely, to assume that those who are passive and compliant at all times are free from personality disturbance.

In this chapter, therefore, a general outline of the main features of personality disorder, its classification, and recognition in clinical practice are first described, followed by a simple identification procedure. This is followed by a discussion of practical steps to be taken to both anticipate problems associated with personality disorder and different lines of management. All these are looked at primarily from the standpoint of primary care.

Initial assessment

Once a patient has been identified as having a personality disorder (or at least suspected of having one) the GP is put in a difficult position. Many studies have been carried out that show that patients with personality disorder, particularly those in the flamboyant group, require much more help from services and make many more demands than those with no personality disorder. In the present economic climate, in which hospitals and general practices have to be run using business methods, the simplest way of dealing with such patients would be to cross them off the practice list. I personally would consider this unethical, but it is certainly legal and economically justifiable. It could also be argued that a patient with a primary personality disorder, and having no other medical or psychiatric pathology, does not, at least in our current state of knowledge, require general practice care for the disorder, because no general practice input has been shown to be successful.

However, personality disorder is often associated with physical illness, and concurrent mental illness is particularly common. The question of whether an individual has a personality disorder or not is not the most pressing initial question for the GP, and it is usually only when management and involvement in care for another disorder are well under way that the possibility of personality disorder is entertained. Early diagnosis is therefore desirable.

Diagnosis of personality disorder

One of the major problems with the use of the term 'personality disorder', or even 'personality problems', is that, until recently, there was considerable confusion and argument over what the label actually meant. For many (e.g. Blackburn, 1988; Lewis & Appleby, 1988) the diagnosis is still a pejorative one which criticises the patient primarily and tells more about the relationship between the diagnoser and the diagnosed than the particular condition in question. However, this view is changing because there is considerable evidence that personality disorder can be diagnosed reliably, and that the attribution of the diagnosis is an excellent predictor of many important aspects of care. Nevertheless, we are only at the bottom rung of the diagnostic ladder; there is still a great deal of argument over issues such as the dividing line between normal and abnormal personality, and between the different categories used in the standard classifications.

Personality is unique, but personality disorder is to some extent stereotyped. People with personality disorders show persistent abnormalities of behaviour and in their relationship with others. There are some (e.g. Rutter, 1987) who maintain that there is insufficient reason to distinguish more than one category of personality disorder from the range of normal personality, as the overlap between them is so great and the fundamental characteristics mentioned above apply to all, but the formal classification (Table 12.1) adopts quite a different position. The 10th revision of the *International Classification of Disease* (ICD–10) (World Health Organization, 1992) and the American classification (DSM–III–R; American Psychiatric Association, 1987) are roughly comparable in identifying eight types of personality disorder, with no fundamental disagreement between them. These are: paranoid, schizoid, anankastic (obsessional), histrionic, dependent, antisocial (dissocial), anxious (avoidant), and borderline personality disorders. The other categories – narcissistic, impulsive, passive-aggressive, sadistic, and self defeating – are represented in only one classification. (Sadistic and self-defeating personality disorders are optional additions to DSM–III–R, and have been excluded from DSM–IV.)

There is little doubt that this classification is not particularly helpful to the working psychiatrist, and even less to the working GP. We are still at the stage of deciding whether certain aberrant types of behaviour are sufficiently distinct to be formulated as separate conditions. It is a reasonable hypothesis

TABLE 12.1
Comparison of current classifications of personality disorder

ICD-10[1]		DSM-III-R[2]	
Description	Code	Description	Code
Paranoid – excessive sensitivity, suspiciousness, preoccupation with conspiratorial explanation of events, with a persistent tendency to self-reference	F60.0	Paranoid – interpretation of people's actions as deliberately demanding or threatening	301.00
Schizoid – emotional coldness, detachment, lack of interest in other people, eccentricity and introspective fantasy	F60.1	Schizoid – indifference to relationships and restricted range of emotional experience and expression	301.20
No equivalent		Schizotypal – deficit in interpersonal relatedness with peculiarities of ideation, appearance and behaviour	302.22
Anankastic – indecisiveness, doubt, excessive caution, pedantry, rigidity and need to plan in immaculate detail	F60.5	Obsessive–compulsive – pervasive perfectionism and inflexibility	301.40
Histrionic – self-dramatisation, shallow mood, egocentricity and craving for excitement with persistent manipulative behaviour	F60.4	Histrionic – excessive emotion and attention-seeking	301.50
Dependent – failure to take responsibility for actions, with subordination of personal needs to those of others, excessive dependence with need for constant reassurance and feelings of helplessness when a close relationship ends	F60.7	Dependent – persistent dependent and submissive behaviour	301.60
Dissocial – callous unconcern for others, with irresponsibility, irritability and aggression, and incapacity to maintain enduring relationships	F60.2	Antisocial – evidence of repeated conduct disorder before the age of 15 years	301.70
No equivalent		Narcissistic – pervasive grandiosity, lack of empathy, and hypersensitivity to the evaluation of others	301.81
Anxious – persistent tension, self-consciousness, exaggeration of risks and dangers, hypersensitivity to rejection, and restricted lifestyle because of insecurity	F60.6	Avoidant – pervasive social discomfort, fear of negative evaluation and timidity	301.82
Impulsive – inability to control anger, to plan ahead, or to think before acts, with unpredictable mood and quarrelsome behaviour	F60.30[3]	Borderline – pervasive instability of mood, and self-image	301.83
Borderline – unclear self-image, involvement in intense and unstable relationships	F60.31[3]	Passive–aggressive – pervasive resistance to demands for adequate social and occupational performance	301.83

1. World Health Organization (1992).
2. American Psychiatric Association (1987).
3. Included under common heading of emotionally unstable personality disorder.

to consider many conditions initially, but the outcome of this sort of exercise is usually that several are telescoped together in the final analysis. Such information that is available suggests that this is already taking place in the case of the personality disorders. This is particularly true of severe personality disturbance.

Essentially, there are three main groups of personality disorder: the antisocial (also called dramatic, emotional, flamboyant, and erratic) group, which tends to have greater effect on society because the abnormal behaviour is antisocial in the broader sense; the withdrawn (sometimes called odd and eccentric) group, in which social isolation, withdrawal and suspiciousness are the main features; and the anxious, fearful group, in which timidity, nervousness, and emotional dependence are most prominent. It is common for the obsessional (anankastic) group of personality disorders to be included in this third group also. However, there is some evidence that this group can be separated from the others, and that hypochondrical and depressive personalities can be linked together with the obsessional one (Tyrer *et al*, 1990). From the point of view of the GP, this grouping of three or four types of personality disorder is of more value than discussing individual members of the groups. In the rest of this discussion, four main groups are described separately; identification and main features are illustrated in Table 12.2.

The reason for making this distinction is clear from the main features outlined in Table 12.2. The antisocial group of personality disorders is represented by the person who causes problems in GPs' surgeries by loudly demanding attention, often in an aggressive and threatening manner, is irritable and angry when thwarted, and who often changes dramatically from day to day and week to week. The withdrawn personalities attract attention by their oddness, although they do not seek the company of others. They have problems in communicating and are often highly suspicious, and this makes assessment of physical problems difficult in the GP's surgery. The dependent personalities may attend surgery frequently, but sometimes are too frightened to venture into what is considered alien territory. They are afraid of being criticised or rejected by others, and are excessively fearful of normal situations that rarely produce anxiety in other people. In an extreme form, such people need to be permanently accompanied by friends or relatives because they feel so insecure.

The last group includes many patients who attend the GP's surgery so frequently that they become 'fat-file' patients. They include people with chronic low-grade depression, which on assessment appears to have been present almost since birth, and also those who complain repeatedly about physical ailments that prove to have no physical basis. Although the notion of a hypochondriacal personality disorder is not accepted in the international classifications, it is only too well recognised by GPs, and as it is a long-term disorder, often beginning in late adolescence and persisting, it can just about be described as a personality disorder (Tyrer *et al*, 1990).

TABLE 12.2
A simplified summary of the main personality disorders

Main group of personality disorder	Individual members	Main features of individual members
Antisocial also called dramatic, emotional, flamboyant and erratic	Histrionic Antisocial Narcissistic[1] Borderline Impulsive	Self-dramatic Shallow mood Insensitivity Aggression Self-importance Lack of empathy Mood swings Identity disturbance Impulsiveness Irresponsibility
Withdrawn also called odd and eccentric	Paranoid Schizoid Schizotypal[1]	Hypersensitivity Suspiciousness Indifference Isolation Odd speech, thinking, and behaviour
Dependent also called anxious and fearful	Avoidant Dependent Passive–aggressive	Self-consciousness – fear of rejection Dependence on others – resourcelessness Procrastination – childish obstruction
Inhibited	Obsessional Hypochondriacal[2] Depressive (dysthymic)[2]	Rigidity Perfectionism Pedantry Health-conscious – disease fearing Pessimism Low self-esteem

1. These are included only in the American classification (DSM–III–R).
2. These are not included in either formal classification, but may be in the future.

The assessment of personality disorder is difficult. Although for many years simple questionnaires were popular – for example, the Maudsley Personality Inventory (MPI; Eysenck & Eysenck, 1969) and the Eysenck Personality Questionnaire (EPQ; Eysenck, 1959) – they do not identify personality disorder adequately. This is partly because patients with severe personality disorder tend to underplay, or even lie about, their personality status, but also because they genuinely do not realise the effect of their personality on others. The other problem is that in the presence of another mental state disorder, such as depression, personality scores on questionnaires are distorted and, once improvement has taken place, the personality apparently changes. In fact, personality is a relatively enduring attribute, and such a rapid change indicates that the questionnaire is, in effect, 'contaminated' by the presence of another mental state disorder.

For this reason, diagnostic interview schedules have been developed to reduce this effect. They include several that are primarily orientated towards the patient, of which the best known are the Structured Clinical Interview for Personality Disorders (SCID–II; Spitzer *et al*, 1987), the Structured Interview for DSM–III–R Personality Disorders (SID–P; Pfohl, 1982), and the Personality Disorder Examination (PDE; Loranger *et al*, 1985). Unfortunately, all of these take at least one hour and sometimes up to four hours to complete, and could not be considered in any general practice.

The two major schedules for interviewing informants (who can often give a more accurate picture of the effect of personality disorder on society) are the Personality Assessment Schedule (PAS; Tyrer & Alexander, 1979) and the Standardized Assessment of Personality (SAP; Mann *et al*, 1981). The SAP is the shorter of these and may only take 15 minutes to be scored completely. In this interview, a check-list of the important qualities of each personality disorder is shown to the informant and those that are positive are followed up with further questions.

However, even these instruments are probably unsuitable for use in general practice, and the author is at present developing a simple set of questions for GPs for the identification of personality disorder in those attending surgeries. This takes only a few minutes to complete but has not yet been fully standardised (copies available on request from the author if desired).

Treatment of personality disorder

Normally treatment and management are regarded as identical in clinical practice, but it is useful to regard them separately in the case of personality disorder. Treatment involves some active therapeutic principle that treats the underlying problem, either temporarily or permanently, and which has been shown in research studies to have specific therapeutic 'value' (as opposed to a placebo effect). Management, on the other hand, involves the day-to-day handling of a problem from the point of view of the service; it obviously can include treatment in the general sense, but also includes emergency action in dealing with the problem, the deploying of staff and other resources, and the general strategy necessary to deal with the disorder.

Antisocial personality disorders

Drug treatment

Treatment can be effective in antisocial personality disorder, and this is one of the few conditions for which randomised, controlled, doule-blind trials have shown treatment to be effective. There have been several studies on the short-term effects of both antipsychotic and antidepressant drugs in the treatment of antisocial personality disorder and its close affiliate, borderline personality disorder. These studies have produced relatively consistent results. Antipsychotic drugs in relatively low dosage (e.g. 5–7.5 mg haloperidol daily; 5 mg trifluoperazine daily) are effective in treating the impulsiveness and aggression of these personality disorders (Soloff *et al*, 1986).

Unfortunately, as one might predict with this group, compliance with treatment tends to be poor, and it is probably unwise to expect the average patient to take any drug by mouth consistently if the primary disorder is a personality one in this group. For this reason, there have been suggestions that the equivalent low dose of a depot antipsychotic drug (e.g. 12.5 mg fluphenazine decanoate every 4–6 weeks) may be an effective alternative for those whose compliance is poor. It is important to realise that improvement does not imply in any way that there is a psychotic element to the disorder. It is much more likely that the instability and impulsiveness of antisocial personality disorders is improved by the antipsychotic drugs probably as a consequence of their effects in blocking dopamine receptors. However, even this is not certain, as improvement is often found in low doses which do not have much effect on dopamine receptors.

Interestingly enough, depression, which is quite commonly found in these personality disorders, is not helped any further by giving antidepressants than by giving antipsychotic drugs (Soloff *et al*, 1986). If the GP comes across a patient with recurrent depression who seems to show little response to antidepressant drugs and shows some of the personality features of antisocial personality disorder, it is reasonable to consider low doses of an antipsychotic drug (e.g. chlorpromazine, haloperidol, trifluoperazine, flupenthixol) as well as psychological treatment.

There is also some evidence that the mood-stabilising drugs lithium and carbamazepine may be effective in controlling the aggressive and impulsive behaviour of antisocial personality disorder (Sheard *et al*, 1976; Cowdry & Gardner, 1988). Lithium may be particularly useful in aggression associated with mental handicap (Tyrer *et al*, 1984), and a new group of compounds, the serenics, of which eltoprazine is perhaps the most promising, may also reduce aggression and impulsiveness in this population.

The major problem with the antipsychotic drugs in treating personality disorders is that, even in somewhat low dosage, there is a danger that tardive dyskinesia, the syndrome of abnormal choreo-athetoid movements, more likely to become manifest after repeated administration, may occur. While it is possible to argue that this syndrome is a justifiable risk when treating patients with severe schizophrenia with antipsychotic drugs, the same argument becomes much less solid in the case of personality disorders. However, to date there is no good evidence of any patient with a primary diagnosis of personality disorder suffering from tardive dyskinesia as a consequence of antipsychotic drug treatment. It is also important to know that tardive dyskinesia is highly correlated with age, and that most people with antisocial personality disorders are relatively young, as they often mature by middle age, and long-term treatment (i.e. life-long) would hardly ever be seriously considered.

Other drugs are best avoided with antisocial personality disorder. In particular, the benzodiazepine group of tranquillisers, which can be associated with paradoxical reactions, including the release of aggression and impulsive paranoid behaviour, should be avoided in this group, as the dangers of provoking an idiosyncratic reaction are considerable.

Psychological treatment

Because of problems of motivation and regular commitment to any form of treatment, psychological treatments often do not succeed in antisocial personality disorder. However, there is no reason in principle why they should not be of some value. In particular, the newer treatment of cognitive therapy (often associated with behaviour therapy) can be particularly valuable because it sets clear targets and goals which can be monitored on a regular basis. As yet, however, this has not yet been formally assessed.

The standard (i.e. traditional) treatment for antisocial personality disorder is the therapeutic community. In such settings the patient is reminded of the effects of abnormal behaviour on others because he/she remains in regular contact with other people with similar disorders, and the negative effects of abnormal behaviour are reinforced constantly. There is some evidence that this has educational value and can be used therapeutically if the professional skills available are good. The conventional alternative of sending such individuals to prison because they offend against society does not appear to be of much value. The pattern of constant re-offending (recidivism) seems to be promoted by constant imprisonment, and there is no evidence that the punishment has an inhibiting or preventing effect on further offences.

Management

Although treatment may be effective for this group, it does not cater for the immediate problems of management when antisocial personality disorders present violent and threatening behaviour in the surgery. Such behaviour often requires emergency treatment purely to prevent damage to property and harm to others.

The most common form of management has been described as 'rapid tranquillisation', and policies for its use are well established in the US but not in Britain (Pilowsky *et al*, 1992). In such situations, drugs with rapid onset of action are usually given intramuscularly in order to produce a calming effect. The most popular drugs are diazepam (dosage range 10–80 mg intramuscularly) and haloperidol (dosage range 10–60 mg intramuscularly) (Pilowsky *et al*, 1992). These drugs are effective within minutes and when given together may act even more quickly. An alternative to these drugs is droperidol (dosage range 10–30 mg intramuscularly), which also acts rapidly and has a much shorter duration of action than other antipsychotic drugs like haloperidol. Although there is no doubt that emergency drug treatment of this nature is effective, it is important not to underplay the importance of psychological forms of management.

In particular, if the signs of aggression are detected early, staff can take avoiding action by isolating the patient and discussing the problem in a neutral setting. It is also important to realise that drugs such as diazepam, lorazepam, and haloperidol can also be given in liquid form and can start to show their effects within 10–20 minutes. A recent review of the subject (*Drugs and Therapeutics Bulletin*, 1991) has concluded that it is preferable to start treatment with a benzodiazepine or haloperidol by mouth, and that more severe disturbance should be treated by intramuscular droperidol or lorazepam (which act more quickly than diazepam by intramuscular administration). If intravenous administration is required, then diazepam in the form of Diazemuls (which does not irritate the veins) is probably the drug of choice.

Withdrawn personality disorders

Unfortunately there are no established psychological treatments for this group of personality disorders. The most widely reported in the literature is a form of psychotherapy, object-relations theory, which may be of value (Guntrip, 1974) but has not been formally tested. In practical terms, most of these patients do not wish to have any long-term therapy, such as a psychodynamic one, and so the issue does not arise. Pharmacological treatment has been evaluated to some extent and the results are somewhat similar to those with the antisocial group of personality disorders. Low doses of antipsychotic drugs may be effective in paranoid personality disorders, but less so in schizoid ones (Goldberg *et al*, 1986).

One of the reasons why treatments have not been properly assessed in this group of personality disorders is that most patients are not motivated to seek treatment. They either regard their behaviour as normal and, although it may cause concern to others, it is quite satisfactory as far as they are concerned (schizoid characteristics), or are abnormally suspicious and do not trust the motives of the therapist or the nature of the treatment (paranoid personality disorder). Such patients are often difficult to treat when they become medically ill, and it helps greatly if the GP or another member of the primary care team already knows the patient and has a reasonable relationship with him/her. The tendency of such patients is to consult late for all types of disorder and then often at the insistence of others rather than because of personal concern.

There is a particular form of paranoid personality which is excessively litigious. Although superficially cooperative, such personalities are extremely rigid and tend to magnify minor problems into major ones. There are many occasions on which such personalities have mortgaged their homes and become destitute through persistent legal action against professionals, including doctors, on issues which are 'matters of principle' but often outside the legal process. However, in view of this attitude, it is important for the GP to be particularly careful in treating such patients and to keep accurate records of all aspects of management.

Anxious personality disorders

Drug treatment

These patients are usually well known to the GP if they have been on the practice list for several years. The normal vicissitudes of life are magnified into major trials and, to cope with them, the patient often seeks help, commonly for what are described as 'nerves'. Anxiety is a prominent symptom, but depression and demoralisation are frequent, and there is often a certain irritability and importuning in the demands for help. Because such patients tend to lurch from one crisis to another, the GP is often faced with requests for emergency treatment for anxious symptoms, particularly panics, 'complaint inability to sleep', or inability to carry out simple tasks.

Under these circumstances the natural tendency is for the GP to prescribe a quick-acting sedative drug such as benzodiazepine, either at night as a hypnotic or during the day as an anxiolytic. If this is done it is important to be aware of the risks. Although treatment may be perfectly appropriate for a few days, patients with this type of personality disorder have more withdrawal problems on stopping benzodiazepines (Tyrer *et al*, 1983; Murphy & Tyrer, 1991), and so there is a danger that long-term prescription will become established.

If benzodiazepines or other sedatives, such as chlormethiazole (Hemi-nevrin), zopiclone (Zimovane), and chloral derivatives (e.g. Welldorm), are prescribed, it is important to emphasise at the outset that they are for short-term use only, and would not be re-prescribed for longer than three to four weeks. However, because such personalities have recurring problems, such short-term treatment is often considered impractical. The practitioner may anticipate this by prescribing antidepressants at the same time as the benzodiazepine tranquilliser or similar drug. All antidepressants have a delay between the initial time of administration and the onset of therapeutic effect, which varies between two and four weeks (up to six weeks with drugs such as the original monoamine oxidase inhibitors such as isocarboxazid and phenelzine). Although antidepressants are not licensed for the treatment of anxiety or the anxious personality disorder it has been known for many years that they are effective in a range of anxiety disorders and their use is becoming increasingly frequent because of concern over the dependence potential of benzodiazepine and similar drugs.

There is no satisfactory evidence that anxious and fearful personality disorders are better treated by antidepressants and other drugs, but there is some evidence that drug treatment is superior to psychological treatments such as cognitive therapy in the long term (one to two years) (Tyrer *et al*, 1992). It is not known which dose range is best for treating these disorders. For many years, GPs have been castigated by their psychiatric colleagues for prescribing antidepressants in 'subtherapeutic' dosage (e.g. 50 mg amitriptyline daily). It remains to be shown that this dosage is ineffective; the possibility remains that it may be ineffective for treating depressed mood as a mental state disorder but not when it is combined with other mood disturbance and personality abnormality.

The choice of antidepressant is also far from clear. There is some evidence that tricyclic antidepressants are more effective than monoamine oxidase inhibitors in treating patients with mood disturbance who also have personality disorder (Shawcross & Tyrer, 1985), but nothing is known about the relative efficacy of the older antidepressants and the new selective serotonin reuptake inhibitors, although there are suspicions that these drugs may be more effective when anxiety is present with depression (e.g. Dunbar *et al*, 1991). There is also one study that suggested that patients with obsessive–compulsive personality disorder responded better to fluvoxamine than those without this personality disorder (Ansseau *et al*, 1991).

The non-benzodiazepine anxiolytic buspirone might also be considered for such disorders. It does not appear to have the potential for dependence (Murphy *et al*, 1989), and although it has a delayed onset of action, this is not so important with these disorders.

If drug treatment is considered appropriate, and shown to be effective, the GP has to decide whether it can be continued long term. Unfortunately, with the anxious personality disorders this position is likely to be encountered more frequently than not. Under such circumstances it is reasonable, at least in a minority of cases, to regard long-term antidepressant therapy (possibly in lower dosage than might otherwise by used) to be justified, together with short-term use of anxiolytic sedatives, when required.

Psychological treatment

Patients with anxious personality disorders are likely to rely heavily on their therapists. Sometimes this can be put to good use, and the doctor then becomes the main treatment for the patient. The only snag with this is that continuous administration of the treatment is usually necessary, and withdrawal symptoms may be marked when the doctor ceases contact. Psychotherapists terms this phenomenon the 'transference cure', in which the patient continues to appear well but only while in therapy. For the GP this need not be a disaster. If the patient is allowed a regular appointment every one or two weeks at times of greater disturbance this can often be enough to stave off emergency calls and other crises from developing.

Sometimes the patient can get completely enmeshed with the doctor in a complicated therapeutic relationship that needs help in disentangling it. Under such circumstances psychiatric help, preferably by direct involvement at the practice, may often be helpful.

Borderline personality disorder

The term 'borderline' has not received much prominence in this account so far. However, if this chapter were being written for a North American audience, it would be dominated by discussion of borderline personality. 'Borderline' is a confusing term that describes the condition that is like a triangle, bordering with schizophrenia on one side, affective disturbance (mainly depression) on another, and antisocial behaviour on the third. The condition is characterised by unstable relationships with others, often of an intense, short-term nature, impulsive behaviour, and brief periods of depression associated with suicidal behaviour. It is easy to see how such patients can cause great distress and disturbance in consultations in primary care, as well as in psychiatric settings. Many such patients abuse alcohol and other drugs, and could also present with addictions to these. Although this borderline group may represent a distinct and homogeneous grouping, I do not think it is sufficiently different to justify separate description.

However, the term will not go away, not least because it describes a form of consultation behaviour – dramatic and crisis-ridden – that the clinician cannot ignore. However, the general principles underlying the management of the antisocial personality disorders still apply, and although their psychological treatments are much better studied (Higgitt & Fonagy, 1992), the average clinician is left with a difficult, often frustrating and demoralising problem in the care of this group.

Conclusions

Although there is an aura of therapeutic gloom around personality disorders, which explains the sometimes excessive avoidance of the term by some practitioners, there are undoubtedly effective short-term treatments for these conditions. In the longer term there are still no unequivocal therapeutic gains. Nevertheless, recognition can at least lead to advice that prevents tragedy and iatrogenic disorder.

References

AMERICAN PSYCHIATRIC ASSOCIATION (1987) *Diagnostic and Statistical Manual of Mental Disorders* (3rd edn, revised) (DSM-III-R). Washington, DC: APA.

ANSSEAU, M. TROISFONTAINES, B., PAPART, P., *et al* (1991) Compulsive personality as predictor of response to serotonergic antidepressants. *British Medical Journal*, **303**, 760–761.

BLACKBURN, R. (1988) On moral judgements and personality disorders. The myth of psychopathic personality revisited. *British Journal of Psychiatry*, **153**, 505–512.

COWDRY, R. W. & GARDNER, D. L. (1988) Pharmacotherapy of borderline personality disorder: alprazolam, carbamazepine, trifluoperazine and tranylcypromine. *Archives of General Psychiatry*, **45**, 111–119.

DRUG AND THERAPEUTICS BULLETIN (1991) Management of behavioural emergencies. *Drug and Therapeutics Bulletin*, **29**, 62–64.

DUNBAR, G. C., COHN, J. B., FABRE, L. F., *et al* (1991) A comparison of paroxetine, imipramine and placebo in depressed out-patients. *British Journal of Psychiatry*, **159**, 394–398.

EYSENCK, H. J. (1959) *The Maudsley Personality Inventory*. London: University of London Press.

—— & EYSENCK, S. B. G. (1969) *Manual of the Eysenck Personality Questionnaire (EPQ)*. London: University of London Press.

GOLDBERG, S. C., SHULZ, S. C., SHULZ, P. M., *et al* (1986) Borderline and schizotypal personality disorders treated with low dose thiothixene versus placebo. *Archives of General Psychiatry*, **43**, 680–686.

GUNTRIP, H. (1974) *Schizoid Phenomena, Object-Relations and the Self*. London: Hogarth Press.

HIGGITT, A. & FONAGY, P. (1992) Psychotherapy in borderline and narcissistic personality disorder. *British Journal of Psychiatry*, **161**, 23–43.

LEWIS, G. & APPLEBY, L. (1888) Personality disorder: the patients psychiatrists dislike. *British Journal of Psychiatry*, **153**, 44–49.

LORANGER, A. W., SUSMAN, V. L., OLDHAM, J. M., *et al* (1985) *Personality Disorder Examination (PDE). A Structured Interview for DSM-III-R Personality Disorders*. White Plains, New York: The New York Hospital, Cornell Medical Center, Westchester Division.

MANN, A. H., JENKINS, R., CUTTING, J. C., *et al* (1981) The development and use of a standardized assessment of abnormal personality. *Psychological Medicine*, **11**, 839–847.

MURPHY, S. M., OWEN, R. & TYRER, P. (1989) Comparative assessment of efficacy and withdrawal symptoms after 6 and 12 weeks' treatment with diazepam or buspirone. *British Journal of Psychiatry*, **154**, 529–534.

—— & TYRER, P. (1991) A double-blind comparison of the effects of gradual withdrawal of lorazepam, diazepam and bromazepam in benzodiazepine dependence. *British Journal of Psychiatry*, **158**, 511–516.

PFOHL, B., STANGL, D. & ZIMMERMAN, M. (1982) *Structured Interview for DSM-III Personality Disorders (SID-P)*. University of Iowa Hospitals and Clinics, Iowa City, USA.

PILOWSKY, L. S., RING, H., SHINE, P. J., *et al* (1992) Rapid tranquillisation: a survey of emergency prescribing in a general psychiatric hospital. *British Journal of Psychiatry*, **160**, 831–835.

RUTTER, M. L. (1987) Temperament, personality and personality disorder. *British Journal of Psychiatry*, **150**, 443–458.

SHAWCROSS, C. R. & TYRER, P. (1985) Influence of personality on response to monoamine-oxidase inhibitors and tricyclic antidepressants. *Journal of Psychiatric Research*, **19**, 31–36.

SHEARD, M. H., MARINI, J. L., BRIDGES, C. I., *et al* (1976) The effect of lithium on impulsive aggressive behavior in man. *American Journal of Psychiatry*, **133**, 1409–1413.

SOLOFF, P. H., GEORGE, A., NATHAN, R. S., *et al* (1986) Progress in pharmacotherapy of borderline disorders: a double blind study of amitriptyline, haloperidol and placebo. *Archives of General Psychiatry*, **43**, 691–697.

SPITZER, R., WILLIAMS, J. B. W. & GIBBON, M. (1987) *Structured Interview for DSM-III-R Personality Disorders*. New York: Biometrics Research Department, New York State Psychiatry Institute.

TYRER, P. & ALEXANDER, J. (1979) Classification of personality disorder. *British Journal of Psychiatry*, **135**, 163–167.

————, OWEN, R. & DAWLING, S. (1983) Gradual withdrawal of diazepam after long-term therapy. *Lancet, i*, 1402–1406.

————, FERGUSON, B., FOWLER-DIXON, R., *et al* (1990) A plea for the diagnosis of hypochondriacal personality disorder. *Journal of Psychosomatic Research*, **34**, 637–642.

————, SEIVEWRIGHT, N., FERGUSON, B., *et al* (1993) The Nottingham study of neurotic disorder: impact of personality status on response to drug treatment, cognitive therapy and self-help over two years. *British Journal of Psychiatry*, **162**, 219–226.

TYRER, S. P., WALSH, A., EDWARDS, D. E., *et al* (1984) Factors associated with a good response to lithium in aggressive mentally handicapped subjects. *Progress in Neuro-Psychopharmacological and Biological Psychiatry*, **8**, 751–755.

WORLD HEALTH ORGANIZATION (1992) *International Classification of Diseases* (10th revision) (ICD–10). Geneva: WHO.

13 Schizophrenia

TOM BURNS and TONY KENDRICK

One in four people with schizophrenia makes an early recovery from the illness. One in ten becomes severely disabled and requires residential care. The remaining two-thirds endure persisting symptoms and social problems, and may be subject to relapses at intervals (Watt *et al*, 1983). These days most sufferers spend nearly all their lives outside hospitals, yet often need continuing support and supervision. Continuing care means care which is planned and organised in anticipation of the illness running a chronic course. This presents a challenge to GPs.

The contribution of GPs, in dealing with the lion's share of minor mental illness, has been central to the early development of a comprehensive mental health service which has been able to give priority to the severely mentally ill and avoid many of the problems experienced in countries like the USA where primary care is not so well organised.

It should not be assumed, however, that this means a simple division of labour, with psychotic patients treated by the specialist services and non-psychotic patients in general practice. A recent follow-up study of patients with schizophrenia discharged from hospital in West Lambeth (Melzer *et al*, 1991) found that only 52% were in contact with a psychiatrist after 12 months, while 57% were in contact with their GP. A similar situation was found by Parkes *et al* (1962) 30 years before, with only 56% of discharged schizophrenics in London in contact with psychiatric services and 70% in contact with their GP in the 12 months after discharge.

In the longer term, many patients with chronic schizophrenia are lost to specialist follow-up altogether. Shepherd *et al* (1966) in their major study of psychiatric disorders in general practice found that only a quarter of patients with psychosis received specialist psychiatric care during their study period of one year. More recently, Pantelis *et al* (1988) found that only 60% of the patients they identified in the course of setting up a register of people with chronic schizophrenia in Camden had any continuing contact with a psychiatrist.

General practitioners have therefore been involved at least as frequently as psychiatrists in the care of patients with schizophrenia since the shift in policy away from long-term hospital care in the late 1950s. While this involvement may often be limited to brief contacts for repeat prescriptions, for many patients such contacts may offer the only opportunity for assessment by a doctor, including a mental state examination.

The contribution of general practice to the management of acute major mental illness has been seriously neglected in the psychiatric research literature. None of the influential studies of alternatives to hospital care has commented on the role of the family doctor (Fenton *et al*, 1979; Stein & Test, 1980; Hoult, 1983). These studies have been conducted in the context of poorly developed or absent primary care services for their patient groups. Even the first replication of these studies in the UK (Muijen *et al*, 1992) does not yet report on input from primary care. This may be because of the higher rate of non-registration with a GP among inner-city populations, or possibly a lower level of organisation of continuing care in general practices in these areas. The most likely reason is that sampling occurred at the 'point of potential admission', after it had been decided that patients had passed to the responsibility of the specialist services.

The central role of the GP

There are a number of reasons why the GP should play a pivotal role in the care of patients with schizophrenia.

(a) The GP has, in many cases, already developed a relationship with the patient before the illness strikes, and is familiar with the patient's home situation, and problems facing the family or other carers, who are frequently the GP's patients too. This is especially important where the onset is insidious or the family's usual behaviour is unknown to the psychiatrist.

Case 1

A 25-year-old man of Ghanaian origin, brought up in London by his devout, very private family, was referred by his GP because of withdrawal and bizarre behaviour since he had lost his job at a local cinema. At assessment he was unforthcoming, but did talk about his disappointment and hopelessness about the future. A diagnosis of depressive disorder with an unusual personality was made.

At a routine liaison meeting, the GP questioned this, suggesting that a change occurred about three years previously, when the patient had dropped out of a course at the local polytechnic. A working diagnosis of a schizophrenic disorder was made and the patient was successfully treated with phenothiazines rather than antidepressants. Over four months he improved markedly and talked about the disturbing blasphemous voices which had tormented him on and off for over two years. Previously, he had been admitted twice to a mental hospital under section 136 of the Mental Health Act, and been discharged both times with no diagnosis. The GP's opinion had not been sought.

Hunter (1978) found that families turned to their GPs more often than to community psychiatric nurses (CPNs) when experiencing difficulties with their relatives with schizophrenia.

(b) Where the GP undertakes the routine review of the majority of patients, particularly those who are in remission, the specialist can concentrate on the more complex problems of diagnosis and management. Our postal survey of one in three GPs in the South West Thames Region found that over 90% of responders agreed that the care of patients with long-term mental illnesses like schizophrenia should be shared between them and the specialist, with the CPN as key worker in regular contact with the patient. An encouraging 41% went further, and thought that care should be primarily organised by the GP with the back-up of the psychiatrist as necessary (Kendrick *et al*, 1991).

(c) The GP needs to be familiar with the patient's usual mental state, and patterns of symptoms which might suggest imminent relapse, to react effectively when problems start to develop. Where regular reviews are the responsibility of the CPN and the GP does not see the patient, then he/she must rely on regular and detailed communication with the CPN.

(d) Patients with chronic schizophrenia suffer increased rates of physical problems, including cardiovascular and respiratory diseases (Allebeck, 1989), which are the proper concern of their GP. They are also entitled, like all other patients, to be offered preventive health care. Psychiatrists or CPNs do not usually listen to patients' chests, take cervical smears, or offer help tackling obesity.

(e) General practitioners are best placed to offer long-term continuing care. They will usually practise in the same place for decades. The advantages of this local service – familiar, easily accessible, non-stigmatising – to patients who may be anxious, disorganised, and diffident are considerable. GPs can apply to their work an established expertise in the management of long-term disorders (Hasler & Schofield, 1984). Continuity of care over long periods, albeit in brief consultations, is well suited to many of these patients. The greater willingness of GPs to accommodate patients' views into management decisions is commented upon by psychiatric trainees in GP training (Burns *et al*, 1991). This more equal relationship is well suited to the 'management of disability'. It generates less anxiety and can help self-esteem.

The syndromes of schizophrenia

Although schizophrenia and its management are used as the paradigm for this chapter, many of the principles and practices are relevant for a wider spectrum of disorders. Whether the patient has attracted a diagnosis of paranoid psychosis, schizoaffective disorder, paraphrenia or schizophrenia will have only a minor effect on the principles of management.

What these disorders have in common is their episodic course, characterised by hallucinations and delusions in the acute phase (the 'positive' symptoms), with variable degrees of social and personal disabilities (the 'negative' symptoms) as a consequence. The acute phases are associated with a break with reality, and the chronic syndromes often with an apathetic, disorganised lifestyle with serious risk for self-neglect.

The classification of acute schizophrenic disorders into 'simple', 'hebephrenic', 'catatonic', and 'paranoid' has little contemporary relevance. The only distinction commonly made is into acute schizophrenia and acute paranoid schizophrenia. The latter tends to start later (in the early 30s rather than the early 20s) and often leads to less personality deterioration. The clinical picture is dominated by suspiciousness and persecutory delusions. Hallucinations are less prominent in paranoid schizophrenia, as are behavioural disturbances and thought disorder.

Psychiatric textbooks concentrate on the presence of the so-called 'first-rank symptoms' to distinguish schizophrenia from the other functional psychoses. These symptoms comprise disorders of logical thinking and a number of 'passivity experiences', where aspects of mental and physical functioning are felt not to be under the patient's control (like telepathy or hypnosis). In practice the course of the illness is usually more important – whether it recurs and the development of negative symptoms and a 'defect state'. Patients with schizophrenia will usually require maintenance medication for several years, whereas those with other functional psychoses may often need no medication between acute episodes.

To maintain motivation and interest in treating patients over many years the doctor needs to have realistic aims. In schizophrenia these are the minimisation of complications, the prevention and prompt treatment of relapse, and the containment of deterioration rather than cure. How should the GP organise such care?

Practice management

A proactive approach

On average, 60–70% of patients (including many schizophrenics) consult their GPs each year. However, many schizophrenics suffer from negative symptoms, including social withdrawal, passivity, inertia, and lack of initiative (Wing, 1989) and cannot be relied upon to seek help. Some chronic schizophrenic patients therefore present only at times of crisis, and GPs may not be immediately aware of how many are on the practice list, or the extent of their problems. There is a need to adopt a *proactive* approach to identify and contact patients with schizophrenia. Left alone, patients' problems can build up to an admission which might have been avoided with earlier recognition and intervention.

This proactive approach involves reversing the usual assumption that if patients stay away from the surgery it is because they are well. When a patient with schizophrenia misses a follow-up appointment the first reason to be excluded is that he/she is relapsing.

Scheduling regular reviews of patients with schizophrenia is no different in principle to policies adopted for other patients at increased risk, such as diabetics. A disease register and call/recall system for patients with schizophrenia can be created quickly. An important first step is to identify all the patients with schizophrenia on the practice list. Just as important is deciding which doctor is going to take personal responsibility for each patient.

Creating a disease register

The average point-prevalence of schizophrenia in England is 3–4 per 1000, yielding around 7 patients per GP, but there is wide variation between areas. The number is likely to be higher in inner-city practices. In Salford, for example, a relatively deprived inner-city area, the prevalence was found to be 6.2 per 1000 (Bamrah *et al*, 1991). Harris & Schofield (1984), reviewing all 8000 case records in their practice, found 28 patients – nearly three times the number they would have expected from the consulting rates reported by the Second National Morbidity Study (Office of Population Censuses and Surveys, 1982), suggesting to them that a proportion of patients with chronic schizophrenia were not receiving continuing care from their GPs.

Reviewing all the case records is time consuming and probably unnecessary. The large majority of patients can be quickly identified, as outlined below (indeed, most patients can be identified from practice and mental health service sources alone).

   (a) *Within the practice*:
      (i) The repeat prescription system, if any, for patients on
         (1) antipsychotic drugs (oral and depot)
         (2) anticholinergics
      (ii) computer records or disease register
      (iii) depot clinics by the practice nurse or practice-based CPN where appropriate
      (iv) appointment lists for the previous three months
   (b) *Mental health services data*:
      (i) CPN clients
      (ii) psychiatric case register, and out-patient records
      (iii) day-hospital patients

(c) *Social services data*:
   (i) social worker caseloads
   (ii) day-centre clients
   (iii) populations of hostels/group homes/sheltered residence
(d) *Voluntary sector*:
   (i) sheltered accommodation
   (ii) drop-in centres
   (iii) churches and other voluntary agencies.

Call/recall systems

Most patients, at least when they are relatively well, can be relied upon to report by themselves every three or six months, sometimes accompanied by a relative or other carer. Others will need to be sought out and sent for, or visited at home. A system is needed to remind the doctor when the patient's next review is overdue. Such a call/recall list will be kept on computer in most practices, but could be a simple diary or card index, one for each month, on which patients' names are entered at the required intervals. The interval between reviews will of course depend on the severity of the problems.

Practice activity analysis data revealed that around half of all prescriptions of phenothiazines were repeat prescriptions where the patient was not seen, and only one-third were given in follow-up consultations (Royal College of General Practitioners' Birmingham Research Unit, 1978). One simple way to improve the regular supervision of patients is to limit the number of repeat prescriptions a patient may have without a mandatory consultation – for example no more than two months' supply. This can be easily programmed into the computer, but again there is no reason why it should not be done using a paper system.

Continuity of care

Continuity is important in the care of patients with chronic disease. For example, compliance with drug treatment has been shown to be greater where the patient knows the doctor well (Ettlinger & Freeman, 1981). The move to group practices has reduced the continuity of care, in terms of the degree to which a single doctor deals with a particular patient, except where a strict policy of personal lists is maintained (Freeman & Richards, 1990).

An explicit policy is needed to maintain a personal-list system. A doctor seeing a patient registered with a partner should ensure that the patient returns to his/her own doctor for follow-up care. Putting the case records for different partners into separate filing cabinets, so that patients have to be asked who their doctor is each time they call, encourages each patient to identify with a particular doctor. In this way Pereira Gray (1979) managed to increase the proportion of personal consultations with his chronic schizophrenic patients from 44% to 100% within a few years. Decisions on practice policy should involve the reception staff, to prevent patients with chronic schizophrenia, who may not cooperate with inflexible appointment systems, being turned away or being seen as 'extras' by the duty partner.

Special sessions

Stott & Davis (1979) pointed out that every consultation provides an opportunity to review the patient's chronic health problems, as well as to deal with the presenting problem, offer health promotion, and modify the patient's help-seeking behaviour. Howie *et al* (1991) found, however, that such consultations were longer, often lasting 15 minutes or more. Fitting regular review into ordinary consultations may be difficult to do properly without either disrupting surgeries or failing to cover important areas of care. The doctor should consider carrying out such reviews at special times.

A home visit is one option which can quickly reveal how well the patient and carer are coping, and provide an opportunity to observe the patient–carer interaction at first hand. Pereira Gray (1978) highlighted the amount of information that can be gathered and the different quality of the doctor–patient relationship on the patient's home territory. He listed schizophrenia as one of the chronic diseases which should be managed at home as much as possible.

Special record cards

The GP sees the patient for all sorts of problems, acute as well as chronic. Important information for the continuing care of a chronic disease may become obscured. It is worth considering having a separate card in the record envelope on which to record the management of chronic schizophrenia (Fig. 13.1). This allows the doctor carrying out regular review to see quickly what has been happening and prompts the next appropriate action. It also makes extraction of data for audit much easier.

The record should have a section on baseline data, including the date of diagnosis, dates of admissions to hospital, the pattern of symptoms during relapses, if known, the names of relatives or other carers, and key professionals involved in the patient's care. A separate section on routine regular review should include a list of checks to be carried out at each attendance, in the main areas of physical, psychological, and social problems.

Periodic review

Mental state

The assessment of mental state is facilitated by using a structured approach, yet it is remarkably easy to forego a systematic assessment of the mental

	Date	Date	Date	Date
Medication				
Anxiety				
Depression				
Hallucinations				
Delusions				
Appearance				
Behaviour				
Preventive				
Cardiovascular				
Respiratory				
Other physical				
Housing				
Finance				
Occupation				
Social life				

Name   Date of birth

First diagnosed   Hospital No.

Hospital admissions

Relatives/other carers

GP   CPN

Consultant   SW

Psychologist   OT

Pattern of relapse

Important notes

(a)   (b)

Fig. 13.1 The special record card used in TK's practice: (a) front, (b) back

state and miss a change in symptoms in a schizophrenic patient one knows well. The failure of mental health workers to question schizophrenic patients about their symptoms has been vividly demonstrated in a study of CPNs and mental health social workers (Wooff *et al*, 1988), but such oversight is unlikely to be restricted to these professionals alone.

Failure to elicit psychopathology may be a consequence of relying too much on open-ended questioning. 'How are you?' will often be answered with 'fine'. The GP will need to be more active in this assessment, and some types of behaviour which an entirely 'patient-centred' approach (Byrne & Long, 1976) might suggest are wrong are actually essential when dealing with patients damaged by chronic schizophrenia. These will include sometimes rejecting patients' offers of explanations, which must be done without alienating them if possible. It is important neither to agree nor explicitly disagree with firmly held delusional convictions. The GP must try to avoid responding too strongly to the patient's feelings, which may be powerful, and try to remain friendly but businesslike. It is important not to get overinvolved. Prolonged silences and a lack of eye contact may have to be tolerated. On the whole jokes are likely to be misinterpreted and should be avoided.

We need to overcome a degree of embarrassment at asking questions about hallucinations and delusions. There is often a lingering suspicion in many of us that talking about them might strengthen them (as if by reminding the patient of them we impede their fading). It is important to word questions about hearing voices in the way that the GP feels most comfortable with:

"Are the voices still troubling you?"
"Are they clear? What do they talk about?"
"Can you ignore them and get on with things?"
"Are they every day/week?"

Long preambles such as "many people with this sort of disorder have strange experiences when they think they hear voices and there is nobody about" can be counterproductive. A matter-of-fact approach often relaxes both patient and doctor.

With delusions (especially with paranoid psychosis or paranoid schizophrenia) direct questioning is even more important. To assess the extent of delusions one needs some indication of their content. It is important when recording in the notes that a patient is deluded to say about what. A mark in the box on the special record card recommended here (Fig. 13.1) will indicate that delusions are present, but such a long-term record does not have much space for the content, which may need to be entered in the normal notes: "Still deluded – neighbours spying, Freemasons sending coded letter." With such a prompt the patient can be asked if he is still worried about the neighbours or Freemasons.

The force of delusions can be measured roughly by the restriction they impose on the patient or the activities they demand: "Deluded about neighbours, keeps curtains pulled"; "Deluded about neighbours, but curtains open and going shopping".

Assessing the level of deficit state in patients who live alone is important. GPs might, however, wonder why they should bother. What can they do about deteriorating withdrawal and apathy? The GP's recognition of a changing level of disability can function as a powerful stimulus to a psychiatric service. Many GPs will have had the experience of referring a chronic schizophrenic for assessment to receive a reply along the lines of:

> "He demonstrates a long-standing schizophrenic defect state but appears well controlled on the fluphenothiazine depot. Perhaps you could request social services to encourage him to attend the day centre which I note they did four years ago. I would be happy to reassess him in the future if required."

This unhelpful reply reflects the difficulty of knowing whether a patient is functioning at optimum level on the basis of one consultation. Increasing withdrawal is a complex issue, and there are a number of possible causes. It may reflect an increase in negative symptoms but may also be due to worsening positive symptoms (the patient may be preoccupied with more persistent hallucinatory voices, for example), or it may be that the patient is depressed. It clearly warrants adequate assessment. If the GP letter states clearly that there has been a substantial deterioration in functioning over a specific period then the psychiatrist or social worker is more likely to pay sufficient attention, for example:

> "This schizophrenic patient has withdrawn from attending his drop-in club just over a year ago. He used to be well nourished and although he kept himself to himself he was never unkempt. More recently he has appeared quite neglected and, I gather, refused his neighbour's customary offer of getting his shopping."

Physical health

A number of studies suggest that between a third and a half of long-term mentally ill patients have significant physical disorders, a proportion of which are either unknown to their doctors or in need of further assessment or treatment (Farmer, 1987; Honig *et al*, 1989; Brugha *et al*, 1989). The relative mortality in schizophrenia is approximately doubled, owing partly to an increased risk of suicide, but also to increased susceptibility to cardiovascular and respiratory diseases (Allebeck, 1989). The side-effects of psychotropic drugs and a sedentary life can combine to cause obesity, and many patients with chronic schizophrenia are heavy smokers, which may have developed during time spent in psychiatric wards.

The physical problems found can usually be dealt with in primary care but are complicated by the patient's mental illness, which can produce inappropriate and counterproductive help-seeking. There is therefore a need for a proactive approach, using closed questions for possible physical symptoms, and regular screening for possible problems.

On this basis we suggest that for patients with long-standing illness, especially for the over-40s, the GP should consider carrying out a battery of examinations and investigations once a year, regardless of a lack of complaints:

(a) full physical examination
    (i) blood pressure
    (ii) chest examination
    (iii) skin examination
    (iv) side-effects
    (v) urinalysis
(b) blood tests
    (i) full blood count
    (ii) erythrocyte sedimentation rate
    (iii) thyroxine tests
(c) chest X-ray
(d) electrocardiogram
(e) vision and hearing testing.

Social needs

Employment

Schizophrenia may strike so early in life that the patient has not had time to gain any qualifications. The illness may also interfere with the person's ability to continue in an established job.

Problems of illiteracy and lack of work skills can be tackled with remedial education and training. The disablement resettlement officer is the person responsible. A telephone call to the local job centre is all that is required of the GP.

Finances

Schizophrenic patients often fail to claim their benefits. A social worker or the Citizens' Advice Bureau can help if requested.

Social network

The involvement of family and friends can be quickly ascertained by questions such as "Is there anyone that you can really count on for help in a crisis?" and "Is there anyone who really counts on you?" As well as revealing important information about the patient, they also show that the doctor is interested in them as a person and their quality of life and relationships. The relatives' need for respite care should be gauged at the regular review.

Antipsychotic medication

Treatment with major tranquillisers (or neuroleptics) is indicated for the 'positive' symptoms of hallucinations, delusions, and thought disorder. Higher doses may be required for severe agitation and restlessness. Neuroleptic drugs vary in their effects, and specialist advice may be needed to find the right one for a particular patient. Chlorpromazine (Largactil), while very effective acutely with an extremely disturbed and psychotic patient, may be too sedating to permit work in the longer term, so a less sedating drug such as trifluoperazine (Stelazine) might be substituted.

The prophylactic role of neuroleptic therapy has been well demonstrated in controlled trials, although compliance may be a problem in a third or more of patients. Depot injections can help to overcome this problem (Hirsch *et al*, 1973; Curson *et al*, 1985). Again, depot neuroleptics vary in their properties; for example flupenthixol (Depixol) may be preferred to fluphenazine (Modecate) for patients who feel sluggish or tend towards depression.

Anticholinergic drugs like procyclidine (Kemadrin) should be prescribed only where Parkinsonian side-effects develop. They should not be used routinely, since they themselves may cause side-effects, are often unnecessary, and may be abused for their stimulant effects. It may be better to try reducing the dose of major tranquilliser or substituting a drug less prone to Parkinsonian side-effects before starting an anticholinergic.

In general, medication should be restricted to one or two drugs, and then at the lowest therapeutic doses. In practice some patients seem to end up taking what may seem to be odd combinations of several drugs, even where two drugs act in the same way. For example, an oral preparation of a major tranquilliser may be prescribed as well as depot injections from the nurse, to allow the patient to titrate medication against symptoms on a day-to-day basis. The degree of compliance is, however, likely to be inversely proportional to the number of medications prescribed.

A range of newer, 'atypical' neuroleptics have recently become available. These atypical neuroleptics have relatively weak affinity for dopamine receptors and appear to exert their effect partly through action at serotonin (5-HT) receptors. The most widely tested members of this class are clozapine (Clozaril, Sandoz) and risperidone (Risperdal, Janssen). Clozapine is not a new drug, having been introduced over 20 years ago but withdrawn in many countries because of safety concerns. It has been re-introduced for treatment-resistant patients and appears to be effective in controlling both positive and negative symptoms in many patients who were previously untreatable. However, it can cause fatal agranulocytosis and, for this reason, all patients have to undergo regular blood tests. Risperidone, a newer compound, is also effective against both positive and negative symptoms and appears to cause far fewer side-effects than other neuroleptics. It does not require the regular blood testing needed with clozapine. At present these new drugs are initiated only by psychiatrists and then only for patients with histories of poor response to conventional neuroleptics. It is highly likely, however, that their use will increase and GPs will become involved in their prescription.

As a general rule, medication requirements should be reviewed every two years. If a patient is stable and symptoms have settled, then a trial of reduced therapy may be considered – in collaboration with the psychiatrist. Long-term medication should continue only where it has been demonstrated that relapse occurs on withdrawal of the drug. There is evidence that patients can remain on excessive doses or inappropriate combinations of drugs for decades without active review (Holloway, 1988).

Audit

Once all patients in the practice are on the disease register and special continuation cards are placed in all their notes, it is simple to gather information quickly to audit the process of care. The process criteria agreed in TK's practice are as follows. All patients with chronic schizophrenia should be:

(a) included in the disease register
(b) see the doctor with whom they are registered each time they consult (accept 8 out of 10 times)
(c) seen by the GP at least once every six months (accept 9 out of 10 if all are seen every year)
(d) be assessed yearly for the psychiatric, physical, and social problems listed on the continuation record (accept 9 out of 10 boxes marked per calendar year)
(e) have recorded in their medical record the following preventive health data
    (i) smoking habit
    (ii) blood pressure within the preceding five years
    (iii) estimate of weight compared with ideal weight
    (iv) alcohol consumption
    (v) cervical smear result within three years for women of child-bearing age
    (vi) method of contraception for women of child-bearing age
    (vii) mammogram result for women aged 50–65.

Conclusions

Setting up a disease register and instituting regular reviews of patients with chronic schizophrenia may involve the doctor in extra work. However, these patients have many problems and really need their doctor's help. The GP's own skills, confidence, and job satisfaction are likely to be improved by getting more involved. These efforts may well *save* time in the longer term, by preempting crises which are time consuming to deal with, often in out-of-hours visits. They also liberate the specialist mental health team to focus on those complex problems which require its resources and skills. We would argue that such a highly disadvantaged group deserves more than most patients the best efforts of a well organised practice.

Acknowledgements

We would like to thank Jean Debono for her help in preparing the manuscript. TK is supported by a grant from the Mental Health Foundation.

References

ALLEBECK, P. (1989) Schizophrenia: a life-shortening disease. *Schizophrenia Bulletin*, **15**, 81–89.

BAMRAH, J. S., FREEMAN, H. L. & GOLDBERG, D. P. (1991) Epidemiology of schizophrenia in Salford, 1974–84. Changes in an urban community over ten years. *British Journal of Psychiatry*, **159**, 802–810.

BRUGHA, T. S., WING, J. K. & SMITH, B. L. (1989) Physical health of the long-term mentally ill in the community. Is there unmet need? *British Journal of Psychiatry*, **155**, 777–781.

BURNS, T., SILVER, T., CRISP, A., *et al* (1994) General practice training for psychiatrists: a study of feasibility and acceptability. *Psychiatric Bulletin* (in press).

BYRNE, P. S. & LONG, B. L. (1976) *Doctors Talking with Patients*. London: HMSO.

CURSON, D. A., BARNES, T. R. E. & BAMBER, R. W. (1985) Long-term depot maintenance of chronic schizophrenic outpatients. *British Journal of Psychiatry*, **146**, 464–480.

ETTLINGER, P. R. A. & FREEMAN, G. K. (1981) General practice compliance study: is it worth being a personal doctor? *British Medical Journal*, **282**, 1192–1194.

FARMER, S. (1987) Medical problems of chronic patients in a community support program. *Hospital and Community Psychiatry*, **38**, 745–749.

FENTON, S. R., TESSIER, L. & STRUENING, E. L. (1979) A comparative trial of home and hospital psychiatric care: one year follow up. *Archives of General Psychiatry*, **36**, 1073–1079.

FREEMAN, G. K. & RICHARDS, S. C. (1990) How much personal care in four group practices? *British Medical Journal*, **301**, 1028–1030.

HARRIS, G. & SCHOFIELD, T. P. C. (1984) In *Continuing Care: The Management of Chronic Disease* (eds J. Hasler & T. P. C. Schofield), pp. 74–75. Oxford: Oxford University Press.

HASLER, J. & SCHOFIELD, T. P. C. (eds) (1984) *Continuing Care: The Management of Chronic Disease*. Oxford: Oxford University Press.

HIRSCH, S. R., GAIND, R., ROHDE, P. D., *et al* (1973) Outpatient maintenance of chronic schizophrenic patients with long-acting fluphenazine: double-blind placebo trials. *British Medical Journal*, i, 633–637.

HOLLOWAY, F. (1988) Prescribing for the long-term mentally ill. A study of treatment practices. *British Journal of Psychiatry*, **152**, 511–515.

HONIG, A., POP, P., TAN, E. S., *et al* (1989) Physical illness in chronic psychiatric patients from a community psychiatric unit. The implications for daily practice. *British Journal of Psychiatry*, **155**, 58–64.

HOULT, J., REYNOLDS, I., POWIS, M. C., *et al* (1983) Psychiatric hospital versus community treatment: the results of a randomised trial. *Australian and New Zealand Journal of Orthopsychiatry*, **17**, 160–167.

HOWIE, J. G. R., PORTER, A. M. D., HEANEY, D. J., *et al* (1991) Long to short consultation ratio: a proxy measure of quality of care for general practice. *British Journal of General Practice*, **41**, 48–54.

HUNTER, P. (1978) *Schizophrenia and Community Psychiatric Nursing*. London: National Schizophrenia Fellowship.

KENDRICK, T., SIBBALD, B., BURNS, T., *et al* (1991) Role of general practitioners in care of long-term mentally ill patients. *British Medical Journal* **302**, 508–510.

MELZER, D., HALE, A. S., MALIK, S. J., *et al* (1991) Community care for patients with schizophrenia one year after hospital discharge. *British Medical Journal*, **303**, 1023–1026.

MUIJEN, M., MARKS, I., CONNOLLY, J., *et al* (1992) The Daily Living Programme. Preliminary comparison of community versus hospital-based treatment for the seriously mentally ill facing emergency admission. *British Journal of Psychiatry*, **160**, 379–384.

PARKES, C. M., BROWN, G. W. & MONCK, E. M. (1962) The general practitioner and the schizophrenic patient. *British Medical Journal*, *ii*, 972–976.

OFFICE OF POPULATION CENSUSES AND SURVEYS (1982) *Morbidity Statistics from General Practice: Second National Study 1970–71*. London: HMSO

PANTELIS, C., TAYLOR, J. & CAMPBELL, P. (1988) The South Camden Schizophrenia Survey. An experience of community-based research. *Bulletin of the Royal College of Psychiatrists*, **12**, 98–101.

PEREIRA GRAY, D. J. (1978) Feeling at home. *Journal of the Royal College of General Practitioners*, **28**, 6–17.

—— (1979) The key to personal care. *Journal of the Royal College of General Practitioners*, **29**, 666–678.

ROYAL COLLEGE OF GENERAL PRACTITIONERS BIRMINGHAM RESEARCH UNIT (1978) Practice activity analysis 4: psychotropic drugs. *Journal of the Royal College of General Practitioners*, **28**, 122–124.

SHEPHERD, M., COOPER, B., BROWN, A. C., *et al* (1966) *Psychiatric Illness in General Practice*. Oxford: Oxford University Press.

STEIN, L. I. & TEST, M. A. (1980) Alternative to mental hospital treatment I. Conceptual model, treatment program, and clinical evaluation. *Archives of General Psychiatry*, **37**, 392–397.

STOTT, N. & DAVIS, R. H. (1979) The exceptional potential in each primary care consultation. *Journal of the Royal College of General Practitioners*, **29**, 201–205.

WATT, D. C., KATZ, K. & SHEPHERD, M. (1983) The natural history of schizophrenia: a 5-year prospective follow-up of a representative sample of schizophrenics by means of a standardized clinical and social assessment. *Psychological Medicine*, **13**, 663–670.

WING, J. K. (1989) The concept of negative symptoms. *British Journal of Psychiatry*, **155** (suppl. 7), 10–14.

WOOFF, K. & GOLDBERG, D. P. Further observations on the practice of community care in Salford. Differences between community psychiatric nurses and mental health social workers. *British Journal of Psychiatry*, **153**, 30–37.

14 Drug abuse

JUDY GREENWOOD

Patterns of drug misuse have changed dramatically in the past 15 years, and continue to alter year by year. Not only has there been an increase in the prevalence of drug-taking, but also a change in the type of drugs misused, and in the age and social background of drug users. Doctors working in primary care, even in rural areas, are increasingly confronted with the challenge of working with drug misusers, and making decisions about drug management for which they are poorly trained.

The recent association of HIV transmission via shared needles among intravenous drug users has complicated the issue still further, and has led to a revision in medical thinking and an increase in the range of intervention strategies considered appropriate for the management of this difficult patient population.

In common with many other medical and behavioural problems, drug misuse is a relapsing condition, yet one from which 30–40% can ultimately emerge, provided they have not developed life-threatening complications. Current medical approaches to management stress the importance of offering help to people while drug misuse continues, in an attempt to limit harm, as well as offering treatment to those motivated to stop.

Drug misusers should be able to choose the type of service that seems relevant to their current needs, and for a variety of reasons, some choose to confide only in their GP. Others have little choice, for despite the range of services described below, they are patchily distributed. Most commonly, a drug user will be involved with several services, of which the GP's is one, necessitating good communication and coordination, to avoid confusion or deceit.

Alcohol and nicotine misuse are not covered in this chapter, although they remain the commonest drugs of misuse with by far the highest mortality and morbidity. Alcohol is discussed in Chapter 9.

Classification

Drug misuse implies drug-taking which is deemed harmful or unsanctioned by the society in which it occurs. Paradoxically, the legal consequences of certain forms of drug-taking, such as smoking cannabis, may prove more harmful than the drug itself. The drugs that are misused can be many and varied, and include a wide range of pharmaceutical products, illicit 'street' preparations, and sometimes common household substances, which may be ingested orally, by inhalation, intradermally, or intravenously.

Drug dependence describes a state of altered tolerance to a drug which produces physical and psychological withdrawal symptoms when the drug is abruptly discontinued. Many misused drugs do not lead to dependence. 'Drug misuse' thus covers the following diverse types of behaviour:

(a) intermittent experimentation with drugs (especially common in teenagers)
(b) regular involvement in illicit drug-taking with its associated lifestyle and social problems
(c) stable dependent use of pharmaceutical or controlled drugs, usually obtained by prescription.

The classification of drug misuse is further complicated by the fact that some drugs are controlled by the Misuse of Drugs Act, and therefore users must be notified to the Home Office by their doctors, whereas others which are equally harmful and misused are not subject to such requirements.

Table 14.1 illustrates some of the common types of drugs misused, whether they have a high risk of dependence, whether they are commonly injected, and whether they are notifiable.

Identification of drug misuse

In all new consultations, doctors should be prepared to inquire routinely about drug use as well as other health-related habits, such as alcohol and cigarette consumption.

Drug users may consult doctors in a variety of ways. Many may be already known to the GP as regular attenders for their conventional benzodiazepine prescription, on which they may have been dependent, for months or years. Some may present with a request for painkillers or tranquillisers for spurious symptoms, without revealing their drug dependence. Others may ask more directly for immediate relief of drug-withdrawal symptoms, or for treatment of their drug problem. They may exhibit sores around nose and mouth if glue-sniffing, puncture marks and scars on forearms, markedly constricted or dilated pupils, and unexplained diarrhoea or constipation, drowsiness or restlessness.

TABLE 14.1
Some commonly misused drugs

Type of drug	Dependency risk	Injectable	Notifiable
Opioids			
heroin	yes	yes	yes
methadone mixture	yes	no	yes
dipipanone (Diconal)	yes	yes	yes
buprenorphine (Temgesic)	yes	yes	no
dihydrocodeine (DF118)	yes	no	no
Benzodiazepines			
temazepam (Normison)	yes	yes	no
diazepam (Valium)	yes	no	no
Stimulants, etc.			
cocaine and crack	yes	yes	yes
amphetamines (speed)	no	yes	no
LSD (acid)	no	no	no
MDMA (ecstasy)	no	no	no
Cannabis	no	no	no
Volatile substances			
butane gas, solvents, glues, fire-extinguisher fluid	no	no	no

Some may present with the medical complications of their drug misuse – overdose, psychosis or withdrawal seizures – or the medical complications of injecting – thrombophlebitis, skin and systemic infections such as abscesses, septicaemia, endocarditis, hepatitis B or HIV infection, etc., many of which are potentially fatal.

A family doctor might also suspect drug misuse from less obvious signs such as breakdown in family or marital relationships, frequent court appearances for criminal behaviour associated with financing a drug habit, a deteriorating work pattern, or truancy from school. Some drug users seek medical help from personal choice, whereas others might be temporarily motivated by an imminent court appearance or the anxiety of a concerned relative.

Clinical ambivalence

Whatever the mode of presentation of a drug user, GPs and psychiatrists working in primary care should establish contact with this often hidden population, and guard against allowing a stereotyped judgemental attitude towards drug users in general to interfere in the quality of medical care offered to a particular patient who happens to misuse drugs.

Clinical ambivalence towards drug users is common, and may be caused by a variety of emotions, including anxiety stemming from inexperience and lack of appropriate medical training in their management, the fear of physical threat, and a lack of rapport and identification with the drug user's age, social situation, and behaviour. Doctors can feel deskilled by the drug user's knowledge of street drugs and their apparent capacity to confound pharmacological principles by the amount of drugs tolerated, and disillusioned by previous encounters with drug users who may have lied, manipulated and relapsed (common in drug dependence). Some doctors feel concerned about colleagues' disapproval if they demonstrate that they are prepared to work with drug users, or unnecessarily anxious that substitute prescribing might be criticised by the Home Office or local medical committee. Some do not realise that a special licence is not necessary in order to prescribe methadone.

Preliminary assessment of a drug user

Whether the initial consultation with a drug user has been because of health problems, a request for help with a drug problem, or a more direct request for drugs, the patient's needs should form the starting point, but often not the end-point, of what the doctor might assess to be appropriate management. The doctor should encourage the drug users to identify what they see as immediate and pressing problems, take a drug history, and attempt to decide what management and supports are needed, and what services are most appropriate to provide them.

The establishment of a sympathetic relationship and the health-education component of the first interview are critical elements in the management of a drug user, and may indeed be life-saving. They will also determine whether the patient returns for further help.

A drug history should include:

(a) type of drug used, quantity, frequency, route taken, and how obtained
(b) degree of dependence and withdrawal symptoms
(c) source of injecting equipment and whether shared
(d) drug-associated past and current health problems
(e) financial and legal problems
(f) family, relationship, and personal problems
(g) daily lifestyle and work
(h) other agencies involved, including past GP if relevant.

At the first interview, urine should be taken for drug-screening to confirm the history (most drugs are identifiable up to three days after ingestion), and information should be sought from other sources, such as relatives or other professionals. If using notifiable drugs (see Table 14.1), the drug user should be notified to the Home Office and, regardless of drugs used, should be reported also to the local drug misuse database.

If possible, physical examination should be performed and arrangements for special investigations or treatment made. Routine screening for HIV infection should not be encouraged without a full opportunity for patients to consider the implications of testing (possible insurance, mortgage or travel restrictions) and their ability to cope with an adverse result. Referral to a specialised HIV counselling and testing service may be possible.

It is usually unwise to prescribe substitute drugs of dependence at a first consultation, although relief of withdrawal symptoms by drugs such as diphenolate and atropine (Lomotil); thioridazine, promethazine or propanolol might be considered.

If other agencies are involved, such as a non-statutory drug agency, social worker or probation officer, it is advisable to seek the patient's permission to make contact with them to coordinate future support. If it is suspected that the patient has a duplicate GP or is masquerading as a temporary resident, this should be investigated further so that the patient can be confronted with this deception and, hopefully, the reasons behind it clarified. Such negative beginnings can be used constructively to promote future honesty, if the patient is not rejected as soon as deception is detected.

Health education

In all cases, the doctor should use this first consultation as an opportunity to ensure that the drug misuser has sufficient information to reduce the harm from drug misuse. This involves education about the danger of taking drugs when alone, the hazards of injecting, and especially the dangers of shared injecting equipment. Users of intravenous drugs should be advised how to obtain clean injecting equipment: sterilisation of used equipment should be undertaken by flushing needle and syringe through first with cold water, then drawing up concentrated bleach or slightly diluted washing-up detergent, and flushing it away – not back into the receptacle – then thoroughly flushing through three times with clean cold water.

The need for safer sex should also be discussed, and advice about where to obtain free condoms offered. The danger of accidental overdose when alcohol is mixed with drugs should also be stressed, together with the danger of driving under the influence of drugs.

Subsequent management of drug users in primary care

Stimulants and solvents

Young and casual experimenters in drug use, whether it be solvents such as glue-sniffing or stimulants such as amphetamines and ecstasy used at the weekend 'rave', may not acknowledge that their drug use is causing problems. But most forms of drug misuse involves law-breaking, excessive expenditure, and danger while under the influence of the drug, such as having unprotected sex, developing a psychosis, or dying from acute cardiac arrest or asphyxia. Drug misuse can also lead to an altered sleep pattern, poor school and work attendance, and a gradual deterioration in relationships and overall functioning. Even occasional injecting can lead to HIV infection. Prolonged experimentation and the regular use of drugs to alter emotions can lead to a wider range of substances being used, and the risk of an inexorable drift into chronic drug-taking and drug dependence with its attendant problems.

Therefore, the doctor should encourage such youngsters to show more concern for themselves (taking on a 'self-parenting' role), to keep an honest account of future drug use, and to follow them up for a few months to determine progress and perhaps uncover family tension which may be undeclared at first, but might be highly relevant to the rebellious teenager's persistent drug-taking. The doctor may be able to deal with this by arbitration at a family interview, taking care to avoid overidentification with the parent's position, or, if more serious, by referral to a local adolescent psychiatric or social service, bearing in mind the risk of adverse labelling and stigmatisation of a youngster at a critical time in development.

Opiates and benzodiazepines

The remainder of this chapter deals with opiate and benzodiazepine users and the management of drug dependence. Such patients often do not present for help until their drug dependence has been established for some years. Their problems are usually a disparate assortment of issues which might include health problems, the daily nightmare of procuring sufficient drugs to prevent withdrawal symptoms, debt and the fear of extortion and violence, criminal charges pending, housing problems, relationship problems, depression, anxiety, and sleeplessness, etc. The doctor might identify more fundamental problems, such as long-standing maturational problems associated with a deprived childhood, or the possibility of HIV infection, which it might not be appropriate to tackle at first.

Management strategies for the dependent drug user

The identification, initial assessment, and health education of a drug user in primary care have already been described, together with the need to identify and deal with current health and social problems and involve other services where relevant.

In addition to this, the family doctor might offer to play a more active role in attempting to alter the patient's drug-taking behaviour. Such an approach has been recommended by the Advisory Council on the Misuse of Drugs (1993) and the Department of Health (1991) in response to the concern about the increasing incidence of HIV infection in intravenous drug users, which is seen as a potentially greater threat to the nation's health than drug use itself.

They argue that medical drug management strategies should be divided into two categories:

(a) minimisation of harm for those unwilling or unable to come off drugs at the present time
(b) drug treatment for those who wish to be weaned from drug dependence.

Minimisation of harm

As drug misuse is a chronic condition, clinical management should aim wherever possible to reduce the harm of drug use, until such time that the patient can be encouraged to stop. In addition to health education and the provision of clean injecting equipment, and condoms, a doctor might also consider the option of offering substitute prescribing of oral opiates or benzodiazepines (or both) under agreed conditions, with the following objectives:

(a) to make and maintain contact with the drug user
(b) to reduce injecting and its dangerous consequences
(c) to reduce the need for criminal behaviour
(d) to stabilise oral drug intake, and lifestyle.

Prescribing guidelines

A GP may choose to prescribe substitute medication directly for a drug user, if the case seems relatively straightforward, or may prefer to refer to a drug consultant, should one be available in the area, for advice. A decision to start prescribing should not be considered until a full assessment of the patient has been made over time. The doctor should try to avoid being hassled into a precipitate decision by the drug user's persistence, sense of urgency, and coercion.

Deciding about the appropriate dosage is not easy, but it is advisable to start with a much lower dose than the drug user alleges he/she is taking, and increase it gradually should clear evidence of withdrawal symptoms be seen. Useful conversion tables of dose equivalents for opioids and benzodiazepines can be found in the Department of Health's (1991) handbook on drug misuse.

Benzodiazepine dependence may occur after a prolonged period of modest therapeutic medication, or as a result of the misuse of illicitly obtained supplies which are often taken in large amounts. Many polydrug users have twin dependencies on opioids and benzodiazepines, and may need substitute therapy for both. It is rarely necessary to give large doses of benzodiazepines to avoid withdrawal symptoms, although even with small doses, many patients report that benzodiazepines are harder to withdraw from than opioids. A longer-acting benzodiazepine such as diazepam should be given if possible. If temazepam is prescribed for night sedation, it should be in the form of hard gel to reduce the risk of injecting, although there is evidence that some drug users continue to inject this form, which can result in tissue damage.

Too little medication leads to manipulations, lies, and a return to the use of street drugs, and possible injecting; too much leads to oversedation and the risk of leakage into the illicit market. Regular consultations are thus necessary in the early stages of substitution therapy, in order to titrate the optimal dose, and, by means of urinalysis, to check that it is being taken by the patient.

Methadone mixture (1 mg in 1 ml), which has a 24-hour action, is more stabilising than dihydrocodeine (4–6 hour action), although it may be easier to withdraw from the latter.

Prescriptions should be written in the GP's own handwriting, with amounts of methadone written in words and figures.

Daily dispensing is to be preferred until the drug use is totally stable. It is often useful to liaise with the local pharmacist over such matters, as he/she will see the drug user even more frequently than the GP.

Terms of an agreement

Linking the prescription to a signed agreement may be helpful and can include:

(a) being seen regularly by one partner only
(b) avoiding harassment of surgery staff
(c) having random urine checks
(d) avoiding street drugs
(e) no replacement of lost medication.

A pragmatic doctor will use these terms in a 'flexibly rigid' way, and may expect occasional lapses but not regular infringements. If chaos persists, it suggests the drug user is not capable of sustaining a harm-reduction programme at that stage, and may need to be reviewed for treatment after a cooling off period without a prescription probably back on street drugs. Experience suggests that younger drug users cope least well with the constraints of harm reduction, yet are the most at risk of harming themselves.

Particularly difficult prescribing decisions may have to be made not only with new and younger drug users, but also with those just out of prison, who are most at risk of accidental overdose, and pregnant women, who may be highly motivated by the pregnancy to deal with their drug problem. A shared decision with her obstetrician to embark on a reduction programme may be the chosen treatment plan.

Drug users who are HIV positive may be particularly helped by the predictability and stability of prescribed drugs, and any approach that reduces their injecting and the risk of contaminated needles being shared must be welcomed. Prescribing for drug users untested for HIV also ensures that they are in regular medical contact, should they unexpectedly develop pneumocystis carinii pneumonia, or other Aids-related symptoms. A drug misuser should be advised not to drive, although, if stable, long-term maintenance is reached, the doctor and drug user may wish to discuss the possibility of medical exemption with the Driver and Vehicle Licensing Centre.

Drug treatment (detoxification or withdrawal from drugs)

Often drug users will express a strong desire to give up their drug dependency, while at the same time admitting that they fear they cannot cope with the emotional stress and possible sleeplessness without recourse to the drugs on which they have learnt to rely. They may be persuaded to contemplate a gradual withdrawal regime over which they can share some control.

Others are more committed and motivated to withdraw from drugs straight away, an objective that may prove more difficult than at first realised. Unrealistic aims by doctor or patient are likely to lead to disappointment and demoralisation and to challenge their subsequent relationship, especially if an inflexible timescale for achieving goals is adopted. A reduction schedule should be tailored to the drug user's motivation rather than the doctor's if it is to have any chance of success.

For many drug users, the desire to withdraw from drugs becomes the natural longer-term result of harm minimisation once the first objectives have been achieved and the drug misuser has become psychologically and physically healthier. They may have learnt new ways of coping with stress, which will need constant reinforcement from the doctor during the reduction programme.

Opioid or benzodiazepine withdrawal programmes can be conducted gradually in the community by means of a reducing prescription, which might involve a reduction in the daily dose of 5 mg at weekly intervals for either drug. If the drug user is dependent on both benzodiazepines and opioids, alternating the reduction of first one drug and then the other can sometimes be useful. If the patient experiences unpleasant withdrawal symptoms at any stage, he/she might be allowed an extra week or two at the same dosage until the symptoms have lessened. Any lapse back to old habits should be discussed and used as a learning experience rather than seen depressingly as a relapse. It is unusual for a drug user to withdraw smoothly without encountering some difficulty.

A more rapid detoxification programme for opioid dependency is possible in a specialist residential drug unit, and this might be followed by a more extended period of residential rehabilitation in a therapeutic community. Withdrawal from even modest amounts of benzodiazepines, however, is often prolonged, and therefore better suited to community management, and preferably accompanied by the support of a local self-help tranquilliser group, if available.

Withdrawal symptoms

Opioid withdrawal symptoms are relatively easy to detect, and begin within 24 hours of stopping regular use, and can continue for up to three weeks. They include vomiting and diarrhoea, restlessness, irritability and anxiety with disordered sleep, joint and bone pains, lachrymation and yawning, shivering and sweating, and dilated pupils.

Benzodiazepine withdrawal symptoms are more subjective and less easily observed by the clinician, but have been clearly documented in the drug treatment of patients with no premorbid emotional problems. They may develop days or even weeks after stopping treatment and can continue for many months. They include anxiety, insomnia, tremor, nausea, feelings of unreality, abnormal body sensations, oversensitivity to noise and light, withdrawal fits, and occasional psychosis.

What other services support drug users?

Generic services

Many of the problems associated with drug misuse, such as housing, legal and welfare, are not primarily medical. Once identified, they can be better dealt with by other, more relevant agencies, although a letter of referral and support from a concerned and interested family doctor may help a socially alienated drug misuser to be treated with more dignity than is often the case. This is particularly so if questions of child custody arise, when the GP, health visitor and social worker each has an important role in ensuring that the needs of the child and its drug-using parents are fully considered. Drug misuse *per se* does not form sufficient grounds for a child's removal into care, and the family doctor may at times be the only advocate of the parents.

Specialist drug services

Community drug agencies

Specialist non-medical drug agencies work with and support drug misusers in many areas, usually working in community projects. The doctor and the patient should become familiar with the services available locally. These might be run by social services, by non-statutory (voluntary) agencies, or as self-help groups led by reformed drug users or concerned relatives. These can offer informal drop-in facilities, family support and counselling, and general help with legal, housing and welfare problems, and many will visit a drug user who is in prison.

Most are prepared to work with drug users while they are still using drugs, although a few are rigorously abstinence-orientated and will only see a drug user highly committed to staying off drugs.

Residential establishments

Non-statutory, religious and private agencies offer long-term drug rehabilitation programmes, which use a variety of differing philosophies and techniques. Most insist that the user has become drug-free before admission, a condition which precludes many well motivated drug users if no local residential drug-detoxification facilities exist in which to become drug-free. Those receiving DSS benefits from the Department of Social Security can usually be funded via social services, while others face a means-assessed charge.

A useful directory of residential establishments (*Drug Problems. Where to Get Help*) is available from the Standing Committee on Drugs and Alcohol (SCODA, 1–4 Hatton Place, London EC1 8ND), and local social services should provide details of drug agencies in each region.

Psychiatric drug services

Many regions in Britain now have specialised psychiatric drug services which run in-patient and out-patient treatment programmes for drug users. Other areas have multidisciplinary community drug teams, which may or may not include a clinician (not always a psychiatrist). Larger cities also have needle and syringe exchange services, which may operate from a fixed site, a mobile bus, or through local pharmacists; doctors working in primary care should be familiar with these local services, also remembering that they too are permitted to provide clean injecting equipment and condoms if necessary.

Does harm minimisation work?

There have been many studies worldwide which show the benefits of methadone programmes in maintaining contact with drug users, reducing injecting and crime, lowering the risk of HIV infection, and improving the quality of life. The prevalence of injecting among Edinburgh's drug users has dropped dramatically since the introduction of a methadone programme which involves shared care of drug users by the Community Drug Problem Service, whose staff see the drug user regularly, usually at home, and the GP, who prescribes for the drug users and therefore also has regular contact with them. Over time, more patients are regaining their self-esteem and dignity, and beginning to risk a reduction in their daily dosage. A few are now drug-free, several on work-training programmes, and most are staying out of prison. But it must be assumed that harm minimisation is a long-term commitment, especially in this era of high unemployment in the areas from which many drug users come. There is little to tempt them back to a more constructive lifestyle at present.

Undoubtedly, in the long term, politicians will have the main role to play in conquering the malaise, the family breakdown, the lack of amenities, and wave of drug-taking that has beset the more deprived areas of Britain. But until these more fundamental social changes occur, the range of services attempting to support those who have become ensnared in chronic drug misuse will not be out of work.

It is a challenge to the medical profession working in primary care and community-based psychiatric services to dovetail their medical contribution into the range of management options available to drug users in the community, while acknowledging the important support offered by the non-statutory sector, and the importance of primary prevention by good drug-education initiatives in schools, and law enforcement policies that help to keep supplies of illegal drugs away from potential new recruits.

References

ADVISORY COUNCIL ON THE MISUSE OF DRUGS (1993) *Aids and Drug Misuse Update.* London: HMSO.
DEPARTMENT OF HEALTH (1991) *Drug Misuse and Dependence, Guidelines on Clinical Management.* London: HMSO.

15 Sleep problems

IAN PULLEN and GREG WILKINSON

Poor sleep is an extremely common complaint, but one that causes a great deal of distress. Many people fear that their health will be compromised if they fail to have eight hours' sleep a night. Such fears appear to be misplaced, as most people do get an adequate amount of sleep. But it is this failure of sleep to live up to expectations that leads so many people to seek help.

Insomnia is not a disease – it is a symptom, a complaint (Oswald, 1988). It may be part of a syndrome requiring specific treatment (e.g. depression), but commonly it is education rather than treatment that is most helpful.

This chapter tackles the question 'What is normal sleep?' before considering the different complaints about sleep and their management.

What is normal sleep?

Just as height and intelligence are normally distributed in the population (represented by a bell-shaped curve), so probably is the duration of sleep for any particular age group. Thus, while the majority of young adults will happily spend six to eight hours asleep each night, there are a minority who regularly sleep for as little as three or four hours, or for as much as 10–11 hours a night. They will be just as happy with their sleep and remain just as healthy. It is normal for them.

The structure of sleep, as denoted by electrical brain waves, develops and changes over time. Pre-school children tend to fall into very deep sleep (stage 4 sleep) almost immediately, during which almost nothing will wake them. They usually have an afternoon sleep and are also likely to wake during the night. By puberty there is still much very deep sleep and wakings are few. Afternoon drowsiness may continue throughout life. With advancing age there is a further reduction in deeper sleep (stages 3 and 4), with an increase in light sleep (stage 2) and drowsiness (stage 1). Older people wake more often, from a generally lighter sleep.

Babies wake and sleep throughout the 24 hours, but children have to learn to fall asleep at the appropriate time of day. This is best achieved by a regular regime and through a calm and reassuring bedtime routine – a drink of milk, a warm bath, a bedtime story, etc. Once a regular 24-hour rhythm is established, sleepiness is reinforced by the routine.

A night's sleep is made up of approximately 90-minute cycles. Each cycle contains a 15–20-minute period of rapid eye movement (REM) sleep, during which active dreaming occurs. The depth of sleep during the rest of the cycle is variable and rated from 1 to 4 (lightest to deepest).

The purpose of sleep

Much is now known about the physiology of sleep, but the function of sleep remains obscure. It is however possible to draw some conclusions. Sleep seems to be more important for the brain than for the body.

Whereas the fine regulation of certain autonomic systems may be affected by prolonged sleep deprivation, psychological testing shows that psychological changes occur quite quickly. Impaired concentration and efficiency can be detected after a night of only three hours' sleep, but complex tests of IQ and decision-making show little effect of sleep deprivation until the second day. After being kept awake for 60 hours or more visual misinterpretations (illusions) and suspiciousness may appear.

Experimental sleep deprivation gives an interesting insight into the 'catching up' process after prolonged loss of sleep. One rather longer night's sleep is all that is required for psychological performance to improve dramatically. The total length of 'extra' sleep over the next few days amounts to only about a third of the total sleep that was lost. However, this extra sleep is made up of stage 4 and REM sleep rather than the lighter sleep (stages 1 and 2) that were lost.

Factors that alter sleep

Many environmental factors will alter sleep length and timing. Some, such as caffeine, are universally recognised, but other equally common factors are less well known and may well seem surprising. These are listed under separate headings below.

Causes of reduced length of night-time sleep

(a) Common – requiring advice
  (i) Sleeping during the day
  (ii) Dieting leading to weight loss
  (iii) Caffeine
  (iv) Nicotine
  (v) Change of routine – shiftwork (jetlag)

(b) Common – requiring counselling
   (i) Increasing age
   (ii) Abuse of stimulant drugs – amphetamines, cocaine, crack
   (iii) Prescribed drugs – antidepressants (selective serotonin reuptake inhibitors (SSRIs), monoamine oxidase inhibitors (MAOIs))
   (iv) Withdrawal of hypnotics, tranquillisers
(c) Less common – requiring treatment
   (i) Depressive illness
   (ii) Alcohol, barbiturate withdrawal
   (iii) Pain
   (iv) Weight loss not due to dieting
   (v) Dementia
(d) Uncommon – requiring treatment
   (i) Hyperthyroidism
   (ii) Hypomania

Causes of increased sleep length

(a) Common – requiring advice
   (i) Boredom associated with unemployment
   (ii) Weight gain
   (iii) Sudden increase in physical exercise
(b) Common – requiring counselling
   (i) Abuse of sedative drugs
   (ii) Starting some medication – tricyclic antidepressants
(c) Less common – requiring treatment
   (i) Depressive illness
   (ii) Hypothyroidism
   (iii) Schizophrenia

Causes of waking too early

(a) Common – requiring advice
   (i) Going to sleep too early
   (ii) Sleeping more by day
   (iii) Alcohol
   (iv) Dieting leading to weight loss
   (v) Bedroom too cold/hot/noisy
   (vi) Change of routine – shift work (jetlag)
(b) Common – requiring counselling
   (i) Increasing age
   (ii) Hypnotics – especially short-acting
   (iii) Daytime benzodiazepines – shorter-acting

   (c) Less common – requiring treatment
       (i) Depressive illness
       (ii) Weight loss not due to dieting
       (iii) Pain
   (d) Uncommon – requiring treatment
       (i) Hyperthyroidism
       (ii) Hypomania

Causes of difficulty getting off to sleep

   (a) Common – requiring advice
       (i) Retiring to bed too early
       (ii) Sleeping too late in the morning
       (iii) Daytime naps
       (iv) No bedtime routine
       (v) Evening stimulants – caffeine (including tea and many soft drinks)
                                  – nicotine
       (vi) Lack of physical exercise
       (vii) Hunger/indigestion
       (viii) Bedroom too cold/hot
       (ix) Fear of not sleeping
       (x) Change of routine
   (b) Common – requiring counselling
       (i) Major life events – bereavement, marriage, promotion, retire-
           ment, etc.
       (ii) Stress – work-related, marital difficulties, financial, exam-
            inations, etc.
       (iii) Withdrawal from hypnotics and tranquillisers
   (c) Less common – requiring treatment
       (i) Anxiety
       (ii) Depression
       (iii) Alcohol withdrawal
       (iv) Opiate, barbiturate withdrawal
       (v) Prescribed drugs – MAOIs, SSRIs, slimming preparations
       (vi) Pain
   (d) Uncommon – requiring treatment
       (i) Hypomania
       (ii) Hyperthyroidism.

Summary

So normal sleep duration and pattern will respond to a variety of environmental changes. Perhaps the most universal is the tendency for sleep length
to be longer in winter months than during the summer. Physiological

changes brought about by losing or gaining weight, through either dieting or illness, produce marked changes to sleep pattern. Increased physical exercise is associated with longer sleep, while smoking is associated with shorter sleep, smokers sleeping on average half an hour less per night than non-smokers.

Once established in childhood, bedtime routines induce preparedness for sleep. This may be upset by the simple alteration to routine resulting from sleeping in a strange bed, to the more dramatic alteration brought about by flying to a different time zone or changing from daytime working to a night shift.

These changes bring about 'normal' adjustments to sleep which, in time, will revert to the individual's new environment. However, any of the above may lead to uncertainty, and the request for help to 'put things right'. The individual is getting the sleep that he/she requires. It is essential that the doctor does not collude with the patient's view that 'a good night's sleep will put everything right'. To do so, would be to fall into the trap of treating symptoms rather than understanding the aetiology and conveying this to the patient.

What then should we make of the legions of patients who complain of 'poor sleep'?

'Poor sleep'

People who complain of poor sleep tend to be dissatisfied with the time it takes for them to fall asleep, the number of times they wake during the night, the time they awake in the morning, and how they feel on waking. They may feel unrefreshed and blame many of their daytime problems on their poor sleep. They are more likely to be women than men, and older rather than young.

Sleep is obviously a very subjective experience. How accurate are people in assessing and reporting their sleep? Oswald (1988) has reviewed people's claims and matched them with objective observation in sleep laboratories. The findings are summarised in Table 15.1.

Studies comparing 'good' and 'poor' sleepers suggest there is considerable overlap between the two groups. Those who complain of poor sleep appear

TABLE 15.1
Observed versus subjective experiences of sleep

Complaint	Laboratory observation
No sleep for days/years	All slept, some up to six hours
Two hours to get off to sleep	Twenty minutes to fall asleep
Only four hours' sleep a night	About six hours' sleep a night

less accurate in their perception of their sleep, but they do on average sleep about half an hour less per night than good sleepers, and wake more often.

Assessment – the sleep history

While it is often possible to recognise the immediate cause (e.g. recent stress), many GPs will find it impossible to assess complaints about sleep in a single seven-minute consultation. It is not possible to do justice to such a complex issue in that time. It is reasonable to explain this to the patient and to defer any management decision until sufficient information has been obtained. Premature decision-making on the basis of inadequate information may result in the prescription of inappropriate treatment, resulting in a longer-term problem for the patient and doctor.

Sleep diary

The patient should be asked to keep a simple sleep diary until the next appointment (probably in a couple of weeks). The patient should record the following each day:

(a) time in bed
(b) time asleep
(c) waking during night
(d) time of final waking
(e) time getting up
(f) daytime sleep

In addition, it would be helpful to have the following recorded for at least one week:

(a) drinks consumed after 6 p.m.
(b) cigarettes consumed after 6 p.m.
(c) time of last meal
(d) drinks/cigarettes consumed during night
(e) mood
(f) any recurrent thoughts on waking in night
(g) timing of any medication (prescribed or otherwise)

Collection of such data may have prevented the misinterpretations illustrated in cases 1–5 (below) from occurring:

Case 1

Miss A, a 70-year-old single woman, was referred for psychiatric assessment because of persistent early morning waking. She could not sleep after 1 a.m. despite taking nitrazepam each night. A simple sleep diary showed that she retired to bed each evening at 7 p.m. because she was bored. She fell asleep almost immediately with the help of the hypnotic and slept for six hours, that is, after a relatively normal night's sleep, but at the wrong time.

Case 2

Mr B, an unemployed teenage youth, demanded sleeping tablets from his GP because he was unable to have a wink of sleep before 6 a.m. The hypnotic made little difference to this situation. The sleep diary graphically pointed out the problem to the patient before he returned to the clinic. He recognised that the problem was not the duration of his sleep, but the timing. He was sleeping each day until 2 p.m., and not getting up until 3 p.m., except on the days that he had to 'sign on'. When he had a reason for getting up he could. On other days he would sleep for as long as he could.

Case 3

Mrs C, a 30-year-old mother of two young children, complained of difficulty getting to sleep and disturbed, unrefreshing sleep. A sleep diary showed that she was going to bed earlier and earlier to try to obtain 'a decent night's sleep'. She would get up at 8 a.m. to get the children off to school, but then return to bed to 'catch up' after a bad night. In fact although she was asleep for only 60% of the time she was in bed, this still amounted to about 8 hours.

Case 4

Miss D, a 20-year-old student, complained of poor sleep. She found that she had difficulty both getting to sleep and staying asleep. Her sleep had dropped from eight hours a night to only five or six. The diary revealed that she was eating nothing in the evening, but consuming large amounts of low-calorie cola drinks as well as smoking excessively. Follow-up questions revealed that she had been actively trying to lose weight by dieting, with considerable success.

Case 5

Mr E, a 50-year-old divorced man, complained of persistent early morning waking, feeling at his worst in the morning, but improving as the day wore on. He was already taking temazepam at night and was asking for something stronger. A diagnosis of depression was considered. A sleep diary showed the extent of a previously unrecognised alcohol problem which led to early waking. He tended to feel less unwell at lunchtime, when he had his first drink of the day.

Interpretation of the sleep diary

The above illustrative case histories were chosen to demonstrate different commonly occurring problems. Even if the diary is not as clear-cut as the above, it should indicate:

(a) total time the patient feels he/she is asleep
(b) total time spent in bed
(c) behaviour during evening.

This should then be compared with the patient's expectations of sleep, the 'normal' sleep for someone of that age and particular situation, and the factors set out above (pp. 222–224).

Education

Much can be achieved by simple education of the patient about sleep. The information given by the doctor may be enhanced by suggesting the purchase of one of the good self-help books available (see reference list). Knowing that most people do get the appropriate sleep for their particular needs is information that most patients require. In addition they need to know which of their behaviours may be contributing to their dissatisfaction with their sleep. (Sample information to be given to patients is given in the Appendix.)

Management plan

Most sleep problems can be helped without recourse to drugs. But to be effective, patient and doctor must understand what is planned and why.

Case 1

Miss A had to acknowledge that no medication would reasonably extend her sleep beyond the amount she was already getting. It was for her to decide when in the 24 hours she wished to be asleep. She reluctantly agreed to go to bed later, but still harboured the wish to be unconscious for half of the 24 hours.

Case 2

Mr B had interpreted the sleep diary correctly. He too was getting the correct amount of sleep but at the wrong time. He decided not to change the pattern – he would get up when he had something specific to get up for, otherwise he would watch television with friends until very late and sleep until he awoke, whenever that was. This pattern changed once he obtained a job.

Case 3

Mrs C fell into the trap of believing that she was unable to sleep because she was 'overtired', hence the decision to retire to bed ever earlier. She accepted that the total time she spent asleep was normal and that her problem was the time she spent in bed awake and wishing she was asleep. She agreed to experiment with going to bed later than ever before, and not returning to bed after the children had gone to school. The result was much less time in bed but not sleeping, and much less distress.

Case 4

Miss D had never heard of the link between dieting and waking early, nor had she realised the increased amount of caffeine she was consuming in the soft drinks. Her attention had been on calories rather than caffeine. She agreed to study the ingredients of soft drinks and to avoid any containing caffeine. She accepted that her sleep would improve once her weight stabilised. In addition she was given a follow-up appointment to check that the dieting was not getting out of hand.

Case 5

Mr E refused to consider reducing his consumption of alcohol and indicated that he did not accept the link between his drinking and his sleep problem. He did agree to reduce his consumption of temazepam, and this was withdrawn without any change to his sleep pattern. It had to be accepted that he was not yet ready to tackle his drink problem, but at least it had been identified.

Not all stories end happily and we cannot solve all problems. But we can try not to compound existing problems by premature drug treatment.

Additional factors to be considered are the level of physical activity, changing sensitivity to stimulants, and drug withdrawal. Most people feel tired after an unusual amount of physical exertion, but even smaller amounts of physical activity improves sleep. As people get older, tolerance to many substances changes. Few recognise that their habitual caffeine consumption may in older age be the cause of their sleep disturbance. Many people who get up in the night and find they cannot get back to sleep make themselves a comforting cup of tea and have a cigarette 'to relax'. Few seem to know that tea contains caffeine or that nicotine, while inducing a sensation of relaxation, is in fact a stimulant. Finally, nor do many patients consider that their remedy for poor sleep, be it hypnotic, alcohol or early night, may be compounding their difficulties.

Hypnotics

The demand for tablets to enhance sleep remains high, despite a general awareness that there are major problems associated with prolonged use of benzodiazepines (see Chapter 16). Recently non-benzodiazepine hypnotics have been introduced, which the manufacturers claim will not lead to similar problems. Other sedative drugs such as low-dose amitriptyline have been suggested as an alternative to hypnotics 'in case the sleep disturbance is secondary to depression'. This practice is illogical, since such a low dose of antidepressant will have little effect on depression.

Traditionally hypnotics have been used in the following situations (clearly described in the *British National Formulary* 1992).

(a) Transient insomnia – this may occur in those who normally sleep well, and is usually related to extraneous factors (e.g. shift work, jetlag).
(b) Short-term insomnia – usually related to an emotional problem or serious medical illness.
(c) Chronic insomnia – often due to mild dependence caused by injudicious prescribing, and may be related to anxiety, depression, drug or alcohol abuse.

It should be borne in mind that many people fail to adjust to shift working, especially as they get older (Waterhouse, 1993). The prescription of hypnotics in all of the above situations has been questioned, particularly their long-term use. More recently concern has been raised about the effect of hypnotics on normal coping. There are theoretical reasons for believing that they may interfere with normal grieving and should therefore be avoided, but such an outlook may be inhumane. Recognition of the cognitive impairment lasting into the next day has led to their abandonment before examinations or driving tests. Primary psychiatric conditions should be treated appropriately.

Tolerance, dependence and withdrawal

Tolerance appears to develop to most hypnotics alarmingly quickly, leading many patients to increase the dose. But for many the original stress will have quickly diminished, removing the need for continued medication. Other people appear to use the same dose for years without encountering problems.

Withdrawal leads to shortened, more disturbed sleep, with more dreaming. Daytime anxiety may also be experienced. Many patients mistake this syndrome for the original symptoms for which the hypnotic was prescribed and assume they should continue the 'treatment'. After trying to withdraw on a few occasions they may exert considerable pressure on their doctor for prescriptions to continue.

There are individual differences, so that while most patients have few withdrawal symptoms, in others disturbed sleep and other symptoms are much more severe for a week or two.

Safe prescribing

Assessment:

(a) the extent of the sleep problem must be clarified
(b) insomnia secondary to treatable conditions (e.g. depression) should have been excluded
(c) non-drug management should have been tried

(d) there must be the prospect of the situation changing (e.g. a date for the move of house; chronic distress and insomnia due to marital disharmony for which neither partner agrees to counselling is unlikely to change).

Before prescription the following must be discussed:

(a) the purpose of the prescription
(b) the duration of prescribing must be fixed
(c) the problems of rebound wakefulness
(d) the desirability of not taking the tablets every night
(e) a ban on any increase above the agreed dose
(f) a ban on taking the tablets during the day
(g) no repeat prescriptions will be issued without an appointment or before an agreed date.

Prescription:

(a) moderately short-acting preparation
(b) small quantities
(c) lowest effective dose
(d) shortest possible time
(e) a review date must be set.

Withdrawal will be aided by:

(a) reducing the dose before stopping
(b) providing support.

These guidelines should apply to all doctors prescribing hypnotics. Hospital doctors (including psychiatrists) should be selective about the prescription of hypnotics and try to withdraw the patient *before* discharge, and not only discontinue the medication as the patient leaves hospital.

While most 'chronic insomnia' is a feature of older people of nervous temperament, much chronic insomnia is iatrogenic or due to psychiatric illness or abuse of alcohol or drugs. These require thorough investigation.

Depression

Most psychiatric textbooks draw attention to depression as a cause of sleep disturbance. Early morning waking (EMW) is one of the cardinal signs of major depressive illness. The discovery of EMW should provoke questions about appetite, weight, mood, mood throughout the day, and energy levels.

EMW on its own does not indicate depressive illness, but may be a pointer to it, to be confirmed by measurable weight loss, lack of energy, diurnal mood variation, and low self-regard. It is important to ask about the thoughts running through the mind in those early hours – happy thoughts, or unhappy thoughts?

It may be that the EMW associated with depression is due to weight loss rather than the depressive illness *per se*. It will improve only when the depression has been adequately treated and weight improves.

Alcohol abuse mimics both physical and psychiatric disorders. It too can produce EMW (see case 5, above).

Other disorders of sleep

This chapter has dealt with the most common sleep problems presenting in general practice, the complaint of 'poor sleep'. A number of other sleep disorders that may rarely be encountered are shown in Table 15.2. Further information on these is given by Oswald (1988).

TABLE 15.2
Other disorders of sleep

Condition	Management
Snoring	Reduce weight, stop drinking alcohol
Nightmares	Support for any anxieties, advice about alcohol/drugs
Night terrors	Support for any anxieties, trial of benzodiazepine
Bruxism	Stop psychotropic or appetite-suppressing drugs
Narcolepsy (recurring daytime sleep)	Specialist advice
Hypersomnia	Reduce weight, caffeine
Sleep apnoea	Specialist advice

Appendix. Information for patients

Sleep

Not everybody needs eight hours of sleep a night. As we get older we often need no more than five or six hours' sleep a night. The older we get, the longer it takes to get off to sleep, the more frequently we wake during the night, and the less total sleep we have. The amount of sleep we need also depends on the amount of physical activity we undertake and our state of health.

In general we get the amount of sleep our body and mind needs, but sometimes it occurs at the wrong time.

Causes of disturbed sleep

Stimulants. Much difficulty sleeping is caused by a high intake of caffeine in tea or coffee, as well as in cola drinks. As we get older we may become more sensitive to this. Nicotine in cigarettes is also a stimulant.

Rebound effect of sedative drugs. Many sedative drugs that induce sleep or reduce anxiety have the opposite effect when their effect is wearing off. Some sleeping tablets have this effect. Alcohol has a similar effect. This results in getting off to sleep quickly, but waking up early with difficulty getting back to sleep.

Changing activities. People who do shift work may find it difficult to adjust to changing sleep and activity patterns. Similar problems may arise on holiday, especially when long-distance travel and changes of climate are involved.

Physical illness. Pain is a common cause of disturbed sleep. In addition to breathing difficulties, a chronic cough or the need to pass water frequently may interrupt your sleep.

Coping with disturbed sleep

It is helpful to make a daily diary of your sleep pattern, because this will show you whether the problem is as bad as you thought and whether it is getting worse, better, or staying much the same over a period. It will also help you to judge whether anything you have tried to improve your sleep has had any effect. Record the times you sleep in each 24 hours. Record the quality of each sleep (e.g. restful, fitful, dozing). Note whether the sleep was in bed, in a chair, or in front of the television. Note whether you used anything to help you sleep (e.g. drug, hot drink, relaxation).

Hints on getting to sleep

► Try not to worry about the amount of sleep you have, this makes things worse.

► Go to bed at a regular time.

► If you find that you have been going to bed too early, go to bed a quarter to half an hour later each evening for a week or so until your sleep improves.

► If you wake tired in the morning, try bringing your bedtime forward a quarter to half an hour until you wake refreshed and not too early.

► Avoid sleeping during the day and reduce the number of naps you have so that you are more tired at bedtime.

► Eat your evening meal at a regular time, several hours before you go to bed.

► Avoid stimulating drinks (including tea, coffee and colas) and tobacco close to bedtime.

► A warm milk drink before bed helps to relax and will stop hunger pangs.

► A warm bath may also help you to relax at bedtime.

► A regular routine at bedtime helps you get into the frame of mind for sleep.

► Try to make the bedroom comfortable and warm.

► Try to avoid reading or listening to the radio in bed unless you have found these are particularly useful ways of helping you relax.

► Avoid sedative drugs (unless specially prescribed by your doctor) and alcohol – these may actually wake you up as their sedative effects wear off.

► Try a relaxation exercise comfortably in bed and repeat this until you drift off.

► If you are unable to sleep because you are worrying and cannot put your problems out of your mind: get up; write down exactly what your problem is; write a list of solutions to the problem; choose a solution that you can begin the next day; plan exactly how you would carry out the plan.

► Do not lie awake for longer than 30 minutes. If you still cannot sleep, get up and find a constructive activity. Read a book or magazine, write a letter, do some housework, play some music, or listen to the radio.

► Return to bed only when you feel sleepy. Get up again if you are not asleep in 30 minutes. Repeat this until you sleep.

► However late you get to sleep, get up at a reasonable hour, no later than 8 a.m. (set the alarm before you go to bed).

► Remember your body will let you have only the amount of sleep you require.

Acknowledgement

The authors are grateful to Professor Ian Oswald for his helpful comments on an earlier draft of this chapter.

References

BRITISH NATIONAL FORMULARY (1992) *British National Formulary, Number 23*. London: British Medical Association/Royal Pharmaceutical Society of Great Britain.

HORNE, J. A. (1988) *Why We Sleep: The Functions of Sleep in Humans and Other Mammals*. Oxford: Oxford University Press.

OSWALD, I. (1988) Sleep disorders. In *Companion to Psychiatric Studies* (eds R. E. Kendell & A. K. Zealley) (4th edn). Edinburgh: Churchill Livingstone.

WATERHOUSE, J. (1993) ABC of sleep disorders: circadian rhythms. *British Medical Journal*, **306**, 448–451.

Further reading

OSWALD, I. & ADAM, K. (1983) *Get a Better Night's Sleep*. London: Macdonald Optima.

16 Benzodiazepines in general practice

KIERAN SWEENEY and
MARGARET CORMACK

When the benzodiazepines were first introduced, with Librium (chlordiazepoxide) in 1960, they replaced barbiturates and were thought to be safe in overdose and non-addictive. There was a steady rise in the prescribing of these drugs until a peak was reached in 1979, when almost 31 million prescriptions were written. By 1985 the number of prescriptions had dropped to 26 million, and by 1988 to 22 million (Department of Health, 1990).

When the benzodiazepines are separated into hypnotic and tranquillising prescriptions, different trends emerge. Benzodiazepines prescribed as hypnotics were prescribed increasingly throughout the 1970s, from under 5 million items at the beginning of that decade, to 13 million at the beginning of the next decade, and then levelled off to remain at 13 million in 1988. In contrast, benzodiazepines prescribed as tranquillisers reached a peak of 18 million in 1978. Since then, there has been a gradual decline to half that amount – 9 million prescriptions in 1988. From separate surveys, Taylor (1987) and Ashton & Golding (1989) calculated that there were 1.2 million users of benzodiazepines in Britain.

Between the two community surveys by Balter (Balter *et al*, 1974; Mellinger & Balter, 1984) there was little change in the numbers of people who took the drugs, but there was an increase in the number of prescriptions issued. This indicated that there had been a move away from new prescriptions towards an increase in the numbers of repeat prescriptions. Many of these long-term users were taking hypnotic benzodiazepines, and most of these people were elderly (King *et al*, 1982; Williams, 1983*a*; Rodrigo *et al*, 1988; Dunbar *et al*, 1989; King *et al*, 1990).

Patterns of benzodiazepine use

In a study by Dunbar *et al* (1989) of over 4000 subjects, 7.7% had taken benzodiazepines within the previous year, with nearly twice as many women as men taking the drugs (9.7% of women and 5.4% of men). Those aged 65 years and over were the highest users of hypnotics, and those aged 45–54 years were the highest users of anxiolytics. Many of the subjects were long-term users: just under half had taken the drugs for more than 12 months and three-quarters of the over 65s had done so. Interestingly, users of benzodiazepines consistently reported more physical illness than non-users. This association between physical ill health and benzodiazepine consumption was also noted by Ashton & Golding (1989).

Ashton & Golding (1989) found that 4.2% of women and 2.1% of men were taking tranquillisers or hypnotics on the day of a household survey of 9000 subjects. This survey found that the prevalence of tranquilliser use was three times higher for people who rated themselves as suffering from physical ill health according to a symptom check-list. Also, unemployed people were three times more likely to take tranquillisers or hypnotics than were those in full-time employment, and those in the manual socio-economic group were higher users of the drugs than those in the non-manual group. These findings are compatible with those of the Black report (Department of Health and Social Security, 1980).

The implications of these patterns of use for GPs are that from an average list size of 2000 patients, 60 of these would be long-term users of benzodiazepines (Holden, 1989). Of these, 45 would be over the age of 60, half of them would have been taking the medication for more than five years, and the majority of these patients would be women.

Patterns of alcohol use

During the time of increase in benzodiazepine prescribing there was a parallel increase in the consumption of alcohol. Between 1960 and 1980 there was a 40% increase in tranquillising benzodiazepine use in Britain, and at the same time there was a 66% increase in per capita alcohol consumption (Taylor, 1987). However, if the trends of alcohol use and benzodiazepine consumption are examined by age and gender, a different picture emerges. Thus, alcohol consumption in the 20–30-year age group tends to be about twice that recorded by those over the age of 65. More men than women drink alcohol regularly (Wilson, 1980): 27% of men but only 3% of women consume more than 21 units per week.

The pharmacology of benzodiazepines

Absorption and fate

Diazepam is completely absorbed from the gastrointestinal tract, and peak plasma concentration is achieved in 30–90 minutes. Following intramuscular injections, absorption is erratic and lower plasma concentrations may be achieved than with the oral dose (Gamble *et al*, 1975). Diazepam is a highly lipid-soluble drug, and it crosses the blood–brain barrier easily; the half-life is biphasic, with an initial rapid distribution phase, and a prolonged terminal elimination phase of up to two days.

The action of diazepam is further prolonged by the longer half-life of its principal active metabolite, desmethyldiazepam, of two to five days, and the relative proportion of this metabolite increases during long-term administration. Diazepam is extensively metabolised in the liver. In addition to desmethyldiazepam, the active metabolites of diazepam, which include oxazepam and temazepam, are extensively bound to plasma proteins and are excreted in the urine. Plasma half-life of these drugs is increased in neonates, in the elderly, and in patients with kidney or liver disease. Diazepam crosses the placental barrier and is excreted in breast milk.

There are two processes identifiable in the metabolism of benzodiazepines: oxidation and conjugation. Among the benzodiazepines, nitrazepam, diazepam, and chlordiazepoxide are oxidised and then conjugated, while oxazepam and lorazepam are simply conjugated before excretion.

Metabolism in elderly people

Appreciation of the biphasic metabolism of some of these benzodiazepines is important in prescribing for older people, in whom oxidation can be impaired, whereas conjugation is relatively unaltered. The impairment of oxidation can slow the elimination of the drug, and the half-life may be doubled. For a patient aged 80, the half-life of diazepam is 90 hours, compared with 20 hours at the age of 20 (Avery, 1969). Rate of clearance does not change with age, probably because of an increase in distribution volume (Koltz *et al*, 1975).

Some surveys have shown that elderly people are more sensitive to the depressant effects of diazepam (Reidenberg *et al*, 1978). The accumulation of benzodiazepine drugs in elderly people can lead to a confusional state. Even 5 mg of nitrazepam taken regularly can be enough to produce a syndrome of disability, with postural hypotension, general deterioration, incontinence, inability to wake, confusion, dysarthria, and disorientation (Evans & Jarvis, 1972).

Swift, in 1981, reported that, despite the evidence linking disturbed behaviour in elderly people to use of psychoactive drugs, nearly 90% of prescriptions for nitrazepam went to patients aged over 65 years of age. Sleep patterns change naturally with age, and advising patients to expect disturbed or reduced sleep at night could be sounder practice than dispensing hypnotics (Chapter 15).

Larson *et al* (1987) found benzodiazepine use to be the most common cause of cognitive impairment in the elderly, and that it exacerbated underlying dementia. In all cases in this study, cognition improved when the drugs were withdrawn and, in general, no ill effects were experienced on withdrawal. The association of benzodiazepine use with falling has been clearly shown by Sorock & Shimkin (1988) in a prospective study, where benzodiazepine users fell twice as frequently as non-users, and the risk of multiple falls was greater for continuous users of the drugs than for those who took them only occasionally.

Interactions with other drugs

Many of the drugs commonly prescribed by GPs interact with benzodiazepines; Table 16.1 shows the mechanism and possible outcome of the interactions.

TABLE 16.1
Interactions of commonly prescribed drugs with benzodiazepines

Drug interacting with benzodiazepine	Mechanism of interaction	Effect of interaction on benzodiazepine metabolism
Antacids	Decreased rate of conversion of metabolites and decreased drug absorption	Diminished effect
Oral contraceptive	Inhibits enzymatic metabolism	Inhibits the metabolism of benzodiazepines, increasing sensitivity to psychomotor impairment
Sodium valproate	Enzyme inhibition and displacement of protein binding	Increased drug side-effects due to diminished metabolism
Theophylline	Antagonism of receptor site	Diminished effect
Disulfiram	Inhibits enzymatic metabolism	Increased effects, particularly psychomotor impairment
Cimetidine	Inhibits enzymatic metabolism	Increased effect
Ethanol	Synergism	Increased sedation

Indications for the use of the benzodiazepines

There are a number of appropriate clinical uses of the benzodiazepines. They are used in anaesthesia, but it is not the scope of this chapter to discuss their use in that context.

In general practice, they are appropriately used for epilepsy and musculoskeletal disorders. Diazepam is the recommended treatment for status epilepticus. In the patient's home, when used rectally in doses not exceeding 20 mg, absorption is rapid and complete. In hospital, intravenous use has a more rapid sedating effect, and a dose rate of 2 mg per minute is recommended. In addition, oral benzodiazepines, particularly clonazepam, nitrazepam and clobazam, are used as second-line drugs in epilepsy.

However, tolerance develops to these drugs and long-term treatment is sometimes disappointing. Small doses of diazepam (e.g. 2 mg three times per day) can be used to assist analgesia in patients with severe muscle spasm.

In general practice, the benzodiazepines are most commonly used for anxiety and insomnia. In the short term, some benefits have been demonstrated, but often these gains are lost through the development of tolerance to certain actions of the drugs, particularly sedative effects (Lader, 1983).

Although benzodiazepines are widely used as anxiolytics, a considerable body of evidence demonstrates their lack of effectiveness in this context. Lader (1981) summarised the long-term use of benzodiazepines as an expensive waste of effort. The drugs have no curative effect in terms of psychoneurotic status (Harris *et al*, 1977) and are not effective in controlling symptoms with patients with low levels of anxiety (Catalan & Gath, 1985), nor are they distinguished from placebo in patients with chronic anxiety reinforced by social, interpersonal, or economic problems (Hollister, 1973).

The benzodiazepines are thought of primarily as anxiolytic agents, but, in recent years, more prescriptions have been issued for hypnotics than for anxiolytics (Taylor, 1987). Tolerance to the sedative action of nitrazepam has been demonstrated after only six nights of ingestion (Tedeschi *et al*, 1985), and the time taken to get to sleep (sleep latency) has been shown to return to baseline levels by the third week of intake (Adam & Oswald, 1982).

A number of studies have shown that benzodiazepines are prescribed for physical illnesses affecting almost every system (Williams, 1978). A survey in the USA, carried out in 1979 (Mellinger & Balter, 1981), indicated that new therapy with an anti-anxiety agent was at least as likely for patients with a primary diagnosis of physical disorder as for those with mental disorder. Cummins *et al* (1982), in a survey of over 7000 middle-aged men, found a strong positive link between tranquilliser use and a doctor-diagnosed physical disease, mostly ischaemic heart disease and hypertension. Similarly, Rodrigo *et al* (1988) noted a correlation between long-term benzodiazepine use and physical illnesses, primarily gastrointestinal, musculoskeletal, cardiovascular, and respiratory. The long-term prescribing of benzodiazepines for physical illness is thus as much an issue as the prescribing of the drugs for psychological problems.

Guidance on the use of benzodiazepines

Guidance on the use of benzodiazepines has been given to doctors by the Committee on Safety of Medicines (1988) and by the Royal College of Psychiatrists (1988) emphasising that the drugs should be used in the short term (maximum four weeks) and only when symptoms are disabling, severe, or subjecting the individual to unacceptable distress. Both bodies stress that benzodiazepines should not be used to treat depression. The *British National Formulary* (1990) advises that benzodiazepines are contraindicated in bereavement, as the drugs may inhibit psychological adjustment.

Dependence

Dependence is characterised by a strong desire to continue taking a drug, combined with a tendency to increase the dose, resulting in a state of dependence with psychological and physical aspects (Martindale, 1989). As with all drugs producing dependence, the withdrawal of benzodiazepines is characterised by a withdrawal syndrome, which may be delayed in onset and may last several days.

The symptoms that have been reported during withdrawal vary in nature and severity. Some of the symptoms reported may appear to be a resurgence of pre-existing symptoms of anxiety or insomnia, but new symptoms are also part of the withdrawal syndrome (Owen & Tyrer, 1983). The most common symptoms reported are perceptual disturbances, particularly hypersensitivity to auditory and olfactory stimuli, sleep disturbance or insomnia, tremor, nausea, vomiting, and muscular problems such as pain, twitching, stiffness, and numbness (Winokur *et al*, 1980; Petursson & Lader, 1981; Tyrer *et al*, 1981; Shader & Greenblatt, 1981; Lader, 1982). Withdrawal should be gradual: abrupt withdrawal can produce a more severe syndrome characterised by confusion, possible convulsions, and a condition resembling delirium tremens.

The effects of benzodiazepines on performance

Studies of the effects of benzodiazepines on performance have consistently noted decrements in simple repetitive tasks, in learning, and in memory (Lader, 1983). Much of this work has involved non-anxious volunteer subjects, and there is an argument that pathologically anxious people may perform better when taking benzodiazepines, as anxiety itself impairs performance on a number of tasks. However, many individuals without any identifiable pathology receive these drugs, and their performance on tasks such as driving can be greatly reduced (Hindmarch, 1979).

Skegg *et al* (1979), in a large study, demonstrated a highly significant association between the use of minor tranquillisers and the risk of serious road accident to drivers. A sobering report by Prescott (1983), using road traffic accident statistics, showed that benzodiazepines contributed significantly to traffic accidents, often in the morning after taking a hypnotic at night. Nitrazepam, flurazepam, and oxazepam are all likely to impair performance the next morning (Nicholson, 1979). The short-acting hypnotic triazolam has also been shown to produce striking memory impairments the day after night-time administration, such that normal activities were disrupted (Bixler *et al*, 1991).

The pattern of decrements for long-term users is different. New learning is significantly impaired (Golombok *et al*, 1988). Visuospatial ability and sustained attention are affected, suggesting deficits in posterior cortical cognitive function, which may be due to lesions in parietal, posterior temporal, and occipital regions.

When patients are referred for psychological therapy which involves learning new behaviour, gains made during a drug state are less stable (Sartory, 1983). Concentration, which is necessary for psychotherapy, is impaired by benzodiazepines. Benzodiazepines can inhibit problem solving and can impair a wide range of intellectual and psychomotor abilities, thus resulting in a deterioration of quality of life. Curran & Golombok (1985) found that patients who withdrew from medication reported improved concentration and increased sensory appreciation, and realised that they had been functioning below par while taking the drugs.

Prescribing in practice

Despite the evidence that benzodiazepines should not be used for bereavement, this is a common use. Even for GPs who prescribe very little, there is a tendency for them to use benzodiazepines in cases of bereavement, although they may offer just a few tablets to last for a few days rather than a longer course of treatment. The pressures on doctors to respond to distress are high: the issues in bereavement involve not only the bereaved person but the relatives and friends of that person, who themselves find difficulty in coping with the individual's distress (see Chapter 5).

There can be problems produced by the act of prescribing benzodiazepines. By prescribing, doctors can imply that a normal human reaction is inappropriate or 'sick', and thus can prevent its normal course and resolution. In 1981, Helman argued that the doctor-initiated solution to a problem, which involves the prescribing of a drug, inhibits patients from confronting problems by suppressing anxiety. Catalan & Gath (1985) reported that benzodiazepines undermined the individual's capacity to draw on personal resources to cope with adversity. They suggested that benzodiazepines should be used only for severe anxiety, and then only for up to three weeks, with concurrent work to investigate the sources of the anxiety.

Prescribing of benzodiazepines may often occur, not because the doctor specifically believes that they are the best treatment available, but because the availability of other forms of therapy is poor. Referral to clinical psychology may mean a long wait; the presenting symptoms may not be sufficiently severe to warrant referral to psychiatric services; there may be no easily available counsellor or social worker; and the doctor may not feel able personally to offer counselling or psychotherapy.

Although the Committee on Safety of Medicines (1988) strongly stated that benzodiazepines should not be used alone to treat depression or anxiety associated with depression, the drugs have been widely prescribed for depression. Interestingly, a study by Clare & Williams (1981) showed that women were more likely than men to be prescribed benzodiazepines when they presented with symptoms leading to a diagnosis of depression. Johnson (1983), in reviewing the literature on the prescribing of benzodiazepines for depression, reported that 20% of benzodiazepine prescriptions were issued for the treatment of depressive symptoms, although there is no evidence that the drugs have any true antidepressant effect.

The act of issuing a prescription is in itself a statement about the patient's problem. It may also indicate a reluctance on the part of the doctor to tackle the patient's problem.

Repeat prescribing

It is widely acknowledged that the repeat-prescribing system itself represents a form of doctor–patient relationship based on anonymity (Balint, 1964). The importance, in prescribing terms, of this anonymous repeat system is that patients can change the reason for taking these drugs over the years. What this means is that to some extent patients are controlling their own medication and the reasons for taking drugs through a repeat-prescription system. In an interview study of 40 long-term users of benzodiazepines, half of them had changed their reasons for taking the drugs (Cormack *et al*, 1989a).

In a survey in Northern Ireland, King *et al* (1982) showed that 60% of prescriptions for tranquillisers were issued as repeats. A study by Dennis (1979) of 13 practices found that benzodiazepines comprised two-thirds of the repeat prescriptions for psychotropic drugs, and that longer repeat prescriptions went to older patients who were less closely monitored by the GP. Varnam (1981), in an audit of prescribing, found that the average length of time on psychotropic therapy was increased if the drugs were issued as repeat prescriptions: 4.3 years as opposed to 2.7 years if the patients were seen. Underlying these differences may be the way in which the doctor copes with the patient's distress. It has been suggested by Melville (1980) that repeat prescribing of minor tranquillisers is linked to the doctor's negative view of the patient's emotional problems. The doctor may be able to create a distance from more difficult patients by allowing them to collect prescriptions when required.

Preventing long-term use of benzodiazepines

One obvious way of preventing long-term use is to prevent the first prescription. There is evidence that doctors are doing this, as there has been a decrease in new prescriptions for benzodiazepines (Williams, 1983*b*). GPs may feel powerless to stop the long-term use of the drugs; however, there are a number of studies which have indicated that GPs can do a great deal to curtail this use.

Hopkins *et al* (1982) requested 78 patients who had taken benzodiazepines for longer than three months to reduce dosage by one-quarter of the original dose weekly, with the intention of stopping taking tablets. During withdrawal, weekly interviews with the GP were offered to the patients. Fifty-eight per cent of patients stopped medication and 17% reduced the dose to less than half. At follow-up three to five months later, 63% had stopped completely. Thus, an intervention requiring very little time and effort proved to be effective. Similarly, Cormack & Sinnott (1983) showed that a letter from a GP requesting that tablets be reduced or stopped was as effective as group treatment in anxiety management by a psychologist, resulting in 40% success in reducing or stopping medication.

A further study, by Cormack *et al* (1989*b*), assessing a letter from GPs to 71 patients requesting that benzodiazepines be reduced or stopped, found that 16 patients stopped benzodiazepine use completely and maintained their abstinence at follow-up a year later, and six patients reduced to less than 100 tablets in the last year of monitoring. Thus the letter produced a 30% success rate. Another study, by Morrison (1990), of 72 patients, used an individual approach agreed between the GP and each patient. After one year, 27 of the patients had stopped benzodiazepines completely and 24 had reduced their previous consumption by more than 50%. This could be viewed as a success rate of 70%.

It is interesting to speculate as to why a letter from a GP may be more potent than the repeated discussions that many GPs had with their patients over the course of time about the long-term use of benzodiazepines. Interviews with patients in the study by Cormack *et al* (1989*a*) indicated that some patients had anticipated (wrongly) that the GP would stop the medication and they therefore had decided to withdraw from the drugs before the event. A number of patients were under the illusion that the doctor had wanted them to take the tablets for a long time and that the letter indicated a change of mind which they obeyed. Certainly, for many patients the doctor's authority, which is clearly demonstrated in a personal letter, is a potent force for change.

An interesting study by Salinsky & Doré (1987), looking at the characteristics of long-term benzodiazepine users in general practice, found coincidentally that the questionnaire for the study had served as a prompt for patients to stop taking their tablets. In the 12 months before the questionnaire was given, 15% of patients had stopped taking tablets. Nine months after the survey, 45% of all those on long-term therapy had given up their drugs. Whether there had been a misconstruing of the correspondence is not known, but it may be assumed that a written communication is at least thought-provoking for patients, and may well lead them to make active decisions about their consumption of drugs.

Guidelines for reducing benzodiazepines

The advice given by the *British National Formulary* (1990) suggests switching from the current drug to diazepam at an equivalent dose as a first step in reduction. Evidence from the work of one of the authors (MAC) and other colleagues suggests that this may be an optimistic first move. Some people may find that the equivalent dose is insufficient, perhaps particularly in switching from lorazepam, thus it may be that the substitution will have to be of a higher equivalent dose. This higher dose may be necessary to deal with the withdrawal effects from the original drug. It may also be that the substitution has to occur over several days or weeks, substituting one tablet at a time. If there are difficulties in substitution, then it may be that there are going to be difficulties in withdrawal, and it could be worth attempting to reduce, at least partially, on the present drug before moving to a substitution.

The fortnightly reductions of 2 mg or 2.5 mg diazepam, which is the maximum recommended rate of withdrawal, also poses problems. The approach assumes that people are taking their drugs regularly, but often people take them intermittently.

The effect of work in small groups

Since the early 1980s there has been a development of self-help and professional-led groups to help people to withdraw from benzodiazepines. The professional-led groups began mostly with anxiety management approaches, combining physical and mental relaxation with problem-solving strategies. Teare Skinner (1984) showed that two-thirds of patients could stop taking anxiolytics after six sessions of group work. Similarly, Stopforth (1986) found that half of the individuals in a group could withdraw from benzodiazepines after eight group sessions.

Another study, combining anxiety management with cognitive techniques (Higgitt *et al*, 1987), demonstrated that seven out of ten people had success in reducing tablet intake after ten weekly sessions. This group work involved sessions on a fortnightly or three-weekly basis for four months after the weekly group, and at follow-up eight of the ten had achieved clinically and statistically significant reductions in drug intake. In comparison, only three individuals out of ten who received treatment by telephone improved to the same extent, suggesting the importance of sharing therapy with others.

The largest project to help people to stop taking benzodiazepines, the WITHDRAW Project (Hamlin & Hammersley, 1989; Hammersley &

Hamlin, 1990), combined information booklets and group treatment for withdrawal with a long-term group offering in-depth psychotherapeutic intervention. At one-year follow-up, 42% of the participants were abstinent, and 22% showed a reduction of between 52% and 99% from baseline. A control group of benzodiazepine users receiving a limited amount of therapeutic contact coupled with information did not show any significant reductions in benzodiazepine intake until they moved on to the group work.

Conclusions

Public concern about benzodiazepine prescribing has resulted in reductions in the prescribing of tranquillisers, but has not had the same effect on the prescribing of hypnotics, especially for elderly people. There are a number of appropriate uses of the benzodiazepines, but specific guidelines now define limitations in their clinical indication and duration of prescribing. Clear evidence shows performance decrements on modest doses of the drugs.

The benzodiazepines continue to be prescribed extensively in general practice, particularly in the form of repeat prescriptions for elderly people. Although doctors have reduced the numbers of new prescriptions issued, they find difficulty in stopping prescribing for long-term users of the drugs. However, there is an increasing body of evidence that people can reduce or stop benzodiazepine medication with minimal intervention, such as a written request from the GP or when they seek help in a small group.

References

ADAM, K. & OSWALD, I. (1982) A comparison of the effects of clormezanone and nitrazepam on sleep. *British Journal of Clinical Pharmacology*, **14**, 57–65.

ASHTON, H. & GOLDING, J. F. (1989) Tranquillisers: prevalence, predictors and possible consequences. Data from a large United Kingdom survey. *British Journal of Addiction*, **84**, 541–546.

AVERY, G. S. (1969) *Principles and Practice of Clinical Pharmacology and Therapeutics* (2nd edn). Edinburgh: Churchill Livingstone.

BALINT, M. (1964) *The Doctor, His Patient and the Illness*. London: Pitman.

BALTER, M. B., LEVINE, J. & MANHEIMER, D. I. (1974) Cross national study of the extent of anti-anxiety/sedative drug use. *New England Journal of Medicine*, **290**, 769–774.

BIXLER, E. O., KALES, A., MANFREDI, R. L., *et al* (1991) Next-day memory impairment with triazolam use. *Lancet*, **337**, 827–831.

BRITISH NATIONAL FORMULARY (1990) *British National Formulary, Number 20*. London: British Medical Association/Royal Pharmaceutical Society of Great Britain.

CATALAN, J. & GATH, D. H. (1985) Benzodiazepines in general practice: time for a decision. *British Medical Journal*, **290**, 1374–1376.

CLARE, A. & WILLIAMS, P. (1981) Factors leading to psychotropic drug prescription. In *The Misuse of Psychotropic Drugs* (eds R. Murray, H. Ghodse, C. Harris, *et al*). London: Gaskell.

COMMITTEE ON SAFETY OF MEDICINES (1988) Benzodiazepines, dependence with withdrawal symptoms. *Current Problems*, **21**.

CORMACK, M. A. & SINNOTT, A. (1983) Psychological alternatives to long-term benzo-diazepine use. *Journal of the Royal College of General Practitioners*, **33**, 279-281.

——, OWENS, R. G. & DEWEY, M. E. (1989*a*) *Reducing Benzodiazepine Consumption: Psychological Contribution to General Practice.* New York: Springer Verlag.

——, —— & —— (1989*b*). The effect of minimal interventions by general practitioners on long-term benzodiazepine use. *Journal of the Royal College of General Practitioners*, **39**, 408-411.

CUMMINS, R. O., COOK, D. G., HUME, R. C., *et al* (1982) Tranquilliser use in middle-aged British men. *Journal of the Royal College of General Practitioners*, **32**, 745-752.

CURRAN, H. V. & GOLOMBOK, S. (1985) *Bottling It Up.* London: Faber and Faber.

DENNIS, P. J. (1979) Monitoring of psychotropic drug prescriptions in general practice. *British Medical Journal*, *ii*, 1115-1116.

DEPARTMENT OF HEALTH (1990) *Health and Personal Social Services Statistics for England.* London: HMSO.

DEPARTMENT OF HEALTH AND SOCIAL SECURITY (1980) *The Black Report: Inequalities in Health.* London: HMSO.

DUNBAR, G. C., PERERA, M. H. & JENNER, F. A. (1989) Patterns of benzodiazepine use in Great Britain as measured by a general population survey. *British Journal of Psychiatry*, **155**, 836-841.

EVANS, J. G. & JARVIS, E. H. (1972) Nitrazepam and the elderly. *British Medical Journal*, *iv*, 487.

GAMBLE, J. A. S., DUNDEE, J. W. & ASSAFT, R. A. E. (1975) Plasma diazepam levels after single dose oral and intramuscular administration. *Anaesthesia*, **30**, 164-169.

GOLOMBOK, S., MOODLEY, P. & LADER, M. H. (1988) Cognitive impairment in long-term benzodiazepine users. *Psychological Medicine*, **18**, 365-374.

HAMLIN, M. & HAMMERSLEY, D. (1989) Drug withdrawal. *Nursing Times*, **85**, 66-68.

HAMMERSLEY, D. & HAMLIN, M. (1990) *The Benzodiazepine Manual: A Professional Guide to Withdrawal.* Birmingham: Hamlin and Hammersley Withdraw Workshops.

HARRIS, G., LATHAM, J., McGUINNESS, B., *et al* (1977) The relationship between psychoneurotic status and psychoactive drug prescription in general practice. *Journal of the Royal College of General Practitioners*, **27**, 173-177.

HELMAN, C. G. (1981) Patients' perceptions of psychotropic drugs. *Journal of the Royal College of General Practitioners*, **31**, 107-112.

HIGGITT, A., GOLOMBOK, S., FONAGY, P., *et al* (1987) Group treatment of benzodiazepine dependence. *British Journal of Addiction*, **82**, 517-532.

HINDMARCH, I. (1979) Benzodiazepines and traffic accidents. *British Medical Journal*, *ii*, 671.

HOLDEN, J. (1989) Benzodiazepine dependence. *Practitioner*, **233**, 1479.

HOLLISTER, L. E. (1973) Antianxiety drugs in clinical practice. In *The Benzodiazepines* (eds S. Garrattini, E. Mussini & L. O. Randall). New York: Raven Press.

HOPKINS, D. R., SETHI, K. B. S. & MUCKLOW, J. C. (1982) Benzodiazepine withdrawal in general practice. *Journal of the Royal College of General Practitioners*, **32**, 758-762.

JOHNSON, D. A. W. (1983) Benzodiazepines in depression. In *Benzodiazepines Divided* (ed. M. R. Trimble). New York: Wiley.

KING, D. J., GRIFFITHS, K., REILLY, P. M., *et al* (1982) Psychotropic drug use in Northern Ireland, 1966-1980. *Psychological Medicine*, **12**, 819-833.

KING, M., GABE, J., WILLIAMS, P., *et al* (1990) Long-term use of benzodiazepines: the views of patients. *British Journal of General Practice*, **40**, 194-196.

KLOTZ, U., AVANT, G. R., HOYUMPA, A., *et al* (1975) The effects of age and liver disease on the disposition and elimination of diazepam in adult man. *Journal of Clinical Investigation*, **55**, 347-359.

LADER, M. H. (1981) Epidemic in the making: benzodiazepine dependence. In *The Epidemiological Impact of Psychotropic Drugs* (eds G. Tognoni, C. Bellantuono & M. Lader), pp. 313-323. Amsterdam: Elsevier.

—— (1982) Benzodiazepine dependence. *Psychiatry in Practice*, **1**, 34-37.

—— (1983) Benzodiazepines, psychological functioning, and dementia. In *Benzodiazepines Divided* (ed. M. R. Trimble). New York: Wiley.

LARSON, E. B., KUKULL, W. A., BUCHNER, D., *et al* (1987) Adverse drug reactions associated with global cognitive impairment in elderly persons. *Annals of Internal Medicine*, **107**, 169–173.

MARTINDALE: *The Extra Pharmacopoeia* (1989) (29th edn) (ed. J. E. F. Reynolds). London: Pharmaceutical Press.

MELLINGER, G. D. & BALTER, M. B. (1981) Prevalence and patterns of the use of psychotherapeutic drugs: results from a 1979 national survey of American adults. In *The Epidemiological Impact of Psychotropic Drugs* (eds G. Tognoni, C. Bellantuono & M. Lader), pp. 117–135. Amsterdam: Elsevier.

—— & —— (1984) Prevalence and correlates of the long-term regular use of anxiolytics. *Journal of the American Medical Association*, **251**, 375–379.

MELVILLE, A. (1980) Reducing whose anxiety? A study of the relationship between repeat prescribing of minor tranquillisers and doctors' attitudes. In *Prescribing Practice and Drug Usage* (ed. E. Mapes). London: Croom Helm.

MORRISON, J. M. (1990) Audit and follow-up of chronic benzodiazepine tranquilliser use in one general practice. *Family Practice*, **7**, 253–257.

NICHOLSON, A. N. (1979) Performance studies with diazepam and its hydroxylated metabolites. *British Journal of Clinical Pharmacology*, **8**, 39s–42s.

OWEN, R. T. & TYRER, P. (1983) Benzodiazepine dependence: a review of the evidence. *Drugs*, **25**, 385–398.

PETURSSON, H. & LADER, M. H. (1981) Withdrawal from long-term benzodiazepine treatment. *British Medical Journal*, **283**, 643–645.

PRESCOTT, L. F. (1983) Safety and benzodiazepines. In *The Benzodiazepines: From Molecular Biology to Clinical Practice* (ed. E. Costa). New York: Raven Press.

REIDENBERG, M. M., LEVY, M., WARNER, H., *et al* (1978) Relationship between diazepam dose, plasma level, age and central nervous system depression. *Clinical Pharmacology and Therapeutics*, **23**, 371–375.

RODRIGO, E. K., KING, M. B. & WILLIAMS, P. (1988) Health of long-term benzodiazepine users. *British Medical Journal*, **296**, 603–606.

ROYAL COLLEGE OF PSYCHIATRISTS (1988) Benzodiazepines and dependence: a College statement. *Bulletin of the Royal College of Psychiatrists*, **12**, 107–108.

SALINSKY, J. V. & DORÉ, C. J. (1987) Characteristics of long-term benzodiazepine users in general practice. *Journal of the Royal College of General Practitioners*, **37**, 202–204.

SARTORY, G. (1983) Benzodiazepines and behavioural treatment of phobic anxiety. *Behavioural Psychotherapy*, **11**, 204–217.

SHADER, R. I. & GREENBLATT, D. J. (1981) The use of benzodiazepines in clinical practice. *British Journal of Clinical Pharmacology*, **11** (suppl. 1), 5s–9s.

SKEGG, D. C. G., RICHARDS, S. M. & DOLL, R. (1979). Minor tranquillisers and road accidents. *British Medical Journal*, i, 917–919.

SOROCK, G. S., SHIMKIN, E. E. (1988) Benzodiazepine sedatives and the risk of falling in a community-dwelling elderly cohort. *Archives of Internal Medicine*, **148**, 2441–2444.

STOPFORTH, B. (1986) Outpatient benzodiazepine withdrawal and the occupational therapist. *Occupational Therapy*, 318–322.

SWIFT, C. G. (1981) Psychotropic drugs and the elderly. In *The Epidemiological Impact of Psychotropic Drugs* (eds G. Tognoni, C. Bellantuono & M. Lader), pp. 325–338. Amsterdam: Elsevier.

TAYLOR, D. (1987) Current usage of benzodiazepines in Britain. In *The Benzodiazepines in Current Clinical Practice* (eds H. Freeman & Y. Rue). Royal Society of Medicine Services International Congress and Symposium Series number 114. London: Royal Society of Medicine.

TEARE SKINNER, P. (1984) Skills not pills: learning to cope with anxiety symptoms. *Journal of the Royal College of General Practitioners*, **34**, 258–260.

TEDESCHI, G., GRIFFITHS, A. N., SMITH, A. T., *et al* (1985) The effect of repeated doses of temazepam and nitrazepam on human psychomotor performance. *British Journal of Clinical Pharmacology*, **20**, 361–367.

TYRER, P., RUTHERFORD, D. & HUGGETT, T. (1981) Benzodiazepine withdrawal symptoms and propranolol. *Lancet*, i, 520–522.

VARNAM, M. (1981) Psychotropic prescribing. What am I doing? *Journal of the Royal College of General Practitioners*, **31**, 480–483.

WILLIAMS, P. (1978) Physical ill health and psychotropic drug prescription – a review. *Psychological Medicine*, **8**, 683–693.

—— (1983a) Factors influencing the duration of treatment with psychotropic drugs in general practice: a survival analysis approach. *Psychological Medicine*, **13**, 623–633.

—— (1983b) Patterns of psychotropic drug use. *Social Science and Medicine*, **17**, 845–851.

WILSON, P. (1980) *Drinking in England and Wales*. London: HMSO.

WINOKUR, A., RICKELS, K., GREENBLATT, D. J., *et al* (1980) Withdrawal reaction from long-term, low-dosage administration of diazepam. *Archives of General Psychiatry*, **37**, 101–104.

Part III. Psychosocial management

17 Communication between general practitioners and psychiatrists

MICHAEL KING and IAN PULLEN

Verbal communication

Over the past 20 years, many psychiatrists have transferred at least a part of their work into primary care. This development, which was not the policy of either government or Royal Colleges, accelerated particularly throughout the 1980s (Strathdee & Williams, 1984; Pullen & Yellowlees, 1988) and has had a profound effect on communication between GP and psychiatrist (Browning *et al*, 1987; Wright, 1991). In fact, the most common reason given by GPs for initiation of liaison schemes is the need to improve communication between primary and secondary care doctors (Strathdee, 1988). Although it would seem indisputable that when psychiatrists work in general practice, discussions between them and the referring GPs take on a more comprehensive perspective, there is little indication of how much communication has changed, or of whether change has resulted in better application of treatment and improved outcome for patients. Regardless of the form it takes (Mitchell, 1985), consultation–liaison psychiatry in general practice should aim to encourage face-to-face meetings between primary care and psychiatric staff, and to establish specific times for informal meetings, in which particular patients and methods of joint working can be discussed and problems in the service can be raised.

Doctors communicate verbally with each other in formal settings, such as lectures and seminars, by telephone, and face-to-face. Family doctors and psychiatrists talk to other members of the mental health and primary care teams. Despite considerable study of the style and content of written communication between GPs and specialists (see below) and of the ways in which doctors communicate with patients, little empirical investigation has been made of how doctors talk to each other.

Formal communication

In recent years formal communication between specialist and GP has changed enormously. The conventional lecture delivered by a psychiatric specialist to a room full of GPs in a postgraduate medical centre is disappearing (see Chapter 20). There is evidence that this didactic form of teaching is an inefficient way of communicating, is patronising to GPs, and too frequently dwells on topics of hospital psychiatry which are of limited relevance to primary care (Lewis & Bolden, 1989).

Changes in funding for postgraduate education of GPs has resulted in increased competition for the provision of teaching facilities to doctors. Far fewer GPs are prepared to sit and be talked at rather than enter into a dialogue in which members of both specialties may learn. Seminars and workshops in which psychiatrists and GPs share ideas and learn together are becoming much more popular. One example is workshops in which doctors and psychiatrists come together in small groups to discuss difficult patients (Corney *et al*, 1988). This can be threatening to some GPs and specialists, but overall attitudes to the workshops are usually positive.

Although there is often opposition by GPs to joint teaching with other members of the primary care team, there has been little attempt to develop self-directed learning for groups containing both GPs and psychiatrists. Problem patients can be discussed, innovations in diagnosis or treatment presented, and the difficulties, problems, and rewards for both sides of the referral fence understood. The format is far less structured than in prescriptive teaching, but much more information is likely to be retained.

A recent example in which verbal communication between psychiatrists and GPs was used extensively to study services in one health district, and begin to modify them, was that of a scheme launched by the Department of General Practice at King's College Hospital in London. Local discussions between GPs and mental health professionals were the springboard upon which innovative changes could be introduced by planners at the level of both district and regional health authority. This is one example of face-to-face discussion between GPs and specialists which led to the introduction and evaluation of important changes in services (Morley *et al*, 1991). Similar work is about to be launched in other areas of Britain under the auspices of the Mental Health Foundation, a charity which supports innovations and research in mental health care. Only in talking directly to each other in a supportive setting can the problems which restrict good working relationships between GPs and mental health professionals be examined and changes introduced.

Telephone contact

Talking on the telephone is the most common form of spoken communication between GP and specialist. Although it does not replace written communication, the telephone is frequently the medium by which information for an urgent referral, or about a patient with complicated problems, is conveyed.

Discourse by telephone also enables exchange of information which neither GP nor psychiatrist wishes to see written into the medical records. This may be of particular importance in the light of changes regarding patients' access to medical records (see below). On occasions doctors might wish to consider diagnostic or therapeutic possibilities without alarming patients. Psychiatry is a specialty in which topics of particular sensitivity may be discussed between referring doctor and psychiatrist. Although it can be argued that resorting to confidential discussion by telephone is patronising to patients and excludes them from taking a full role in their investigation and treatment, it may allow more candid discussion between referring and consulting doctor before a definitive diagnosis or management plan is decided upon.

For sensitive issues, such as the possibility of HIV infection, which may involve third parties, it is sometimes preferable not to record certain aspects of the diagnosis or treatment. In these circumstances, verbal communication between doctors must be clear and unambiguous.

Telephone communication between family doctor and specialist is sometimes frustrating and difficult. There is much anecdotal evidence that GPs find psychiatric consultants and junior staff difficult to reach by telephone, and mutual understanding may not be easily reached unless GP and psychiatrist have some knowledge of each other. Conversely, many psychiatrists and their trainees often fail to contact their GP colleagues when patients have been discharged from care and treatment plans need to be agreed. Although written discharge summaries and letters are essential, a telephone call provides a crucial interim form of communication before letters are typed and post arrives.

Regular telephone conversation between consultant and GP also encourages the development of their working relationship. Little work has been carried out into the *process* of this form of communication. How often and in what circumstances are telephone calls between specialist and GP made? Even less investigation has been conducted into the potential *benefits* which accrue. For example, it should be possible to compare the uptake of treatment plans and short-term outcome for patients whose GPs are contacted by the psychiatrist by telephone and followed up by letter, with those for whom only a letter is used to convey the treatment plan.

Telephone contact may also enable the psychiatric specialist to verify information provided by the patient. Although relatives and close friends of patients are frequently consulted by psychiatrists in order to confirm and extend their knowledge of the patient's history and symptoms, it is less usual that the family doctor is consulted in order to confirm points of history or mental state. Whether or not the patient's GP has made the referral, he/she is in a pivotal position to advise the psychiatrist on the patient's background and ways of responding to difficulty.

There is one caveat concerning telephone communication between psychiatrist and GP. All too infrequently the GP or psychiatrist verifies that he/she is indeed talking to a colleague. Although a rare event, it is not unknown for reporters or others with a similar interest in investigating patients' affairs to masquerade as medical specialists. Despite careful maintenance of confidentiality in other circumstances, it is occasionally surprising how readily information about a patient is given by telephone without any attempt to confirm the source of the inquiry. A simple return call may be enough to verify the claims of the caller. Although a small point, it highlights the need for psychiatrist and GP to be on familiar speaking terms with each other. Unfortunately, time in a particular service for trainee psychiatrists or GPs may be too short to allow this process to take root.

Face-to-face contact

When psychiatrists work directly in general practice, they and the referring GPs encounter a useful mode of communication. They talk to each other. It would appear that a desire among family doctors for regular face-to-face communication with psychiatrists is one of the driving forces behind the development of general practice psychiatry (Brown & Tower, 1990). Mitchell (1985) has characterised the diverse ways in which psychiatrists conduct their work in general practice (see also Chapter 2). All of them, including the model whereby the psychiatrist merely transfers his/her out-patient department into the family-practice setting, entail more face-to-face communication with the referring doctor. Where psychiatrists discuss patients and advise on management without actually consulting, communication may need to be more detailed and protracted (Creed & Marks, 1989).

How do doctors talk together in this setting, and does it make any substantial difference to the process of patient care or to clinical outcome? Again, there is too little information to give a clear answer. Many psychiatrists visit the practice at a time in the week when they can join in a practice meeting, as well as consult with patients. In this format, communication is efficient but, with the continuing changes in government contracts with family doctors, there is a danger that psychiatric topics may be squeezed out by more pressing concerns of practice management. Advantages are that detailed discussion may cover wider psychological issues of patient care, and members of the primary care team may raise difficult topics, knowing the rest of the team and the psychiatrist are available for support. In this venue, the referral process itself may be modified (Creed & Marks, 1989). Discussions may cover the usefulness or otherwise of a referral, precise reasons for referral can be given, and appropriate information passed to the psychiatrist.

Most psychiatrists will communicate with their GP colleagues in the corridors or offices of the health centre or over coffee. Although at times it may seem that discussion is less that adequate, even in these fleeting venues the concerns of the GP will be communicated and may be of greater application to the patient's difficulties than lengthy details of history. The consultant or senior trainee psychiatrist who delivers the consultation–liaison service has an unparalleled opportunity to gauge the GP's reaction to the patient and the GP's principal concerns about the patient's current mental or social state. There is also an opportunity for the psychiatrist to talk informally with other members of the primary care team, such as practice nurses, manager, and receptionists, who may all be valuable sources of information never available in letters to the hospital. Receptionists in particular see all patients who attend the practice, regardless of which GP is consulted. They have observed and interacted with the patient in the less formal setting of the waiting area, and are often sensitive to changes in their emotions and behaviour. They should never be overlooked by the liaison psychiatrist as an important source of common-sense information.

It is just as crucial that the psychiatrist gives adequate verbal feedback to the primary care team after an assessment of the patient. Although there is a need for a short summary to be typed and attached to the patient's record, verbal feedback, preferably as soon as possible after the assessment, may prove to be the most useful to the GP, and will allow discussion of treatment options. When the case is complicated or when referral to yet another mental health professional, such as a psychologist, is suggested, communication between GP and psychiatrist is vital if recommendations are to be followed (Gask, 1986).

Much will depend on the time at which patients are seen. It is often the case that for reasons of space the psychiatrist works in the practice at a time, such as the middle of the working day, when there is less demand on consulting-rooms. Although this may allow adequate facilities for the consultation, and patients may be able to wait with the added privacy of there being few others in the waiting area, it can also mean that the GP is absent from the practice at the time the psychiatrist has completed the assessments. In these cases it is essential that contact is established by telephone later the same day. Verbal communication about the patient by the psychiatrist may be most germane when conducted soon after the consultation.

Although there has been extensive study of the ways in which GPs and psychiatrists communicate with their patients in developing empathy, eliciting a history, and arriving at a diagnosis, there has beeen little analogous study of verbal communication between doctors. One exception is a recent study of personal contacts between psychiatrists and primary care staff in a series of psychiatric clinics held in general practice surgeries and health centres in an inner-city area of Nottingham (Darling & Tyrer, 1990). All face-to-face contacts between psychiatrists and primary care staff were recorded during one calendar year. There were 351 contacts between three psychiatrists and up to 33 GPs and their teams. The majority of contacts were about specific patients, and almost 90% of them took place between psychiatrists and GPs. More than two-thirds of verbal exchanges lasted less than five minutes, and few were longer than 15 minutes. Perhaps surprisingly, clarification of the role of staff was the subject most commonly discussed. This was followed, in descending order of frequency, by giving information about a patient, general management and advice, and medication. Twenty-six per cent of contacts concerned patients not in psychiatric care, implying that considerable liaison was taking place, without direct consultation. Contacts between psychiatrists and other members of the primary care staff showed a similar pattern, except patients were present more often during the discussions, which tended to be longer, and often involved family and social issues.

Thus, face-to-face contacts were common and sought by both family doctor and psychiatrist. Their brevity is typical of the pattern of working in British general practice, but short discussions such as these must be regarded within the broader context of continuing care. Thus it is clear that consultation–liaison psychiatry in general practice allows considerable contact, at least between doctors, and follows a pattern quite distinct from that inherent in traditional psychiatric practice.

Although such work informs us about the process and content of communication between psychiatrists and GPs, it does not indicate the value of such communication and whether it can be improved. The development of effective communication skills between doctors may be as influential on overall patient care as those developed for consultation between doctors and their patients. In general practice psychiatry, the need for adequate and informative communication between referrer and specialist is even more important if this source of liaison is not to be wasted. One empirical question which might readily be addressed is whether there is any significant difference in clinical outcome between those patients for whom the GP receives advice from the psychiatrist in a strictly liaison format, and those for whom the psychiatrist makes a direct assessment of the patient. Another question is whether talking with the GP is helpful for the psychiatrist, as reflected in uptake of treatment recommendations and patient outcome, over and above simply having direct access to GP records. Finally, there has been little exploration of joint audit by psychiatrists and GPs. Once a consultation–liaison clinic has been established and the respective professionals are cooperating, it may be possible to carry out joint audit exercises to assess process of referral, implementation of treatments, and patient outcome.

Conclusions

Perhaps because it is so much part of our everyday experience, there has been little attempt to make empirical observation of the ways in which family doctors and psychiatrists communicate verbally with each other. With the continuing developments of community psychiatry and the move of psychiatric practice into primary care, communication between GP and psychiatrist is becoming more direct and personalised. Changes are occurring whether verbal contact is in a more formal teaching atmosphere, by telephone, or face to face. Hypotheses about the purpose and value of the various forms of verbal communication between psychiatrists and GPs are testable, and require a greater emphasis in the expansion of audit and health services research.

Written communication

Despite the trend for psychiatrists to move into the community and work alongside GPs in primary care, the letter remains the main mode of communication between them; it also forms the permanent record for the case notes. While doctor–patient communication skills form an important part of undergraduate and postgraduate training, doctor–doctor communication has not been so well examined. New doctors learn their letter writing 'skills' from the correspondence they come across in case notes, and frequently construct their letters to record their findings for the hospital case record rather than as a communication to another doctor. No wonder Bussy (1960), with a feeling of exasperation, observed "medical communication is a wide-ranging, undisciplined, chaotic and highly unscientific business".

The elements of good written communication

Excellent advice is offered by Kessel (1984), who sets out five elements of good communication:

(a) communicators must themselves acquire the information that is to be passed on
(b) they must not be too lazy or too busy to convey it
(c) they must keep in mind exactly what they need to tell
(d) they should always consider what the recipient will want to know
(e) the door should always be kept open for further communication.

Letters

In recent years some attempts have been made to improve the situation, and written communication is a prime target for simple, but worthwhile audit. One-way communication between GPs and a routine psychiatric clinic was studied by de Alarcon & Hodson (1964), and Birley & Heine (see Kaeser & Cooper, 1971) considered referral letters to an emergency psychiatric clinic were an "ineffective means of communication". Margo (1982) found that

GPs appeared to be satisfied with the letters from one psychiatrist. It is perhaps unfair to criticise the letters received by a particular service without exposing one's own letters to scrutiny.

Two-way communication between GPs and psychiatrists has also been studied. Williams & Wallace (1974), assessing referral letters to a psychiatric clinic in Cardiff and the psychiatrists' replies, concluded that "the standard of communication in letters needs improvement on both sides".

A similar study conducted in Edinburgh ten years later (Pullen & Yellowlees, 1985) set out to discover whether communication had improved over the decade. Psychiatrists were asked to indicate the five most important items that they considered a GP should include in a referral letter, and GPs were asked for the five 'key items' that a psychiatrist should include in a report on one of their patients. Altogether 120 referral letters and replies were rated for the presence of 'key items', length, and legibility, from two years a decade apart (1973 and 1983).

Referral letters – what psychiatrists want

The key items that psychiatrists identified as being of greatest importance for the GP to include in a referral letter were:

(a) medication prescribed so far
(b) family history – especially sensitive information
(c) main symptoms or problems
(d) reason for referral
(e) psychiatric history.

To this list may also be added:

(f) expectations of outcome.

Not only is it necessary to include the names of all drugs prescribed, but the dosage and duration of each is required. Patients are often unreliable when it comes to recalling this information in sufficient detail.

The GP may hold a wealth of accumulated knowledge about patients and their social situations by dint of continuity of care. There is a complex association between this accumulated knowledge and the process of consultation (Hjortdahl & Borchgrevink, 1991). What the psychiatrist is requesting is that the GP include in the letter any sensitive issues, particularly the sort of thing that a patient might be reluctant to discuss on a first (and perhaps only) visit to the psychiatrist.

The reason for referral may appear obvious. But, if the GP is to receive an appropriate response from the consultation, the psychiatrist needs to know the *real* reason for the referral. "Please see and advise" conveys next to nothing about the referrer's hopes or intentions. The referring doctor may have in mind a number of specific questions and outcomes:

Please confirm my diagnosis
Please confirm my treatment plan
Please clarify what is going on   } I wish to continue
Please suggest a management plan   managing this patient
Please assess suicide risk

Please share the care of this worrying/stressful patient
Please take over the care of this patient for a while   } Do not refer
Please use your specialist skills to treat this patient   straight back
Please use your specialist facilities for this patient

Referral letters – what psychiatrists get

The Edinburgh study found that while the main symptoms or problems were given in almost all letters and a reason for referral mentioned in over 80%, medication was mentioned in only two-thirds of letters. While three-quarters of these mentioned dose, less than half gave the duration. A minority of letters contained anything about the family in 1983, a significant drop from a decade earlier, but information about psychiatric history was more likely to be included. The decline in the amount of information about the family may represent a decline in accumulated knowledge of families or may merely reflect a change of attitude on the part of GPs.

Reasons for referral tended to be couched in general terms. Few hints were given about expectations. Were referring doctors keen to continue managing the patient after receiving advice, or were they looking for some continuing help? It was usually impossible to tell.

To be effective, letters must be legible. Over two-thirds of them were typed, and of the remainder only 9 (out of 120) were difficult to read.

Relationships between doctors appear to be reflected in the letters written. Letters written to a named consultant contained significantly more key items than letters addressed to an anonymous clinic. Doctors seem to try harder when they know who is going to read the letter.

Psychiatric replies – what general practitioners want

The key items identified by Edinburgh GPs for psychiatrists to include in their reports after seeing a new patient were:

(a) diagnosis
(b) treatment
(c) follow-up

(d) prognosis
(e) concise explanation (formulation).

To this list may be added:

(f) what the patient has been told
(g) an answer to any specific question in the referral letter.

It is clearly important to communicate not only what treatment is recommended, but who is to take responsibility for its prescription, in what dose, and for how long.

The 'concise explanation' refers to what psychiatrists sometimes call a formulation, a brief statement pulling the elements of the case together to postulate why this particular person has become ill in this particular way at this particular time. While the nosological diagnosis will indicate the choice of medication, the formulation will often point to non-drug management. For example, the concise explanation may state ''Major depressive illness in a man with a strong family history of depression and two recent major life events, redundancy and marriage''. While the depressive illness is receiving appropriate antidepressant therapy, this man would also benefit from the opportunity to talk about the redundancy and the impact of this (and the depression) on his new wife and their relationship. She should also be seen.

Psychiatrists always read the referral letter before seeing the patient, but may well dictate their reply without reminding themselves of precisely why the GP had decided to make the referral and whether he/she had asked any specific questions.

Psychiatric replies – what general practitioners get

While almost all letters gave clear follow-up arrangements, a diagnosis was not always given (88%). Treatment was usually included, but prognosis was rare (27%). Perhaps this is excusable, as the letters were written after a single interview. Even when no further sessions were planned, prognosis was seldom mentioned. Over the ten years there had been a significant improvement in the number of letters containing a concise explanation (60%), but few mentioned what the patient had been told.

A common complaint is about the length of psychiatrists' letters. Consultants wrote letters that were half the length of those written by senior house officers and registrars. They contained the same number of key items, but these were often submerged in the verbiage of the longer letters. The use of headings can be helpful.

Williams & Wallace (1974) commented that ''as regards the psychiatrists' letters the function of case summary and specialist opinion is not satisfactorily fulfilled in one letter'', but they were unable to suggest a workable solution. The argument that the letter acts also as a case summary is not a valid excuse for long, rambling letters, but is merely a smokescreen to hide a poorly conceptualised case. The hospital record requires no more information than is contained in a well considered letter to a GP. The positive findings from the history and examination of the mental state, together with important negative findings, should be arranged succinctly to form a concise explanation of the condition and hence management recommended and the likely outcome. Any questions raised by the GP must be answered.

How long should a letter be?

Anybody who has worked in general practice knows the constraints of time and the quantity of hospital letters received every day. After scanning the letter for action to be taken, the letter is filed, only to be seen again when the file is opened and the patient in the room. Long letters without paragraphs or headings are of little use. Structure and length must be considered.

A group of psychiatrists were asked to select their 'ideal' GP letter from six sample letters all referring to the same patient and containing the five key items (Blaney & Pullen, 1989). They were of varying length, both with and without headings. They chose a letter that covered one side of A4 paper with two headings. This is longer than the usual referral letters.

A similar exercise, with GPs selecting psychiatrists' letters (Yellowlees & Pullen, 1984), suggested that psychiatrists should aim at a similar sort of letter – one page with two headings. This is similar to the letters written by many consultants, but not those of junior psychiatrists. It appears that while consultants have evolved a way of communicating that meets the needs of GPs, they do not pass this on to their junior staff.

Follow-up correspondence

Much valuable time is wasted by either the failure to convey up-to-date information or the receipt of unnecessary correspondence. Neither side is blameless.

In Pullen & Yellowlees' (1985) study of 120 referral letters, not one follow-up letter from the GP was received, although this does not necessarily mean that no fresh information was given verbally. Frequently the psychiatrist will suggest a particular drug. At review a month later the medication may have been changed by the GP on more than one occasion because of side-effects or some other problem. No indication has been given to the psychiatrist, who might make incorrect deductions on the assumption that the medication is what was suggested, or may discover the change of tablet without being able to discover from the patient just what the new preparation and dose are. This is both frustrating and inefficient, and yet GP follow-up letters are as rare as hens' teeth.

Psychiatrists go to the other extreme. Many junior psychiatrists will write a letter every time they see the patient, out of habit or a misguided belief that this represents good practice. These letters fill both general practice and hospital case notes, making it more difficult to find significant information. Psychiatrists should write letters, after the first report, only when there is a significant change in the patient or the treatment, or to remind the GP after a gap of many months that the patient is still being seen.

Hospital admissions, discharges, and deaths

Psychiatrists should remember that the GPs should be informed by letter (and preferably by telephone) of any admission. GPs require enough information to be able to support other family members and the patient, who may consult them while out on pass. During a prolonged admission, periodic updates are useful, with a suitable summary on discharge or death.

A discrepancy exists between the type of discharge summary required for hospital notes and that preferred by GPs (Craddock & Craddock, 1989). A Birmingham study showed that while GPs overwhelmingly preferred a summary of one side of A4 paper ending with pertinent information without headings, psychiatrists chose a 2¼-page 'summary' with information under 11 headings. One solution is to send a hospital summary with a covering note to meet the GP's needs.

Day-hospital patients require similar consideration.

Notes fit for patients to read

The Access to Health Records Act 1990 came into force on 1 November 1991, and gave patients the right to see any information held in the medical case record after that date (with the exception of third-party information or where the information might cause serious mental or physical harm to the patient or someone else), and to obtain a photocopy. This puts a particular onus on doctors to write as though the patient were looking over their shoulder. Jargon should be kept to a minimum, and personal comments and potentially offensive remarks avoided.

While it is too early to assess the effect of this legislation on case notes and correspondence, GPs and psychiatrists have indicated that they would feel inhibited about recording opinions about a patient's personality (McShane *et al*, 1992).

It may well be that if psychiatrists do indeed try to write letters fit for patients to read, then they will also be writing letters that make more sense to GPs. Perhaps this will also make referral letters less cryptic. Since these letters contain information 'owned' by the patient, should we not be giving patients responsibility for their notes? Gilhooly & McGhee (1991) considered the ethics of patient-held records, while Essex *et al* (1990) assessed a shared-care record card held by 84 patients with severe mental illness. The cards were acceptable to the patients, increased their autonomy, and improved communication and the effectiveness of shared care. However, the obstacles to further development of the approach were the attitudes and anxieties of the doctors, nurses, and managers.

Education and training

Much is now known about the inadequacies of written communication between doctors. Doctors have a tendency to write to their agenda, forgetting Kessel's elements of good communication – to think what it is that the recipient will want to know.

Since 1983 the Edinburgh postgraduate psychiatry course has contained a session on letter writing. Such discussion should be a part of all postgraduate training and induction courses. Sensible advice on using a dictating machine is available (Windle, 1979) to help trainees avoid the many pitfalls for the novice. For a common-sense approach to doctor–doctor communication, all hospital and practice libraries should include *Doctor to Doctor* (Walton & McLachlan, 1984).

References

BLANEY, D. & PULLEN, I. M. (1989) Communication between psychiatrists and general practitioners: what style of letters do psychiatrists prefer? *Journal of the Royal College of General Practitioners*, **39**, 67.

BROWN, L. M. & TOWER, J. E. C. (1990) Psychiatrists in primary care: would general practitioners welcome them? *British Journal of General Practice*, **40**, 369–371.

BROWNING, S. M., FORD, M. F., GODDARD, C. A., *et al* (1987) A psychiatric clinic in general practice. A description and comparison with an out-patient clinic. *Bulletin of the Royal College of Psychiatrists*, **ii**, 114–117.

BUSSY, R. K. (1960) *Journal of the Albert Einstein Medical Center*, **8**, 249.

CORNEY, R., STRATHDEE, G., KING, M., *et al* (1988) Managing the difficult patient: practical suggestions from a study day. *Journal of the Royal College of General Practitioners*, **38**, 349–352.

CRADDOCK, N. & CRADDOCK, B. (1989) Psychiatric discharge summaries: differing requirements of psychiatrists and general practitioners. *British Medical Journal*, **299**, 1382.

CREED, F. & MARKS, B. (1989) Liaison psychiatry in general practice: a comparison of the liaison–attachment scheme and shifted outpatient clinic models. *Journal of the Royal College of General Practitioners*, **39**, 514–517.

DARLING, C. & TYRER, P. (1990) Brief encounters in general practice: liaison in general practice psychiatry clinics. *Psychiatric Bulletin*, **14**, 592–594.

DE ALARCON, R. & HODSON, J. M. (1964) Value of general practitioners' letters. *British Medical Journal*, **ii**, 435–438.

ESSEX, B., DOIG, R. & RENSHAW, J. (1990) Pilot study of records of shared care for people with mental illnesses. *British Medical Journal*, **300**, 1442–1446.

GASK, L. (1986) What happens when psychiatric out-patients are seen once only? *British Journal of Psychiatry*, **148**, 663–666.

GILHOOLY, M. L. M. & MCGHEE, S. M. (1991) Medical records: practicalities and principles of patient possession. *Journal of Medical Ethics*, **17**, 138–143.

HJORTDAHL, P. & BORCHGREVINK, C . F. (1991) Continuity of care: influence of general practitioners' knowledge about their patients on use of resources in consultations. *British Medical Journal*, **303**, 1181–1184.

KAESER, A. C. & COOPER, B. (1971) The psychiatric patient, the general practitioner and the outpatient clinic. *Psychological Medicine*, **1**, 312–325.

KESSEL, N. A. (1984) Hospital consultant's view. In *Doctor to Doctor* (eds J. Walton & G. McLachlan). London: Nuffield Provincial Hospitals Trust.

LEWIS, A. P. & BOLDEN, K. J. (1989) General practitioners and their learning styles. *Journal of the Royal College of General Practitioners*, **39**, 187–189.

MARGO, J. L. (1982) Letters from psychiatrists to general practitioners. *Bulletin of the Royal College of Psychiatrists*, **6**, 139–141.

MCSHANE, R., ROWE, D. & JULIER, D. (1992) Will the information recorded in psychiatric notes change when patients have the right to read them? *Psychiatric Bulletin*, **16**, 404–405.

MITCHELL, A. R. K. (1985) Psychiatrists in primary health care settings. *British Journal of Psychiatry*, **147**, 371–379.

MORLEY, V. EVANS, T. & HIGGS, R. (1991) *The Camberwell Report – A Case Study in Developing Primary Care*. London: King's Fund Centre.

PULLEN, I. M. & YELLOWLEES, A. J. (1985) Is communication improving between general practitioners and psychiatrists? *British Medical Journal*, **290**, 31–33.

—— & —— (1988) Scottish psychiatrists in primary health-care settings. A silent majority. *British Journal of Psychiatry*, **153**, 663–666.

STRATHDEE, G. (1988) Psychiatrists in primary care: the general practitioner viewpoint. *Family Practice*, **5**, 111–115.

—— & WILLIAMS, P. (1984) A survey of psychiatrists in primary care: the silent growth of a new service. *Journal of the Royal College of General Practitioners*, **34**, 615–618.

WALTON, J. & MCLACHAN, G. (eds) (1984) *Doctor to Doctor – Writing and Talking About Patients*. London: Nuffield Provincial Hospitals Trust.

WILLIAMS, P. & WALLACE, B. B. (1974) General practitioners and psychiatrists – do they communicate? *British Medical Journal*, **i**, 505–507.

WINDLE, H. (1979) Be a dictator. In *How To Do It* (ed. S. Lock). London: British Medical Association.

WRIGHT, A. (1991) General practitioners and psychiatry: an opportunity for cooperation and research. *British Journal of General Practice*, **41**, 223–224.

YELLOWLEES, A. J. & PULLEN, I. M. (1984) Communication between psychiatrists and general practitioners. What sort of letters should psychiatrists write? *Health Bulletin (Scotland)*, **42**, 285–296.

18 Teamwork in the community

TONY KENDRICK, ANDRÉ TYLEE and TOM BURNS

Primary care and mental illness

In our two-tiered system of medical care there are a number of tasks to be accomplished in primary care:

(a) primary prevention requires the identification and modification of known risk factors for the development of illness
(b) acute illnesses must be identified, classified into those which require specific interventions and those which do not, treated where possible in primary care, or referred for advice or care to the specialist services where necessary
(c) continuing care and support must be provided for patients with chronic illnesses, including those referred back from the specialist service, with the aim of tertiary prevention of the progression of the illness and development of complications
(d) for illnesses which have resolved but are likely to recur, the task is one of prevention of further bouts where possible.

Mental illnesses present a formidable challenge to the primary medical care system (Chapter 3). One in four people suffers from psychological problems at any one time (Goldberg & Huxley, 1980, and see also Chapter 3). Most of these people present to their GPs over the course of a year, and psychological problems are the second commonest type of problem seen among adults in general practice, being outranked only by respiratory problems.

Overall GPs identify just over half of the psychological problems among the patients presenting to them, but there is wide variation in the proportion of disorders detected, and psychiatric problems associated with physical disease are less likely to be acknowledged as in need of treatment in their own right. Training GPs in interviewing skills can improve their accuracy in the diagnosis of psychiatric disorder (Gask *et al*, 1987).

The bulk of psychological problems presenting in general practice are minor disorders of anxiety and depression and personal problems, which, while they do not require specialist referral, may make considerable demands on primary care. Research continues to shed light on the natural history of the common symptoms of mental illness and the thresholds of severity required for the identification of 'cases', which by definition are likely to respond to an increasing number of possible interventions, including drug therapy and psychological treatments (Copeland, 1981).

About 1–2% of patients are referred to the psychiatric services. The main responsibility for the continuing care of patients with severe mental illness such as schizophrenia after discharge from hospital has always rested with primary care, and the consequent workload has been increasing since the shift in policy away from long-term hospital care (Parkes *et al*, 1963; Melzer *et al*, 1991). Patients who have recovered from major depressive illness are at increased risk for further episodes and may benefit from targeted surveillance and support.

It seems probable that the primary care of mental illness should be most efficient and effective where members of the primary health care team besides the GP are involved, including district nurses, health visitors, and practice nurses. These professionals are in frequent contact with many patients and could work in concert with the GP on the tasks of preventing, identifying, and managing mental illness in primary care. The World Health Organization working party on psychiatry and primary care (1973) concluded that "the primary medical care team is the cornerstone of community psychiatry".

Opportunities for teamwork – primary and secondary teams

Major changes in general practice have taken place in recent years which have in principle increased the scope for effective teamwork in the primary care of mental illness in the community.

The 1990 GP contract introduced payments for health promotion clinics, and this has contributed to a large increase in the number of practice nurses employed to run them. The contract also gave family health service authorities more discretion to approve reimbursement of some of the cost of employing and training a range of professionals, including psychologists and counsellors (Department of Health, 1991).

At the same time opportunities are increasing for direct contact between the primary care team and members of the community mental health team. Many psychiatrists now spend part of their time working in general practice (Strathdee & Williams, 1984). Some have simply shifted their out-patient clinics to be more accessible to patients, but an increasing number of psychiatrists are involved in liaison-attachment schemes (Mitchell, 1985), where the psychiatrist meets regularly with GPs to discuss the patients they have in common and advise about other patients who need not be referred. Strathdee & Williams' (1984) survey found that in 45% of schemes a community psychiatric nurse (CPN) had joined the attachment, in 24% a clinical psychologist, and in 10% social workers had also become involved.

A national survey of a random sample of practices in England and Wales stratified by size and family health service authority has recently been carried out from St George's Department of General Practice. The 1542 practices sampled had the following professionals working on site: practice nurses (97%), health visitors (83%) CPNs (34%), counsellors (17%) clinical psychologists (12%), psychiatrists (9%), psychiatric social workers (6%), and psychotherapists (3%) (Kendrick *et al*, 1993). These professionals tended to cluster together with a preponderance in larger training practices, reflecting a tendency for them to work in teams within practices which can provide them with space and workload.

What is teamwork?

Much of the literature on teamwork emphasises that members of the team should share a common goal. Thus Gilmore *et al* (1974) suggested primary care teams should have the following characteristics.

(a) The members of a team share a common purpose which binds them together and guides their actions

(b) Members of the team have a clear understanding of their own functions, appreciate and understand the contribution of the other professions represented on the team, and recognise commonness of interest and skill

(c) The team pools knowledge, skills and resources, and all members share responsibility for the total outcome of their decisions

(d) The effectiveness of the team is related both to its capabilities to carry out its work and its abilities to manage itself as an interdependent group of people.

How much teamwork goes on?

In practice there are a number of problems standing in the way of such teamwork in the care of mental disorder in the community. The care of any one person may involve professionals working in three different teams: the primary care team, the community mental health team, and social services. Communication between the different teams may be poor, members of one team often having no contact at all with members of the others.

Within each of the three teams the level of teamwork which is practised varies widely too.

A joint working party of the Royal Colleges of General Practice and Nursing identified a number of problems in teamwork within the primary care team (Royal College of General Practitioners, 1986). District nurses and health visitors, unlike practice nurses, are not employed by the GP, and are accountable to nurse managers. GPs, as independent contractors, may be reluctant to work in a team. They sometimes act entirely independently, and can confuse and frustrate the other professionals. Such problems are compounded by differences in educational attainment, status, and rewards.

Measuring teamwork in terms of the sharing of goals and responsibilities is not easy; collaboration is easier to measure, in terms of the degree of two-way communication of information and subsequent interaction between professionals. Gregson *et al* (1991) used a five-level model based on the taxonomy of Armitage (Table 18.1) to measure collaboration among 148 doctor–community-nurse pairs and 161 doctor–health-visitor pairs, in 20 representative health districts. Overall, collaboration was low, with professionals 'communicating' with one another rather than 'collaborating'. A large proportion of the doctor–health-visitor pairs did not even communicate regularly. It appears therefore that, despite repeated exhortations in the primary care literature over the last 20 years or more, in practice full collaboration in highly integrated teams is uncommon.

This is not to deny that much joint and interactive work goes on, however. In order to play a central role in the provision of effective and efficient community mental health care, it is important for GPs to be aware of the respective roles of different professionals and the potential benefits to patients of their intervention. What is possible in practice, and what can be done to increase interprofessional collaboration?

TABLE 18.1
A five-level model of collaboration

Stages of collaboration	Definitions
(1) Isolation	Members who never meet, talk, or write to one another
(2) Encounter	Members who encounter or correspond with others but do not interact meaningfully
(3) Communication	Members whose encounters or correspondence include the transfer of information
(4) Partial collaboration	Members who act on that information sympathetically, participate in patterns of joint working, subscribe to the same general objectives as others on a one-to-one basis in the same organisation
(5) Full collaboration	Organisations in which the work of all members is fully integrated

After Gregson *et al* (1991).

Health visitors

The training of health visitors emphasises the prevention and early detection of problems, as well as health education. By virtue of their regular contacts with young families, health visitors are in a good position to practise the prevention and early identification of many psychosocial problems (Briscoe & Lindley, 1982). Health visitors have a statutory duty to visit all new babies at home in the first few weeks of life. Postnatal depression affects 12–15% of mothers, and the health visitor is ideally placed for its early detection, which is important for the mother and may prevent an array of deleterious effects on her children, including behavioural, intellectual, and emotional problems.

The health visitor can help persuade a woman who feels unable or unwilling to attend for assessment and management of depression by the GP. She can allay misconceptions that the woman may have about, for example, depression being caused by a 'lack of moral fibre', particularly as the time after childbirth is supposed to be a time of great joy. She can reassure the mother that antidepressants can be used even when breastfeeding, and that they are not addictive. The best management approach may be a combined strategy using pills from the doctor for symptoms, and counselling from the health visitor for problems.

Interventions by health visitors have been shown to be effective in managing non-psychotic postnatal depression (Holden *et al*, 1989). Benefit was achieved after eight weekly counselling sessions by health visitors who had been given a short training in Rogerian non-directive methods.

Health visitors in the West Midlands have been collaborating directly with CPNs to support women with postnatal depression (Jebali, 1991). Once the health visitors have identified difficulties they arrange a joint assessment with the CPN and a treatment plan is arranged that avoids unnecessary duplication of effort. Either can be the key worker, and this is said to work because of the good communication that exists. Unfortunately, no empirical evidence was provided to support the effectiveness of this arrangement. An important question is whether health visitors can tell which patients require specialist psychiatric nursing, and which do not.

Health visitors can practise primary prevention by targeting longer-term support for high-risk groups for depression, such as single mothers with several preschool children at home. Work with such a patient group might include arranging social activities and child-care for the mother. They can practise secondary prevention by being alert to the early 'cues' of depressive illness, both verbal and non-verbal, including psychomotor retardation and neglect of housework or child-care.

District nurses

District nurses regularly visit old people who are physically ill or disabled, often isolated, and therefore at increased risk of depression. Such visiting may continue for months, and the nurse may become very familiar with the home situation. It has been suggested that district nurses could identify depression and bring it to the attention of the GP.

A study has recently been carried out in Wandsworth of the ability of 60 district nurses to detect depression among their elderly housebound patients. Accuracy measured against the results of self-report questionnaires was generally poor (Gilleard, 1993). District nurses, like GPs, probably need training in interviewing skills if they are accurately to identify depression in their patients. Given the high incidence of depression reported among the elderly, such training might be cost-effective, although district nurses may have time to do little more than carry out the physical nursing tasks required of them.

Practice nurses

The rapid increase in the number of practice nurses has increased the potential for teamwork in the care of mental disorders in general practice. However, so far there is little evidence that practice nurses are involved at all in the management of psychiatric problems, except in a few cases where they administer depot injections to patients with chronic schizophrenia. Tudor-Hart (1985) has pointed out that they are an under-used resource, who could be valuable if trained properly, given enough time, and allowed to maintain skills by continued experience.

The potential of trained nurse-therapists is considerable. Marks (1985) randomly assigned 25 patients with phobic and obsessive–compulsive disorders to receive either six one-hour sessions of behavioural treatment with exposure therapy from a trained nurse-therapist in primary care or routine treatment from the GP. Patients treated by the nurse did better according to self-rating scales and fear questionnaires. Nurse treatment was also thought to be less expensive when patients' time off work was taken into account.

A pilot study carried out in three urban group practices has demonstrated the feasibility of providing practice nurse support as an adjunct to GP treatment (Wilkinson *et al*, 1993). The practice nurses were used to enhance adherence to treatment by discussing side-effects and encouraging patients to continue with antidepressants. Large-scale randomised controlled trials are in progress to assess the effectiveness of such interventions.

Counsellors

Counsellors have been increasingly recruited into general practices, perhaps because of the large numbers of patients who seek help with situational crises or interpersonal difficulties, who want time to talk that the GP feels personally unable or unwilling to provide. At present there is no requirement for such counsellors to undergo formal accreditation in order to work in general practice, although many arrange this voluntarily with organisations such as the British Association of Counselling and the British Psychological Society. Counselling may be offered in general practice by CPNs, psychologists, or 'practice counsellors'. It is likely that some are referred problems for which they are not trained (Sibbald *et al*, 1993).

Marriage-guidance counsellors have a specific training. They have been found to be happy to work in general practice as opposed to their usual setting (Waydenfeld & Waydenfeld, 1980), and GPs with an interest in psychotherapy were pleased with the outcomes achieved by attached marriage-guidance counsellors (Corney, 1986). However, there is a lack of evidence for the effectiveness of counselling in terms of patient outcome. Many of the problems counsellors tackle may be short-lived and self-limiting. The natural history of the more minor psychological problems is uncertain, and the need for intervention is therefore open to question.

Working with members of the secondary care services

General practitioners and psychiatrists

General practitioners and psychiatrists are being asked to work together more frequently in this era of community care, in situations such as emergency admissions and meetings to plan for hospital discharge. The Mental Health Act 1983 has strengthened patients' rights and placed more pressure on approved social workers to avoid the use of emergency assessment orders whenever possible. This means that the social worker will try strenuously to get two medical recommendations rather than one.

Where possible one of these should be from a GP who has prior knowledge of the patient. Often the GP will have been called in first by the family or neighbours. Such prior knowledge can help the psychiatrist to gain access. Despite the fraught nature of the situation, patients often accept the status of the GP, even if they reject his/her judgement on the need for admission. The psychiatrist, on the other hand, is usually unknown to the patient and carries the overtones of stigma and fear that so often attach to mental hospitals.

Where the GP is prepared to capitalise on this prior relationship and stay in role, the admission is often accomplished smoothly. Psychiatrists will focus on eliciting the pathological aspects of the mental state and the patient's recent experiences. Their appeal to the patient to accept admission will be based mainly on an explanation of how the symptoms can be alleviated. It is often most effective when the GP takes a differing but complementary tack, often much more 'familiar' than the psychiatrist. Some examples of powerful, non-psychiatrist interventions include:

> "You've always trusted me in the past and I think you should trust me now."

> "You know what a gossip the woman downstairs is. If this doctor has to get the police and all that then it'll be all round the estate."

> "Look Mary, I know you don't agree but this man has been perfectly reasonable with you. There is simply no excuse for shouting like that. Stop being so rude and come along now!"

Multidisciplinary meetings to plan discharge are mandatory under section 117 for all patients admitted under the treatment sections (sections 3 and 37) of the Mental Health Act, but should also be held for any patients regarded as vulnerable and in need of long-term coordinated care. The Royal College of Psychiatrists (1989) has recommended that consultants should keep responsibility for discharged patients, delegating care to a named key worker and discharging them to GP care only when after-care is no longer necessary. In response, the Royal College of General Practitioners (1990) has emphasised, however, that GPs are responsible under their terms of service for the continuing care of patients registered with them. A postal survey of one in three GPs in South West Thames Region carried out from St George's found that 90% of GPs favoured a shared care plan for long-term mentally ill patients, with the CPN as key worker (Kendrick *et al*, 1991).

The presence of the GP at section-117 meetings is therefore desirable, given the likely involvement of the primary care team after discharge. It is sometimes possible to schedule meetings so that two or three patients with the same practice are discussed together, which is a more efficient use of the GP's time. GPs may be unaware that they can request such a meeting, for any of their patients who are receiving specialist care, at any time.

A regular informal liaison meeting between the community mental health team and the primary care team can do much to resolve issues of roles and responsibilities for mental illness. One of us (TB) has been involved in such a scheme with three group practices in Wimbledon for the last eight years.

Increasing contact with the psychiatric team helps GPs and other members of the primary care team to develop and use their own skills in managing patients. It benefits the psychiatric team also because, as well as developing good working relationships, they are likely to be made aware of patients with more severe problems earlier in their illness and less often as emergencies.

A joint working party of the Royal Colleges of Psychiatry and General Practice (1993) made a number of recommendations aimed at establishing or increasing such collaboration between primary care and mental health teams.

Clinical psychologists

Psychological treatments have been sought as an alternative to drugs, and can reduce both prescriptions and demands on the GP's time (Earll & Kincey, 1982; Robson *et al*, 1984). Cognitive therapy has been shown to be of value (Chapter 20), particularly for patients with depression who are unable or unwilling to take antidepressants.

Clinical psychologists are a scarce resource in many areas, and some have advocated alternative roles for themselves, such as consultation–liaison, following the lead of psychiatrists. They may offer education, research, and supervision of psychotherapy by other professionals, as well as direct contact with patients, in order to use psychological treatments more appropriately (Salmon, 1984). Such liaison exists in the practice of one of us (AT) in the form of monthly meetings with the catchment-area clinical psychologist, who takes direct referrals. Case discussion provides opportunities for GPs to learn the range of interventions that can be provided and improve the appropriateness of referrals. In some cases the psychologists have seen patients together with the GPs, in order jointly to assess the need for therapy.

Community psychiatric nurses

Community psychiatric nursing developed in response to the need for after-care for patients discharged from psychiatric hospital. Hunter's (1978) survey for the National Schizophrenia Fellowship showed that a large part of their job was to follow up patients with schizophrenia who were stabilised on medication and give regular depot phenothiazine injections.

Community psychiatric nurses frequently accompany the consultant psychiatrist on domiciliary visits, and are responsible for follow-up visits and the administration or supervision of medication. They may be familiar with standardised psychiatric rating scales and play a part in gathering data and research. They usually give continuing support and health education to the patient and to the relatives or other lay carers, as well as practical advice on medication. Such support may continue for years.

There is good evidence of the effectiveness of CPN follow-up for patients with chronic problems of the severity found among psychiatric out-patients. Paykel *et al* (1982) compared CPN follow-up with psychiatric out-patient attendance for 71 chronic neurotic patients. No difference was found between the two types of service in outcome for patients' symptoms, social adjustment, or burden on the family. However, the patients favoured the CPN follow-up, in particular home visits, and expressed a greater satisfaction with the amount of information given.

Some GPs have argued the case for attaching CPNs to general practice, to avoid having to refer patients via a consultant psychiatrist (Harker *et al*, 1976). Some CPNs have welcomed such attachments, for the benefits of closer liaison and feedback, and greater understanding of their role by other members of the primary care team (Dyke, 1984).

However, problems have arisen from the move towards giving GPs direct access to CPNs. There is evidence that GPs use the opportunity to refer patients with minor disorders of anxiety and depression, situational crises, and interpersonal difficulties, who would not previously have been referred to the specialist service. Wooff *et al* (1986) found that the CPN services in Salford took on many more patients directly from GPs between 1976 and 1982, and were concerned that by treating the morbidity found in primary care, the service was being diverted away from the severely mentally ill. In a further study they suggested that nurses attached to primary care services became isolated from the specialist psychiatric team, received little supportive supervision from their managers, and lacked training in the assessment and treatment skills required for their changing role (Wooff & Goldberg, 1988).

The five-yearly survey of CPNs in Britain (White, 1991) showed that referrals from psychiatrists fell from 59% to 42% between 1985 and 1990, while GP referrals increased from 23% to 36%. Many long-term mentally ill patients have no contact with CPNs, while many CPNs work where their services are needed least, in practices with lower rates of mental illness where other mental health professionals already work. The government is concerned that specialist services such as community psychiatric nursing should be targeted appropriately to patients with more severe problems (Department of Health, 1988).

Social workers

Given the frequency with which social problems are associated with psychiatric disorders in general practice, collaboration between GPs and social workers would seem highly desirable, yet is often extremely limited.

Social workers can play a number of roles in the primary care of mental disorder (Corney, 1984*a*). They can carry out a detailed social assessment, which can help other members of the team plan their management, provide practical help through their access to local authority resources (such as home-helps, temporary or permanent residential care, and day nurseries), advise on benefits and rights, and they can carry out counselling, crisis intervention, and group work.

Cooper *et al* (1975) measured the effect of a social worker attached to a primary care team in the management of a group of 92 patients with chronic neurotic illness over 12 months, compared with a matched group of

97 patients attending neighbouring practices without such an attachment. The outcome was better for the intervention group in terms of symptoms and the need for continuing medication and supervision. An analysis of the social workers' activities (Shepherd *et al*, 1979) found that they dealt with practical problems in two-thirds of cases and gave psychotherapy in one-third. There was more evidence of benefit from the practical help than from psychotherapy. However, 16% of the patients declined to see a social worker, preferring continuing support from the doctor.

Corney (1984*a*) conducted a randomised controlled trial of social-worker intervention versus routine GP care for 80 acutely depressed women aged 18–45, over six months. She found no overall difference in clinical or social outcome between the two groups. On analysing results for subgroups of patients, however, it seemed that women with acute-on-chronic depression associated with marital difficulties fared significantly better with the help of a social worker.

Attachments of social workers to general practice are usually welcomed by the GPs, as well as being potentially beneficial to patients. Williams & Clare (1979) found that GPs particularly appreciated the social worker's help with patients with financial, employment, housing, and criminal problems.

Collaboration has decreased since the Seebohm reorganisation of 1970, however, when the three social-work departments of child care, welfare, and mental health were combined into the social services department, with generic social workers based in area offices with strict catchment areas. Corney (1984*b*) found that social workers attached to general practices had many more contacts with the primary care teams than intake social workers based in a local-authority department, yet the intake social workers tended to see the same sorts of people, with a similar range of problems, including mental or physical health problems, which might have benefited from the primary care team's help.

The Community Care Act may increase the interaction between primary care and social services. The new legislation makes social-service authorities responsible for ensuring that multidisciplinary assessments of need are made, and calls on GPs to contribute to these. The government has reminded GPs that under paragraph 13 of their terms of service they are obliged to refer patients needing specialist care and to give advice to those patients who might benefit from local-authority social services. Where close working relationships are not already in place, the government wishes to see the development of clearly agreed local arrangements between GPs and social services (Secretaries of State, 1989).

How can teamwork be improved?

A joint working party of the Royal College of General Practitioners (1986) and the Royal College of Nursing set out a number of suggestions for enhancing teamwork within primary care. They stressed that communication is essential to teamwork and that members must give communication high priority. Formal and structured meetings should be held at intervals to define the needs of the practice population and to construct objectives for the team. On a day-to-day basis, members should be available to each other at short notice – it is unacceptable to keep another professional waiting longer than one is prepared to wait oneself. Each team member should have access to a desk and telephone, and adequate common-room facilities. Shared records can improve teamwork, although different members may wish to keep separate records as well, to maintain confidentiality where necessary.

Interdisciplinary education, in both vocational training and continuing education, is seen by most of the proponents as the best way to increase teamwork in the future. Joint training initiatives between GPs and social workers (Samuel & Dodge, 1981), and GPs, social workers, and nurses (Jones, 1986), were set up with the aims of improving recognition of each other's roles, encouraging attitudes of mutual trust, and increasing collaboration as a result. Small but positive changes in attitude were reported.

Pritchard (1981) suggested that established teams should set aside time to take a look at their own processes – and ask a number of questions:

Goals/tasks	What are we trying to achieve?
Roles	Who does what?
Procedures	How do we go about it?
Relationships	Do we get on well together?

Interdisciplinary training seems to be on the increase. A survey by the Centre for the Advancement of Interprofessional Education (CAIPE), carried out between 1987 and 1988, revealed that shared learning activities were numerous and distributed broadly across Britain. GPs were involved in 37% of the examples, and social workers in 46%. Over 50% of the reported initiatives included as objectives the promotion of teamwork or the advancement of interprofessional understanding, or both (Horder, 1992).

Unfortunately, there is a paucity of empirical evidence to support the effectiveness of teamwork in terms of outcome for patients. There is a need for a rigorous evaluation of the effectiveness of teamwork, particularly in mental illness, taking into account the views of the sufferer. Research is needed comparing the outcome for patients in practices with high levels of collaboration with that for practices with low levels.

It is usually assumed that more teamwork will lead to better care for patients. However, Dingwall (1979) has pointed out that this is not necessarily the case. Patients may be better off with a range of different approaches from which to choose, some of which may be more sympathetic to their particular personality and beliefs, and may even exploit differences between professionals to advantage, rather than being faced with a cohesive team presenting a united front. Studies of the effectiveness of teamwork are therefore awaited with great interest.

Meanwhile, the burden of mental illness will continue to disadvantage many patients living in the community. GPs and their co-workers could do more in many cases to relieve that burden, by undergoing training where necessary and organising themselves so that, between them, they can offer a range of interventions in primary care.

Acknowledgements

We are grateful to Professor Paul Freeling for his invaluable comments on the manuscript. TK is supported by a grant from the Mental Health Foundation.

References

BRISCOE, M. E. & LINDLEY, P. (1982) Identification and management of psychosocial problems by health visitors. *Health Visitor*, **55**, 167–169.

COOPER, B., HARWIN, B. G., DEPLA, C., *et al* (1975) Mental health care in the community: an evaluative study. *Psychological Medicine*, **5**, 372–380.

COPELAND, J. (1981) What is a case? A case for what? In *What Is a Case; The Problem of Definition in Psychiatric Community Surveys* (eds J. K. Wing, P. Bebbington & L. N. Robins), pp.9–11. London: Grant McIntyre.

CORNEY, R. H. (1984*a*) The effectiveness of attached social workers in the management of depressed female patients in general practice. *Psychological Medicine*, **14** (Monograph Suppl. 6), 1–47.

——— (1984*b*) The mental and physical health of clients referred to social workers in a local authority department and a general practice attachment scheme. *Psychological Medicine*, **14**, 137–144.

——— (1986) Marriage guidance counselling in general practice. *Journal of the Royal College of General Practitioners*, **36**, 424–426.

DEPARTMENT OF HEALTH (1988) *On the State of the Public Health. The Annual Report of the Chief Medical Officer of the Department of Health for the Year 1987*. London: HMSO.

——— (1991) *On the State of the Public Health. The Annual Report of the Chief Medical Officer of the Department of Health for the Year 1990*. London: HMSO.

DINGWALL, R. (1979) Problems of teamwork in primary care. In *Teamwork in the Personal Social Services and Health Care* (eds S. Lonsdale, A. Webb & T. L. Briggs). London: Croom Helm.

DYKE, B. (1984) CPNs and primary health care team attachment. *Nursing Times*, 7 March, 55–57.

EARLL, L. & KINCEY, J. (1982) Clinical psychology in general practice: a controlled trial evaluation. *Journal of the Royal College of General Practitioners*, **32**, 32–37.

GASK, L., MCGRATH, G., GOLDBERG, D., *et al* (1987) Improving the psychiatric skills of established general practitioners: evaluation of group teaching. *Medical Education*, **21**, 362–368.

GILLEARD, C. (1993) *The Housebound Elderly Project*: Final Report to the South West Thames Regional Health Authority Research and Development Committee, St George's Hospital Medical School, London.

GILMORE, M., BRUCE, N. & HUNT, M. (1974) *The Work of the Nursing Team in General Practice*. London: Council for the Education and Training of Health Visitors.

GOLDBERG, D. & HUXLEY, P. (1980) *Mental Illness in the Community, the Pathway to Psychiatric Care*. London: Tavistock.

GREGSON, B. A., CARTLIDGE, A. & BOND, J. (1991) *Interprofessional Collaboration in Primary Health Care Organizations, Occasional Paper 52*. London: Royal College of General Practitioners.

HARKER, P., LEOPOLDT, H. & ROBINSON, J. R. (1976) Attaching community psychiatric nurses to general practice. *Journal of the Royal College of General Practitioners*, **26**, 666–671.

HOLDEN, J. M., SAGOVSKY, R. & COX, J. L. (1989) Counselling in a general practice setting: controlled study of health visitor intervention in treatment of postnatal depression. *British Medical Journal*, **298**, 223–226.

HORDER, J. (1992) A national survey that needs to be repeated. *Journal of Interprofessional Care*, **6**, 65–71.

HUNTER, P. (1978) *Schizophrenia and Community Psychiatric Nursing*. London: National Schizophrenia Fellowship.

JEBALI, C. (1991) Working together to support women with postnatal depression. *Health Visitor*, **64**, 410–411.

JONES, R. V. H. (1986) *Working Together, Learning Together*. Exeter: Royal College of General Practitioners.

KENDRICK, T., SIBBALD, B., BURNS, T., *et al* (1991) Role of general practitioners in care of long-term mentally ill patients. *British Medical Journal*, **302**, 508–510.

——, SIBBALD, B., ADDINGTON-HALL, J., *et al*, (1993) Distribution of mental health professionals working on site in English and Welsh general practices. *British Medical Journal*, **307**, 544–546.

MARKS, I. (1985) Controlled trial of psychiatric nurse therapists in primary care. *British Medical Journal*, **290**, 1181–1184.

MELZER, D., HALE, A. S., MALIK, S. J., *et al* (1991) Community care for patients with schizophrenia one year after hospital discharge. *British Medical Journal*, **303**, 1023–1026.

MITCHELL, A. R. K. (1985) Psychiatrists in primary health care settings. *British Journal of Psychiatry*, **147**, 371–379.

PARKES, C. M., BROWN, G. W. & MONCK, E. M. (1962) The general practitioner and the schizophrenic patient. *British Medical Journal*, **ii**, 972–976.

PAYKEL, E. S., MANGEN, S. P., GRIFFITH, J. H., *et al*, (1982) Community psychiatric nursing for neurotic patients. A controlled trial. *British Journal of Psychiatry*, **140**, 573–581.

PRITCHARD, P. M. M. (1981) *Manual of Primary Health Care. Its Nature and Organisation*. Oxford: Oxford University Press.

ROBSON, M. H., FRANCE, R. & BLAND, M. (1984) Clinical psychologist in primary care: controlled clinical and economic evaluation. *British Medical Journal*, **288**, 1805–1808.

ROYAL COLLEGE OF GENERAL PRACTITIONERS (1986) *Prevention and the Primary Care Team*. Exeter: Royal College of General Practitioners.

—— (1990) *Comments on the Working Party Report on Good Practice in Discharge and Aftercare Procedures for Patients Discharged from Inpatient Treatment*. London: Royal College of General Practitioners.

—— (1993) *Shared Care of Patients with Mental Health Problems* (Occasional Paper 60). London: Royal College of General Practitioners.

ROYAL COLLEGE OF PSYCHIATRISTS (1989) *Good Practice in Discharge and Aftercare Procedures for Patients Discharged from Inpatient Treatment*. London: Royal College of Psychiatrists.

SALMON, P. (1984) The psychologist's contribution to primary care: a reappraisal. *Journal of the Royal College of General Practitioners*, **34**, 190–193.

SAMUEL, O. W. & DODGE, D. (1981) A course in collaboration for social workers and general practitioners. *Journal of the Royal College of General Practitioners*, **31**, 172–175.

SECRETARIES OF STATE FOR HEALTH, SOCIAL SECURITY, WALES AND SCOTLAND (1989) *Caring for People. Community Care in the Next Decade and Beyond*. London: HMSO.

SHEPHERD, M., HARWIN, G. G., DEPLA, C., *et al* (1979) Social work and the primary care of mental disorder. *Psychological Medicine*, **9**, 661–669.

SIBBALD, B., ADDINGTON-HALL, J., BRENNEMAN, D., *et al*, (1993) Counsellors in English and Welsh general practices: their nature and distribution. *British Medical Journal*, **306**, 29–33.

STRATHDEE, G. & WILLIAMS, P. (1984) A survey of psychiatrists in primary care: the silent growth of a new service. *Journal of the Royal College of General Practitioners*, **34**, 615–618.

TUDOR-HART, J. (1985) Practice nurses: an underused resource. *British Medical Journal*, **290**, 1162–1163.

WAYDENFELD, D. & WAYDENFELD, S. W. (1980) Counselling in general practice. *Journal of the Royal College of General Practitioners*, **30**, 671–677.

WHITE, E. (1991) *The 3rd Quinquennial National Community Psychiatric Nursing Survey*. Department of Nursing, University of Manchester.

WILKINSON, G., ALLEN, P., MARSHALL, E., *et al* (1993) The role of the practice nurse in the management of depression in general practice: treatment adherence to antidepressant medication. *Psychological Medicine*, **23**, 229–237.

WILLIAMS, P. & CLARE, A. (1979) Social workers in primary health care: the general practitioner's viewpoint. *Journal of the Royal College of General Practitioners*, **29**, 554–558.

WOOFF, K., GOLDBERG, D. P. & FRYERS, T. (1986) Patients in receipt of community psychiatric nursing care in Salford 1976–1982. *Psychological Medicine*, **16**, 407–414.

—— & —— (1988) Further observations on the practice of community care in Salford. Differences between community psychiatric nurses and mental health social workers. *British Journal of Psychiatry*, **153**, 30–37.

WORLD HEALTH ORGANIZATION (1973) *Psychiatry and Primary Medical Care*. Copenhagen: WHO.

19 Counselling and psychotherapy

MICHAEL SHELDON

Medicine has a long history and tradition which mould and affect the beliefs and actions of the doctor. Change is slow, but this is held to be a good thing as it is so easy to be persuaded by the latest fashionable treatment, and end up doing harm to patients. Within my own professional lifetime there have been several major disasters through too hasty acceptance of the latest wonder drug. The slow process of careful testing is not an establishment ploy to hold back medical advances, but a necessary protection for patients, who may be extremely vulnerable. Of course, helpful advances are also slowed down, and innovators have to suffer the rejection of their peers as they seek to change accepted beliefs and practices. However, I would not advocate changing the vetting procedures, and recommend that the talking therapies are scrutinised as closely as any new drug, so that patients are helped effectively and efficiently, and not harmed in any way.

All doctors have to learn to relate well to their patients, encouraging them to talk and reveal their hidden problems. But most have not the time, skill, nor inclination to provide the psychotherapeutic help which may benefit a large proportion of patients. Often in the doctor's mind is the unspoken question as to whether the talking therapies actually do any good. Perhaps they just make the patient feel a little better, so they put up with their problems with a smile rather than a frown? Most doctors still prefer to give physical treatment with drugs, diet, or surgery, which they feel they understand, rather than a 'talking treatment', the effectiveness of which is not so easy to measure.

What about the patients? Do they want counselling and psychotherapy? If you ask people what they want from their doctor they will include such attributes as 'kind and warm personality', 'always available', 'makes an accurate diagnosis', 'gives the correct treatment', or 'quickly refers to the appropriate specialist'. They usually do not appreciate being told that their problem is in the mind, or that they need a psychiatrist to help them. They can respond with statements like ''Are you saying that there is nothing wrong with me?'' Few patients welcome the idea that their problem is not physical, but somehow within themselves. The identification of the value of the person with their mind and emotions is strong. They are prepared to say ''My lungs are letting me down'', but less happy to admit ''My thoughts and emotions are letting me down''.

In summary we need to acknowledge that the beliefs and opinions of both doctors and patients have played a large part in the resistance to the introduction of the talking therapies into medicine. There have of course been pioneers such as Michael Balint (1964), who helped doctors to understand the value and potential of the use of their own personality as a part of the therapeutic process. With increasing understanding of the role of stress in producing illness, and the importance of the patient's beliefs and attitudes in the treatment, the talking therapies are at last taking their rightful place as an essential part of general practice. But as this area is still relatively new, there are many problems and questions which will need answering before they are generally accepted as a routine part of general practice.

This chapter looks at the different types and the effectiveness of counselling before considering its place in primary care, and in particular whether GPs should do the counselling themselves, or whether the attachment of a counsellor to the primary care team is more appropriate. Finally, the practical issues in counselling attachments are discussed.

The 'talking therapies'

The term 'talking therapies' covers a wide range of activities which focus on the interaction between the patient and a caring professional as the main part of therapy. The range of such therapies is wide and, as shown in Fig. 19.1, includes patient self-help groups at the bottom of the 'ladder', up to psychiatry at the top. In Fig. 19.1 the therapies on the left of the ladder would normally take place within primary care, and those on the right outside primary care.

Many professionals use the skills of counselling within their work, and in primary care health visitors, nurses, and doctors all exercise these skills daily. Some GPs go further and set aside extended consultations in order to provide more in-depth therapy for their patients, using the skills of counselling and psychotherapy.

'Medical counselling' is a term which covers the specialist nurses who are attached to hospital clinics and provide advice and counsel for patients with such illnesses as colostomies, diabetes and cancer. 'Primary care' counselling includes all counselling which is short term (usually around six sessions), and which involves the core skills and beliefs of counselling rather than a particular school or therapeutic approach. 'Specialist' counselling will normally be situated outside the practice and use special therapeutic

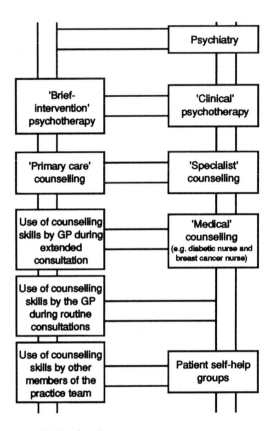

Fig. 19.1. The ladder of talking therapies

techniques such as drama and group therapy. Brief-intervention psychotherapy is similar to primary care counselling in that it uses straightforward intervention therapy to effect a change in the patient in a few sessions. It is therefore different from other psychotherapeutic approaches, which would normally go more deeply into the patient's background and personality rather than simply focus on the current problems presented.

Counselling and psychotherapy

Sometimes the terms 'counselling' and 'psychotherapy' are used as if they were interchangeable, but although there are many similarities between them, there are also key differences. As far as the client is concerned they overlap rather more than they diverge. The counsellor does not usually work explicitly with the transference of feelings between the counsellor and the client, whereas a psychotherapist does. Psychotherapy tends to deal with deep-seated personal issues, and consequently is more long term and greater in depth. Counselling, on the other hand, tends to focus on how to deal with specific current life problems. Training in psychotherapy takes longer than counsellor training and often includes personal analysis, which is less common with counsellors. However, many psychologists offer counselling and are happy to offer a limited number of sessions to deal with specific problems. Some counsellors are also trained and experienced in offering more long-term, deep psychotherapeutic exploration. To a large extent, the similarities and differences depend on the needs of the client and the training and orientation of individual practitioners, rather than being inherent in the activities themselves.

Counselling skills in primary care

The basic skills of counselling centre around communication between the patient (or client) and the carer at a deep personal level. They involve the ability to create a warm relationship and listen in an encouraging way which enables patients to talk freely about feelings, thoughts, beliefs, and attitudes. The ability to understand patients' situations and personal responses (which includes appropriate sympathy and empathy) is extremely important. Finally, carers need to summarise and clarify patients' situations to enhance their own understanding of their difficulties, and then encourage them to seek their own solutions and activities to resolve difficulties. These skills are therefore effective and useful in a wide variety of situations, and all members of the primary care team should have basic instruction in their use.

The real problems associated with the use of counselling skills centres on the issues of lack of time and expertise. Listening to people and keeping a 'patient-centred' approach takes time. Also, not all doctors have the natural ability and training to focus on patients in the required way and then allow them to set the pace and direction of an interview.

Formal counselling

All counselling uses these basic skills of counselling, but within a certain belief and value structure. This may be summarised as follows:

> Clients are at the centre of the process and their beliefs and values are respected. The counsellor creates a relationship of trust and acceptance in which he/she listens, without making judgements, and reflects back to clients an objective view of their subjective experience so that they can clarify thoughts and feelings, thereby helping them grow in understanding themselves and gaining new perspectives on their situation. This enables clients to obtain more control over their own lives by recognising problems and discovering appropriate solutions for themselves.

The counsellor would seek to help a client to address and resolve feelings of inner conflict, improve relationships, cope with crises, and make decisions. Counsellors should avoid giving advice, but should help clients to reflect on any advice they had received from others in order to assess its value for them personally.

The most important part of the counselling process is the therapeutic relationship that develops between a counsellor and the client. The counsellor structures the counselling process in order to allow clients both the time and the freedom to explore their thoughts and feelings in an atmosphere of trust and respect. Counselling aims to help people accept and come to terms with their difficulties and identify ways of coping more effectively and resourcefully.

Stages of counselling

The counselling process thus follows a series of stages which Egan (1986) has described as problem exploration and clarification, solution finding, and action and resolution. While other models may differ from this categorisation, Egan's three-stage skills model is well recognised, and is structured as follows.

Stage 1. Problem exploration and clarification. The counsellor, within the context of a warm, accepting relationship, enables clients to explore their problems from their own frame of reference, and then to focus on specific concerns. This stage requires attention-giving, listening, and 'active-listening' skills. The latter includes the counsellor's communication of empathetic understanding, by non-critical acceptance and genuineness, using paraphrasing, the reflection of feelings, summarising, focusing, and helping the client to be specific.

Stage 2. New understanding to find solutions. Clients are helped to see themselves and their situations in new perspectives, and to focus on what might be done to cope more effectively. They are thus helped to see what strengths and resources are available to them. This stage requires all of the skills mentioned in stage 1, along with what Egan calls 'challenging' skills which comprise:

(a) the communication of deeper empathetic understanding, including such intuitive techniques as the use of 'hunches', and trying to discern what clients are really trying to say behind the words and problems they present

(b) helping clients to recognise themes, inconsistencies, behaviour patterns, and feelings

(c) giving feedback of what the counsellor has discerned, including appropriate sharing of both the counsellor's and client's feelings and experiences; this aims to help clients understand what is happening between themselves and the counsellor

(d) finally, the setting of realistic goals is encouraged.

Stage 3. Action and resolution. Finally, clients are helped to consider ways in which they are going to act, to look at the costs and consequences involved, to plan action and how to implement and evaluate it. The skills involved are all of the above, and in addition focusing on creative thinking, problem-solving and decision-making, and the planning and evaluating of actions.

Egan's three key stages illustrate the steps in counselling and identify a range of skills the counsellor uses to facilitate the process and to help the client resolve his/her problems. While the counsellor's approach and interventions will depend on the theoretical model adopted, most methods of counselling will be underpinned by a structure similar, but not necessarily identical to this.

'Specialist' counselling

There are said to be over 250 different models of counselling, although the main ones involve a person-centred, humanistic approach. Many counsellors additionally use a variety of therapeutic techniques such as behavioural therapy, transactional analysis, Gestalt therapy, and cognitive therapy. Besides different schools of counselling, there are counsellors who concentrate on particular needs such as abortion, bereavement, and marriage guidance. Usually, these counsellors have had specific experience and training in their special area of expertise, in addition to their basic training in counselling.

'Medical' counselling

This term covers a more directive type of advice and help for people with specific long-term or terminal medical conditions. They may be considered as the medical answer to the self-help group. Help is usually provided by a trained nurse with special knowledge and understanding of the particular illness. She/he is available to the patient to answer questions, direct to resources, provide reassurance, and generally help patients cope with fears and anxieties as they adapt to the new situation. Such counsellors have been especially helpful in such areas as breast cancer, colostomies, genetic illnesses, and diabetes.

'Brief-intervention' psychotherapy

This type of psychotherapy has many similarities to counselling and is also used to help a patient cope with specific presenting problems rather than undertake an in-depth analysis of the patient, which can be a lengthy process.

Often a straightforward model of behaviour modification may be used to achieve a specific short-term objective. Group therapy is also used to help relaxation and stress management, to stop smoking or other addictive behaviour. A limited number of sessions is usually offered, and help is given in a specific rather than a general way.

'Clinical' psychotherapy

This includes the whole range of psychotherapeutic help, where deeper analysis is used to increase patients' self-understanding and so help them to resource long-term changes in their beliefs and behaviour which have been producing the presenting problems. Therapy usually takes longer than other types of counselling, and may involve several team members, from psychiatric nurses to psychiatrists as well as psychologists. This chapter concentrates on the counselling in primary care, and so these therapies are not elaborated upon.

Do the talking therapies work?

While it is important to conduct trials to determine the effectiveness of the talking therapies, it is difficult to organise satisfactory clinical trials because of their personal and individual nature. There is also a large range of theoretical approaches to counselling, each one having dedicated practitioners who accept that their approach is effective and, in the right hands, without harmful effects. Only a few clinical trials have been attempted on the use of psychotherapy and counselling attachments in general practice, and the results have not been decisive.

Several studies have attempted to evaluate the effectiveness of counselling by assessing changes in patients' behaviour and health through an examination of medical records before and after therapy. Details of numbers of attendances, prescriptions written and referrals made have been collected from the medical records. Such studies (McLeod, 1988) have shown a reduction in visits made to the doctor after counselling when compared with a similar period beforehand. Other studies have found a reduction in the number of psychotropic drugs prescribed or in the number of psychiatric referrals.

It has been argued that not only has the patient's health improved after counselling, but also that counsellor attachments are cost-effective in reducing the workload of GPs and by decreasing prescriptions needed. Results using such retrospective record analysis must be treated with caution, and it must be recognised that in a successful counsellor attachment there may be other factors which use up any time saved, and other costs which may increase. Although we might confidently assert that patient care has improved, it may not be easy to assert that money or time has also been saved.

What of the dangers of counselling? Firstly, because of the extended time needed for counselling consultations, the patient may deteriorate mentally without the doctor seeing the patient until the therapy is finished. The counsellor may not be skilled enough to recognise dangerous symptoms and signs, and so harm may occur to the patient. The counsellor and doctor need to work closely together to avoid this. Secondly, the counsellor may affect the patient's behaviour on the surface, but concealing deeper psychological problems, which may deteriorate unnoticed and so medication may not be given at the appropriate time. Thirdly, appropriate referrals may be delayed by an overoptimistic attitude of the counsellor in reporting back to the GP.

Which patients benefit from counselling?

The main aim of counselling is to identify emotional problems with ineffective coping at an early stage, and by appropriate actions prevent more serious disturbances developing. Some of the common problems which may be helped are anxiety, stress, and malaise provoked by difficulties and conflicts in marriage, the family, and other relationships. Likewise, mental and emotional illnesses such as depression and phobia, and addictive behaviour such as drug and alcohol abuse, may also benefit from counselling. Patients suffering from problems such as personality disorders, severe mental disturbance, or those with psychotic tendencies usually need more help than counselling can offer. Such problems will usually need the use of medication and are properly considered the province of the GP and psychiatrist rather than the counsellor.

Counselling in general practice

If counselling and psychotherapy are to be widely accepted in general practice, we need to face certain problems and issues which arise, and seek for answers which satisfy both doctors and counsellors. One of the main questions concerns whether the doctor is the best person to provide this, or whether there is a need for professionally trained counsellors to come into practices to take on this task.

Can the GP provide counselling?

Although most GPs have not received formal training in counselling, their personality and life experience usually make them well suited to it. They are often good listeners, who find that patients will reveal their more personal problems with little encouragement. Whatever the experience and competence of GPs in counselling, their professional role puts them in touch with a large number of people who will turn to and confide in their doctor when they are in trouble. Many studies have indicated that up to a third of patients who present in general practice have problems that are largely emotional or psychosocial in nature (Chapters 1 and 3).

Every working day the GP deals with relationship, marital and family problems, problems at school and at work, sexual and reproductive difficulties, illness and disability, and the problems of dying. Doctors in primary care are in a unique position to help patients in times of trouble. They will often have known their patients for a number of years, enabling the practitioner and patient to build up a relationship of trust and confidence, and thus giving the doctor an insight into the patient's personality, family, and situation. The GP may use this on-going therapeutic relationship to 'counsel' the patient, helping him/her come to terms with a distressing event, such as a bereavement, by encouraging the patient to talk about the feelings engendered by the loss. Many doctors find this a rewarding aspect of their work and will set aside extended consultations for those patients who need more time to talk.

Unfortunately there are some patients who never seem to get better, whose problems seem insoluble, and who present again and again without seeming to deal satisfactorily with the underlying issues in their lives. The GP thus needs to learn when his/her 'counselling' the patient within the brief or extended consultation will suffice, and when the patient would benefit from more formal counselling.

Is counselling appropriate within the consultation?

When the GP uses counselling skills, the situation arises out of the normal consultation and is an extension of it. Many GPs are aware of the psychological aspects of patient's presenting problems, and will attempt to examine these issues in the course of the consultation. It is important to stress that the use of counselling skills does not make the GP a counsellor. There is a difference between counselling within the confines of the consultation by the use of counselling skills to facilitate the consultation process, and counselling in the formal sense outlined above. While few doctors take on formal counselling, most will inevitably find themselves in situations every day where counselling skills are needed.

The use of counselling skills by the GP

The doctor's use of counselling skills benefits both the doctor and patient. There is good evidence to show that using counselling skills in a clinical consultation improves medical management. The outcome of patient care is likely to be improved if the doctor actively involves the patient in his/her treatment through discussion and explanation. Exploring the patient's beliefs, emotions and concerns, in addition to specifying the nature and history of the presenting problem, has been shown to facilitate diagnostic skills and to increase patient cooperation in following advice, thus leading to improved patient care (McLeod, 1988). Moreover, the clinical consultation is ideally conducted in an atmosphere not too different from that of counselling – the doctor sharing with the patient the task of solving a problem, bringing his/her expertise as a resource as they work together on the problem.

The GP as counsellor

While the simple use of counselling skills during the course of a normal consultation rarely leads to difficulties, more formal counselling in inexperienced hands may actually cause harm. Whether or not the GP should offer formal counselling to patients is open to some debate. Although the problems and practicalities facing the doctor as counsellor can be overcome, it is worth drawing the attention of interested GPs to some of the issues that need to be addressed if he/she is to practise counselling.

Although counselling skills help the GP in the clinical consultation, the main focus of the doctor's work is often different from that of the counsellor. The aim and function of counselling is to encourage the client to help him/her to clarify difficulties and attempt to resolve them. Rather than giving advice, reassurance or medication, the counsellor systematically attempts to avoid long-term dependency by putting the responsibility for their lives back into the patients' hands.

The GP's role, however, is more that of an expert, with knowledge not generally available to the patient. The doctor's job is to listen to the patient, attempt to diagnose any disorder, and to prescribe treatment to ease or cure. GPs are seen as authoritatiave helpers who define and resolve problems, direct the course of treatment, and give advice and support. Thus the doctor and patient would need to make a mental shift in the way they see each other before formal counselling could begin. Many patients see the doctor more as a father figure than as an equal, and could find the change from the doctor role to the counsellor role difficult to accept. Even so, the relationship between doctor and patient is unlikely to be purely that of counsellor and client, since the doctor will frequently be called upon to give practical help and directive advice, which would be inappropriate in formal counselling. The dual role of doctor/counsellor can therefore be a difficult one for both the patient and the practitioner.

Counselling is centred on the patient, and so takes more time than a doctor-centred consultation. Counsellors usually allow up to an hour per session and see the client for six to ten sessions. If offering counselling in the formal sense described here, it is unlikely that a doctor could satisfy the demands of patients for counselling without adversely affecting the time needed for clinical work. Some doctors who have tried to offer psychotherapeutic assistance in general practice have found that their personal and home life suffers. Counselling is often stressful, and the effective counsellor needs to be able to listen to clients' problems without over-defending or identifying too closely with them.

Need for supervision

It is becoming increasingly accepted that counsellors need a supervisory relationship, preferably with a more experienced counsellor. The counsellor should meet with a supervisor regularly, to discuss both cases and personal problems raised by the counselling load. Supervision enables counsellors to have an overview of a case, identifying personal feelings and professional bias which may be hindering rather than helping the client. Supervision is a form of consultation with a peer, which involves a continuing process of learning and an opportunity for counsellors to reflect on their work and some of the feelings engendered by it. Many GPs would not see the need for this type of supervisory relationship, but it is helpful and important where the nature of the counselling activity concentrates on emotional areas which can drain the energy of the doctor and adversely affect his/her personal life.

Issues of training

Being aware of the difference between formal counselling and counselling skills will help the GP to recognise when a patient needs more formal counselling, and when one or two brief consultations in the surgery may suffice. For the GP committed to counselling, the problems of the dual role of doctor/counsellor are not insurmountable but need some forethought. In the interests of the therapeutic relationship and effective counselling, those doctors wishing to undertake counselling in general practice will need specific training, and should also enter into a continuing supervisory relationship with another counsellor. The GP's training may well have included counselling issues, but the whole thrust of training in counselling is to allow the counsellor to be comfortable and effective in a 'client-controlled' environment, where advice and help is given in such a way that the client can modify or even reject it without damaging the relationship. This attitude is not one in which doctors have normally received training and experience.

Should counselling be provided in primary care?

Is counselling an activity which can usefully become a routine part of primary care? Some may argue that counselling services should be independent of general practice, but to others it seems appropriate to make a resource which is beneficial to the patient more widely available by including it within the primary care team. It has been suggested that there are many advantages for both counsellors and GPs when they work closely together. A referral to a practice counsellor within the same building is usually more acceptable to the patient and produces a more fruitful cooperation between the doctor and counsellor. A counsellor who builds a good relationship with all the other members of the primary care team can have a much greater effect on patient care than solely through the patients he/she counsels directly.

Sheldon (1992) discusses these issues further in a 'counselling information folder' produced by the Royal College of General Practitioners in conjunction with the British Association for Counselling, which includes practical experience and applications in the attachment of counsellors.

Practical issues in counselling attachments

Which counselling theory is best?

Despite many basic differences between counselling methods, it has been suggested that a positive outcome and the deliverance of effective counselling depend more on certain characteristics in the counsellor than on the theory of counselling used. Counsellors who offer warmth and acceptance and exhibit genuineness and empathy are consistently the most effective.

This raises the question of the importance of the theories of counselling, and yet there is evidence from both the applied and research fields to support the argument for counsellors to have worked out a clear theoretical model for themselves. Basing their counselling on a theory of understanding can provide grounding for the counsellor in face of the client's occasional intense distress. Many counsellors use a variety of sources in their work and develop a method of working most suited to their personality and beliefs, honed by experience.

Assessment of training and qualifications of counsellors

General practitioners who work with a counsellor need to ensure that the counsellor is competent and adequately trained. The British Association for Counselling (see Appendix) gives guidance about the qualifications and accreditation of counsellors.

Responsibility for the patient

The GP has the final responsibility for any patient referred to a practice counsellor, so procedures for referral and consultation, note-keeping and reporting back, all need to be clearly defined at the start of an attachment. It is advisable to write down the agreed procedures and then review them regularly, as the issue of confidentiality may create problems if not faced openly. All counsellors should also have their own professional insurance cover, as they have to take responsibility for all that happens within the counselling relationship.

It is advisable for a practice counsellor to become a full member of the practice team, and attend team meetings. There should be a regular review of the methods of referral, issues of confidentiality, and the appropriateness of referrals.

Confidentiality and record-keeping

It is normal for any counsellor to have and respect a code of confidentiality equivalent to that of doctors. The problem comes with access to a patient's notes by the counsellor, and then the keeping of confidentialities which the counsellor has received from the patient and of which the doctor may not be aware. Some practices allow the counsellor full access to the medical records, while others provide only a written referral note and expect the counsellor to ask the GP for any further information required. Likewise, the counsellor may make his/her notes available to the GP, but more usually a report would be provided which could be placed in the patient's medical records. It must now be recognised that the patient has access to most records, so care should be taken with what is committed to writing. At all times patients should be kept informed of confidentiality procedures, and their permission asked if there is any change in these rules.

Conclusions

Many would now argue that the case for counselling attachments to general practice has been made, and patients can only benefit from the addition of counselling and psychotherapy to the range of therapies offered in primary care. While this belief may be correct, we still need to encourage careful studies of the positive and negative effects of such attachments. While I believe that all good GPs should learn about counselling, and practise the use of counselling skills within their consultations, I do not see how large numbers of GPs can become effective in counselling without disrupting their working practices.

Let us welcome well trained and competent counsellors into general practice, and give them the same status as we give to nurses, midwives and those of the team who minister to the physical needs of our patients. The illnesses of the mind and heart are usually much more devastating than those of the body, and GPs and their teams are ideally placed to help and support people in their times of difficulty.

Appendix. Resources

The British Association for Counselling (BAC) has many books, leaflets and other resources concerning counselling. There is a specific division for Counselling in Medical Settings, which has produced many helpful leaflets. The address of the BAC is: 1 Regent Place, Rugby, Warwickshire CV21 2PJ (tel. 0788-578328, fax. 0788-562189).

Michael Balint (1964) describes his theories and findings, which contain many insights into the doctor/patient interaction. Egan's (1986) textbook describes the theories and stages of counselling which he recommends and practises. McLeod (1988) describes and evaluates the work of counsellors attached to 14 general practices. Many practical problems are discussed, and references to relevant work are provided.

The information folder edited by Sheldon (1992) and produced by the Royal College of General Practitioners is a collection of articles by counsellors and doctors with practical experience in general practice counselling. This arises from a joint working party between the College and the BAC. It contains many references and is a useful resource pack for anyone contemplating bringing counselling into the practice. The BAC has produced two guides to counselling in general practice (Irving & Heath, 1991; Rowland & Hurd, 1991). These two booklets, available from the BAC, provide an introduction to the potential and problems of GP attachments in counselling.

Rowland *et al* (1989) discuss the differences between the use of counselling skills and the formal practice of counselling. It is an excellent paper to read to convince doctors that they do not in fact undertake counselling within normal consultations, and so encourage them to value and work with counsellors for the benefit of their patients.

References

BALINT, M. (1964) *The Doctor, His Patient and the Illness* (2nd edn). London: Pitman.

EGAN, G. (1986) *The Skilled Helper* (3rd edn). Pacific Grove, CA: Brooks/Cole.

IRVING, J. & HEATH, V. (1991) *Counselling in General Practice – A Guide for GPs*. Rugby: British Association for Counselling.

MCLEOD, J. (1988) *The Work of Counsellors in General Practice. Occasional Paper 37*. London: *Royal College of General Practitioners*.

ROWLAND, N., IRVING, J. & MAYNARD, A. (1989) Can general practitioners counsel? *Journal of the Royal College of General Practitioners*, **39**, 118–120.

—— & HURD, J. (1991) *Counselling in General Practice – A Guide for Counsellors*. Rugby: British Association for Counselling.

SHELDON, M. G. (ed.) (1982) *Counselling in General Practice*. London: Royal College of General Practitioners.

20 Cognitive behaviour therapy

JANINE SCOTT

Cognitive behaviour therapy (CBT) is a short-term, problem-solving form of psychotherapy which has gained wide acceptance on both sides of the Atlantic. CBT has been applied to a wide variety of psychological problems:

(a) depression
(b) generalised anxiety disorders
(c) panic disorders
(d) phobias
(e) obsessional disorders
(f) hypochondriasis and somatisation
(g) eating disorders
(h) drug and alcohol problems
(i) chronic pain
(j) distress secondary to cancer
(k) bereavement
(l) personality disorders.

For some disorders, its use has been described only in case reports (e.g. post-traumatic stress disorders) or open studies (e.g. borderline personality disorder); nevertheless, the outcome of such interventions appear to be sufficiently promising for more sophisticated treatment trials to be planned. Specific outcome research has been undertaken on depression, anxiety, hypochondriasis and panic disorders, and the results suggest that CBT is an effective alternative to both pharmacotherapy and other non-pharmacological treatments (Murphy et al, 1984; Clark et al, 1985; Beck, 1988). A review of 81 outcome studies of the treatment of neurotic disorders suggested that "cognitive therapy is the most powerful specific psychological treatment for depressive neurosis and for some personality disorders" (Andrews, 1991).

In Britain, several CBT studies have focused specifically on its use with depressed patients seen in primary care (Blackburn et al, 1981; Teasdale *et al*, 1984; Ross & Scott, 1985; Scott & Freeman, 1992); again, the results confirm the efficacy and acceptability of this psychological approach. However, the fact that CBT is applicable to many of the psychological problems encountered in primary care does not mean it can be promoted as an alternative treatment without question. The realities of day-to-day clinical practice suggest a number of issues which still need to be resolved. For example, in the research studies quoted, the CBT was undertaken by therapists with special training in this approach. As yet no study has looked at the use of CBT *by* members of the primary care team as opposed to its use by cognitive therapists working *in* primary care. A major difficulty for primary care professionals is the lack of specialist cognitive therapists in many parts of Britain. This means that referral has to be more restricted than might be desirable. In addition, lack of access to a therapist is often mirrored by a similar lack of access for primary care staff to appropriate training to develop their own skills in CBT. Even if such training were available, CBT requires more time to be spent with the patient than does drug treatment. To justify the use of this approach it would be necessary to show either that CBT uniquely benefits certain subgroups of patients, or that CBT produces lower relapse rates (hence being more cost-effective in the long-term). There is minimal evidence for the former, but tentative support for the latter: naturalistic treatment follow-up studies tend to suggest a better prognosis for patients treated with CBT as opposed to other approaches (Clark, 1990).

Having noted all these issues, this chapter begins by reviewing why CBT may be an important component of the therapeutic armamentarium available in primary care. This is followed by a description of Beck's (1976, 1979) model of the cognitive theory and therapy of emotional disorders. The chapter ends with a discussion of possible adaptations of the CBT approach for use by primary care staff.

Why use cognitive behaviour therapy?

If a primary care team has ready access to a trained cognitive therapist then the most appropriate referrals will be for neurosis (particularly anxiety, panic, somatisation and obsessional disorders), mild to moderately severe depression (particularly where psychosocial factors appear to have a causal role), eating disorders and post-traumatic stress disorders. In addition, CBT can be attempted for patients with personality dysfunction or whose psychological problems have failed to respond to any other form of therapy (such as chronic depression).

Even when access to a therapist is more restricted, there are several reasons why CBT may become the treatment of choice for certain patients. A significant and increasing number of them do not wish to be prescribed medication for psychological problems. As well as patient preference for non-drug treatments, the GP or liaison psychiatrist may also wish to avoid medication. Such situations arise where the distress does not fit neatly into the category of a recognised disorder with an obvious indication for drug treatment (which is often the case in primary care), or because a non-pharmacological approach is simply more appropriate. Lader (1975) has questioned the use of medication in some crises, suggesting that drugs may inhibit patients' efforts to organise themselves and merely give an inappropriate 'message' about how to resolve stress.

Alternatively, CBT may be required as an adjunct to pharmacotherapy. Patients with post-traumatic stress disorder (e.g. victims of physical or sexual violence) often fall into this category. Pharmacotherapy may be required to relieve the immediate feelings of distress (and indeed may be necessary to allow the patient to settle sufficiently to engage in a psychological approach). However, overcoming the trauma and resolving problems may equally require a focused psychological intervention such as CBT. In other cases, doctors may be wary of prescribing drugs because of potentially dangerous interactions between psychotropic and any other medications being used, because the patient is particularly sensitive to drug side-effects, or because the patient is at risk of deliberate self-harm and the medication provides a means by which this can be achieved.

A number of research studies suggest that poor compliance with pharmaco-therapies is a major problem. Johnston (1981) showed that 8% of patients did not even take their prescription to the chemist, while a further 44% failed either to complete the course of treatment or to take the medication as prescribed.

Finally, non-response to all other appropriate therapies may mean that CBT is the only option untried.

The above discussion highlights an important role for psychological approaches in the management of mental health problems seen in primary care. The cognitive approach is popular for a number of reasons. The model on which the therapy is based is readily understood by both doctors and more importantly by patients of different intellectual capacities (including those with learning difficulties (Williams & Moorey, 1989)). The therapy is by definition short term, giving it a cost–benefit advantage over many psychological therapies. The problem-solving, goal-directed approach is particularly attractive for GPs: clear targets can be set and change can be monitored more readily than with less specific counselling approaches. Finally, the therapy is amenable to empirical testing and has generated more process and outcome research than has been undertaken with most psychological approaches. The research data have certainly influenced and generally increased clinical support for CBT.

The cognitive theory of emotional disorders

The cognitive theory of the emotional disorders (Beck *et al*, 1979) states that:

"An individual's emotional response to an event or experience is largely determined by the conscious meaning placed upon it."

Thus, it is not simply what happens to people, but how they perceive what has happened to them that becomes critical. It is hypothesised that early learning experiences lead to the development of underlying beliefs or rules (termed 'schemas' or 'assumptions') which the individual uses to construct subjective reality (Scott, 1984). It is suggested that people vulnerable to emotional disorders have developed dysfunctional schemas (usually because the 'rules' are extreme and rigid). These schemas may be activated by critical events or incidents that mesh with the person's belief system, and once this occurs, the schemas give rise to negative automatic thoughts (Fennell, 1989). These cognitions (which are involuntary but conscious) play a crucial intermediary role between day-to-day events and the emotional response to these events. The therapy aims to expose 'event–thought–feeling' links and the way these influence (and are influenced by) the individual's behaviour.

It is hypothesised that the depressed individual frequently interprets external events in terms of loss or deprivation or both. Negative attitudes towards themselves, their world and their future have an adverse impact on their mood and make the individual more depressed and more prone to interpret all events (positive, neutral or negative) in a negative way. Thus, as shown in Fig. 20. 1, a vicious cycle develops which maintains the depressive episode.

Vulnerability to develop anxiety disorders is characterised by the tendency to interpret situations in a threatening way, over-estimating danger or underestimating potential rescue factors (Clark, 1989). Clark suggests that the underlying dysfunctional schemas in anxiety often relate to acceptance, competence, responsibility, or control. Common cognitive distortions in panic disorder relate to catastrophic misinterpretations of bodily symptoms which are perceived as indicators of impending physical or mental disaster (Clark, 1989). Although ongoing research frequently leads to subtle modifications to these theories, knowledge of the specific cognitive model of the disorder being treated is vital to the development of the therapy package.

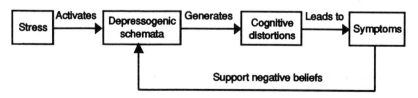

Fig. 20.1. Diagrammatic representation of the cognitive model of the development of depression

Overview of cognitive behaviour therapy

General characteristics

Cognitive behaviour therapy is described as "an active, directive, time-limited, structured approach" (Beck *et al*, 1979). The core characteristics of this form of psychotherapy are:

(a) it is time-limited – a course of therapy lasts approximately 6–20 sessions (of about 45 minutes each)
(b) it is structured – each session has an agenda, and homework tasks are always negotiated
(c) it is collaborative – the therapist and patient are seen as equal partners in the therapeutic relationship
(d) it is problem-oriented and focused on 'here and now' issues
(e) it is a scientific approach – automatic thoughts are regarded as hypotheses to be tested
(f) it is an educational approach – the aim is to teach the patient specific skills that can be applied to present and to future problems
(g) it is based on a coherent theoretical model.

Misconceptions about CBT are firstly that it is some form of positive thinking and secondly that it is simply a collection of cognitive and behavioural techniques that can be applied in 'cook-book' style (a little of this, a splash of that) to emotional disorders. The therapy (as opposed to individual techniques) actually comprises a specific package of verbal and behavioural interventions with a unifying rationale (Fennell, 1989). This means that interventions differ not only with the type of disorder being treated, but also with the conceptualisation of the specific problems and the hypothesised underlying assumptions identified for that particular patient. At different points of therapy, a variety of interventions may appear possible. In cognitive therapy the choice of intervention is not random, the decision as to which particular technique will be used is made on the basis of the cognitive behavioural formulation (constructed from the assessment and history data).

The goals of CBT

Behavioural and verbal procedures are used to:

(a) define and detect cognitions (automatic thoughts)
(b) examine and test these cognitions
(c) develop alternative constructions of day-to-day events
(d) record dysfunctional thoughts
(e) develop alternative, more flexible schemas

(f) rehearse both cognitive and behavioural responses based on these new assumptions.

Cognitive behaviour therapy also aims to explore the underlying belief system that has rendered a person vulnerable to reacting in a dysfunctional way. The aim here is to modify the assumptions to prevent future relapse. Thus, CBT differs significantly from the more superficial 'problem A = technique A' level of intervention. This is not to suggest that the latter is never beneficial, but merely highlights that these approaches must be recognised as quite separate.

Engagement in therapy

The preliminary CBT sessions have two important goals: to jointly define the patient's problems and to socialise him/her into the cognitive model. Patients are first encouraged to identify all of their perceived problems. At this stage the therapist should take a questioning stance, intermittently taking the opportunity to summarise the information and feed it back to the patient to ensure that they have clearly understood the patient's problems. It is vital to be specific about the issues described. It is also helpful to use subheadings for any symptoms noted such as cognitive, behavioural, affective, motivational, and somatic.

Having identified all the relevant problems, the therapist helps the patient undertake a 'problem reduction' exercise. Many problems are different components of a single issue. Problem reduction brings together these linked components and classifies them under one heading, such as 'difficulty socialising' or 'low self-esteem'. Issues may be usefully divided into internal (intrapersonal difficulties such as self-image, self-esteem) and external categories. The latter can be further subdivided into interpersonal (e.g. relationship problems) and situational (e.g. financial problems) categories. The final version of the problem-list must be agreed collaboratively and key issues may then be prioritised at this point. The therapist must ensure that the patient does not dwell only on problems; the assessment should also identify personal resources and assets as well as difficulties.

Throughout the assessment session, the therapist should take the opportunity to introduce the relevant components of the cognitive model, specifically taking the opportunity to demonstrate 'event–thought–feeling' links. Useful strategies may be to ask patients how they were feeling when they were sitting waiting to meet the therapist. Having established the event and the feeling, the therapist now asks "What went through your mind at that moment in time?", thus trying to identify and demonstrate to the patient their automatic thoughts (or images). Alternatively, if a patient shows a sudden mood shift in the session, for example, becoming weepy, it is again useful to break into the dialogue to try to establish the automatic thoughts just experienced.

Throughout CBT, the therapist should adopt a collaborative, questioning style, using summarising and feedback. It is vital not to lecture patients or try to persuade them that they have a particular problem. Nor should the therapist try to guess at automatic thoughts. The aim is for self-discovery by the patient using the techniques taught to them by the therapist.

The types of patient who seem to do well with cognitive therapy have been reviewed by Twaddle & Scott (1991). Such patients show a desire to be an active participant in their therapy, and have an internal locus of control. They are psychologically minded, are able to distinguish thoughts and feelings, adapt to a problem-solving stance, and are both accepting of and show some confidence in the model put forward.

Session structure

Cognitive therapy sessions always follow the same format, commencing with the setting of a collaborative agenda, where the goals of that specific session are agreed. Sessions begin with a review of the previous week's homework, particularly focusing on what has been learnt from that task. Patient and therapist then identify one or two key issues to be explored in the main part of the session. The latter stages of the session focus on defining between-session homework tasks. These should follow logically from the discussions undertaken within the session (Scott, 1984), but it is important that the patient and therapist agree the precise goals of the task. Homework tasks should allow hypotheses to be tested and also promote the transfer of skills from the therapy sessions to the patient's own environment. The session ends with feedback from the patient about all aspects of the session, and both patient and therapist review and reinforce what has been learnt.

While the structure of the sessions is relatively fixed, the content changes throughout the course of treatment. Initially the focus is on behaviour and identifying logical errors in thinking. As the therapy progresses, the focus shifts gradually from the acute problems and automatic thoughts associated with the initial presentation, to more complex concepts such as underlying assumptions. The identification and modification of dysfunctional schemas and the development of problem-solving strategies represent an attempt to prevent relapse, and to prepare the patient for discharge.

Core therapy techniques

While CBT draws on a wide variety of techniques, it is possible to identify core interventions that any exponent of CBT should be able to employ. These techniques, listed below, are described briefly in the section that follows:

(a) behavioural techniques
  (i)   weekly activity scheduling
  (ii) mastery and pleasure ratings
  (iii) graded task assignment
  (iv) task assignment
(b) cognitive techniques
  (i)   eliciting automatic thoughts
  (ii) testing automatic thoughts
  (iii) identifying and modifying schemas.

Behavioural techniques

Behavioural techniques are often more prominent in the early stages of therapy (particularly in those with severe symptoms). These interventions are 'action-oriented', focusing on how to act or cope, as well as serving the purpose of allowing automatic thoughts associated with different situations and activities to be identified. Patients are encouraged to use their time more adaptively and to learn specific procedures to deal with concrete situations. Four core strategies are described below.

Weekly activity scheduling

The therapist helps the patient to develop self-monitoring of daily activities. Initially, any differences between the patient's perception of his/her level of activity and the actual level of activity recorded by data collection are explored. The diary may be used to monitor all activities or may focus particularly on drinking or eating patterns, depending on the types of problems being explored.

Having established the patient's baseline activity level, the diary can now be used for forward planning. Providing a planned structure to the day often helps overcome inertia and hopelessness. In addition, a realistic level of activity can be planned, incorporating pleasant events as well as basic day-to-day activities. The schedule can then be used to test automatic thoughts by exploring cognitions associated with particular events recorded in the schedule.

Mastery and pleasure ratings

As well as monitoring activities carried out, patients are encouraged to rate each activity for mastery (how well they achieved the activity given how they felt at that moment in time) and for pleasure (how much they enjoyed it). These ratings usually help patients to overcome misconceptions regarding their ability to perform or enjoy tasks undertaken.

Graded task assignment

This technique uses a 'step-by-step' approach to goals which the patient currently considers difficult or impossible. The task is broken down into manageable subunits which are undertaken in sequence. The aim is to provide concrete evidence that a task previously regarded as insurmountable can be undertaken successfully. By breaking the task down and reinforcing completion of each subunit, the therapist helps patients overcome their procrastination and inertia. This approach may be used for day-to-day basic tasks such as home management or helping people develop a social network.

Task assignment

Simple tasks may not be amenable to division into subunits. Such tasks are often used as homework assignments early in therapy to give the patient the experience of success. Later in therapy, complete tasks (both simple and more complex) may be assigned to allow collection of automatic thoughts related to a specific behaviour, for example, attending a social function. 'Cognitive rehearsal' during a session may be used in an attempt to explore and overcome any potential barriers to successfully undertaking the planned task.

Cognitive techniques

By definition, CBT is aimed at identifying and testing automatic thoughts. The patient is encouraged to see automatic thoughts as hypotheses to be tested rather than as the absolute facts. Core cognitive techniques focus initially on teaching individuals to identify automatic thoughts, then on how to challenge these cognitions and finally on how to modify maladaptive assumptions.

Eliciting automatic thoughts

As mentioned earlier, to help the patient understand the links between events, thoughts and feelings, it is useful initially to explore examples of mood shifts that occur within the session. Having educated the patient in what automatic thoughts are, and their influence on feelings, additional techniques are used to identify the thoughts.

Increasing awareness. Many patients initially find it difficult to identify automatic thoughts. Simply setting the task of counting how many they are aware of in a particular time, or asking them to try to note cognitions when their mood state changes is helpful in the early stages.

Role plays. Getting the patient to replay particular events in the therapy session can be particularly useful for identifying automatic thoughts associated with interpersonal situations.

Imagery. The patient is encouraged to relax and re-create in detail the event under investigation. In so doing it is often possible to identify the associated thoughts and feelings.

Guided discovery. The style of CBT requires the therapist to engage in inductive questioning in order to help patients discover for themselves the thoughts being investigated. To this end, 'what' questions are more appropriate than 'why' questions. As highlighted by Fennell (1989), the latter invariably lead patients to give an explanation of a situation rather than to recount the specific thoughts associated with it. "What went through your mind when you felt anxious?" is therefore preferable to "Why were you anxious?"

Dysfunctional thought record (DTR). The DTR is used to allow accurate recording of 'event–thought–feeling' links. A five-column technique is used, as shown in Table 20.1, firstly to identify the thoughts and feelings and secondly to develop rational responses to these ideas and note any subsequent changes in mood state. Patients are initially taught how to use the form by practising filling it in during the CBT sessions. When they have mastered this the patient is then encouraged to use it to keep a systematic record of their cognitive and emotional state between sessions. Clark (1989) often adds a 'sixth column' to the record which is entitled 'action'. The patient is encouraged to note here any specific problem-solving tactics that can also be used to challenge the thought.

Testing automatic thoughts

Having helped the patient to begin to identify thoughts associated with anxiety or depression or that may lead to maladaptive behaviours (e.g. bingeing, deliberate self-harm), the therapist now tries to help the patient begin to develop rational responses to his/her ideas. The key questions (Fennell, 1989) are:

(a) What is the evidence for this thought?
(b) What kind of thinking errors are being made?
(c) What alternative interpretations are there?
(d) What are the advantages/disadvantages of thinking this way?
(e) If the automatic thought is accurate, is the situation as bad as it is being portrayed?

Additional details of the techniques are described below.

Examining the evidence. The patient and therapist examine the evidence for and against the identified automatic thought. What information is available to confirm or disconfirm the idea? What effect does this have on the patient's emotional state? Sometimes there is insufficient evidence available within the session, and so an experiment is devised as a homework task. The patient

TABLE 20.1
Example of a dysfunctional thoughts record

Date	Situation	Emotion(s)	Automatic thought(s)	Rational response	Outcome
	Describe: (a) Actual event leading to unpleasant emotion, or (b) Stream of thoughts, daydream or recollection leading to unpleasant emotion.	(a) Specify sad/ anxious/angry etc. (b) Rate degree of emotion 1–100	(a) Write automatic thought(s) that preceded emotion (b) Rate belief in automatic thought 0–100%	(a) Write rational response to automatic thought(s) (b) Rate belief in rational response 0–100%	(a) Re-rate belief in automatic thought(s) 0–100% (b) Specify and rate subsequent emotions 0–100%
	At a party where people know I've been off work because of my nerves. A friend asks "How are you feeling?"	*Anxious. 75%*	*I must look really bad for her to be so concerned. 80%* *She must think I am totally inadequate. 70%*	*She cares enough about me to ask how I'm getting on. 80%* *She has probably noticed that I'm looking better than when I last saw her and wants to know if I feel better. 65%* *She's never expressed any ideas that I am inadequate and indeed only recently told me that she would never be able to cope with the stress of my job. 70%*	*Belief in automatic thought. 30%* *Anxious. 25%*

Explanation. When you experience an unpleasant emotion, note the situation that seemed to stimulate the emotion (if the emotion occurred while you were thinking, daydreaming, etc. please note this). Then note the automatic thought associated with the emotion. Record the degree to which you believe this thought: 0% = not at all; 100% = completely. In rating degree of emotion: 1 = a trace, 100 = the most intense possible.

and therapist agree on the hypothesis to be tested and data are gathered for and against the idea (e.g. by canvassing the views of others). Alternatively, a specific behavioural experiment is devised.

Generating alternatives. The patient is encouraged to understand that just because the automatic thought may be the first idea that came into their mind in a given situation, this does not mean it is the most accurate interpretation of what has occurred. The patient and therapist therefore develop rational alternative responses to the automatic thoughts recorded on the DTR. Each rational response is then examined to test its validity, to see how it affects the patient's belief in the original automatic thought and its effect on how the patient is feeling.

Reattribution. For patients who personalise issues it is often useful to use reattribution techniques. This may be particularly helpful in preventing a patient taking excessive responsibility for events. Asking the patient to apportion responsibility to everyone else involved is an important strategy in trying to reduce damage to self-esteem.

Decatastrophising. In some situations, the automatic thought recorded by the patient will be an accurate interpretation of the situation. However, the patient has often not considered the specific implications of such a situation. For example, if it is really true that a colleague at work does not like them, what are the implications of this? Should it be assumed that the patient is unlikeable? How could the difficulties that may be encountered be managed? By asking for specific information and using a problem-solving approach it is often possible to reduce the negative effect of such realities.

Identifying and modifying schemas

The identification of underlying assumptions is not as easy as identifying automatic thoughts. Often patients have no real knowledge of the rules they have used to govern their interpretations of the world. While the therapist must avoid reaching premature conclusions about the types of schemas operating, it is helpful to be aware of the assumptions commonly identified in anxiety and depressive disorders. This information allows the therapist to pinpoint important themes and topics in the patient's dialogue, so increasing the chances of uncovering the individual's belief system.

The DTR sheets may be useful in initially identifying schemas. It is often fruitful to set patients the task of picking out the recurrent themes or specific logical errors that they use. Assumptions regarding issues of control, acceptance and achievement are often central (Beck *et al*, 1985). Verbal techniques used to explore automatic thoughts within therapy may also uncover discrete assumptions.

Having established the nature of a specific problem, vertical questioning (referred to as the 'downward arrow' or 'what if?' technique) is used. Rather than exploring the automatic thought, the therapist essentially explores the meaning of the situation by repeatedly asking the same question, "If that were true, what would that mean?" (or a slight variation). In this way, the dialogue progresses from the specific automatic thought through a sequence of statements, which usually leads to the identification of the underlying general belief.

Once a number of schemas have been identified, it is important to try to challenge or modify those which are maladaptive. Again, questioning and behavioural experiments, along with the use of flashcards (Clark, 1989) are useful techniques. The latter comprises a file card on which the patient is encouraged to note specific information about the dysfunctional schema. Firstly, the assumption is recorded; underneath, the origins of the belief are briefly noted (including why it is understandable that the patient holds this belief) and the reason why the belief is dysfunctional is also written down. A plan of behavioural and cognitive methods to be used to undermine the dysfunctional schema are noted, along with a statement of a more adaptive schema. Patients are encouraged to put these brief notes on a small card that is readily accessible to them. In this way they can easily remind themselves of what has been noted down, and the card prompts them to carry out tasks aimed at reducing the strength of belief in the original schema.

Figure 20.2 gives a diagrammatic representation of the course of CBT with a depressed patient, highlighting the gradual shift in the nature of the interventions over time, and showing that the balance between predominantly cognitive or behavioural interventions is also influenced by the severity of the presenting symptoms.

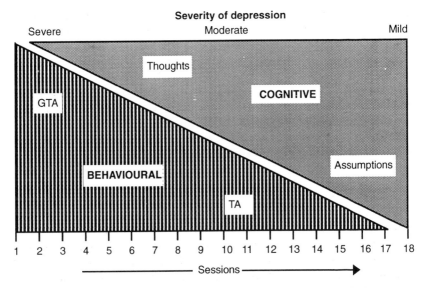

Fig. 20.2. Diagrammatic representation of CBT for depression

Adapting cognitive behaviour therapy to primary care

To be able to develop a shorter version of CBT that would be attractive for use in primary care, it would first be necessary to identify the 'active ingredients' of the therapy. Twaddle & Scott (1991) have reviewed the important factors, and found that the therapist's CBT skills, adherence to the CBT model, the degree of change achieved in automatic thoughts, and the patient's beliefs in the likely success of the therapy were important components. A study is currently underway in Newcastle upon Tyne using an abbreviated model of CBT (six sessions of 20 minutes each) to explore whether shorter treatment programmes can be effective in treating depression in primary care. Although the results of the pilot study suggest this approach may be effective (Scott *et al*, 1993), it is unlikely to be perfected for some time. In the interim, what aspects of CBT can be used in primary care by the professionals working in that setting? Some components of the package that may be used to good effect are:

(a) using the CBT approach in interviews
(b) 'bibliotherapy'
(c) using specific techniques in adjunct to pharmacotherapy
(d) using a brief CBT package.

Interview style

Socratic questioning and a collaborative approach to problem definition are core components of CBT which are applicable in primary care. Such an approach has many aspects in common with the 'problem-based interviewing' style advocated by Lesser (1985). Educating patients about the nature of their disorder, ensuring that both doctor and patient agree about the nature of the problem, identifying a list of target symptoms to be treated and exploring automatic thoughts about proposed medication, are techniques likely to increase patient satisfaction and improves treatment compliance. Such approaches do not need to be restricted to psychological problems, but can be used to assess factors that impede recovery from somatic problems.

'Bibliotherapy'

While the primary care team may not be able to spend long periods of time undertaking CBT, the use of educational books is of potential benefit. Several researchers (Teasdale *et al*, 1984; Twaddle & Scott, 1991) have commented on patients who have rapidly adapted to the CBT approach after a small number of sessions supplemented by reading material. Many patients are able to understand and begin to use the techniques with minimal explanation.

Alternatively, it may be possible to allocate the patient specific chapters of self-help books to read as 'homework assignments'.

Adjunctive techniques

Minimal interventions using single techniques can be used by GPs without extending the consultation session. Depressed patients receiving pharmaco-therapy often find using activity schedules and thought diaries of great benefit. Several patients have spontaneously commented that making a daily timetable reduces tension and distress and helps overcome inertia. It seems that simple structuring of the day can be of great benefit. Likewise, keeping a thought diary allows exploration of links between mood shifts and specific negative ideas. Writing the thought down seems to distance the patient from the thought, and allows a more objective approach to challenging it. Using individual techniques and a problem-solving approach allows the clinician to assess progress on a number of parameters.

Conclusions

It is possible to use cognitive and behavioural approaches in primary care, but these must be clearly distinguished from the specific therapy package that constitutes CBT. The latter requires more formal training, and interventions are selected on the basis of an underlying rationale. In order to begin to develop an understanding of cognitive models of emotional disorders, GPs are directed towards the increasing body of clinical texts on this subject (Beck *et al*, 1979; Hawton *et al*, 1989; Scott *et al*, 1989).

To pursue training, it is helpful to obtain supervision by an experienced therapist and, where possible, to record therapy sessions in detail (preferably on tape), to allow review of skills development.

Extensive outcome research suggest that CBT is an effective treatment for non-psychotic out-patient psychological disorders, a population obviously seen extensively in primary care and liaison clinic settings. In addition, as cost–benefit analysis becomes a major concern of health service purchasers and providers, the short-term, time-limited nature of this approach is likely to lead to an increase in its use in the future.

Books of interest to patients

BECK, A. T. & GREENBERG, R. L. (1974) *Coping with Depression*. A brief introductory booklet available from: Center for Cognitive Therapy, 133 South 36th Street, Philadelphia, USA.
BLACKBURN, I. (1987) *Coping with Depression*. Edinburgh: Chambers.
BURNS, D. (1980) *Feeling Good: The New Mood Therapy*. New Jersey: Signet.

Recommended reading for clinicians

BECK, A. T. (1976) *Cognitive Therapy and the Emotional Disorders*. New York: International Universities Press.
—— , RUSH, A. J., SHAW, B. F., *et al* (1979) *Cognitive Therapy of Depression*. New York: Guilford Press.
HAWTON, K., SALKOVSKIS, P. M., KIRK, J., *et al* (1989) *Cognitive Behaviour Therapy for Psychiatric Problems: A Practical Guide*. Oxford: Oxford University Press.
SCOTT, J., WILLIAMS, J. M. G. & BECK, A. T. (1989) *Cognitive Therapy in Clinical Practice*. London: Routledge.
WILLIAMS, J. M. G. (1984) *The Psychological Treatment of Depression: A Guide to the Theory and Practice of Cognitive-Behavioural Therapy*. London: Croom Helm.

References

ANDREWS, G. (1991) The evaluation of psychotherapy. *Current Opinion in Psychiatry*, **4**, 379–383.
BECK, A. T. (1976) *Cognitive Therapy and the Emotional Disorders*. New York: International Universities Press.
—— (1988) Cognitive approaches to panic disorder. In *Panic: Psychological Perspectives* (eds S. Rachman & J. D. Maser), pp. 91–110. Hillsdale: Lawrence Erlbaum.
—— , HOLLON, S. D., YOUNG, J. E., *et al* (1985) Treatment of depression with cognitive therapy and amitriptyline. *Archives of General Psychiatry*, **42**, 142–148.
—— , RUSH, A. J., SHAW, B. F., *et al* (1979) *Cognitive Therapy of Depression*. New York: Guilford Press.
BLACKBURN, I., BISHOP, S., GLEN, I. M., *et al* (1981) The efficacy of cognitive therapy in depression: a treatment trial using cognitive therapy and pharmacotherapy, each alone and in combination. *British Journal of Psychiatry*, **139**, 181–189.
CLARK, D. M. (1989) Anxiety states. In *Cognitive Behaviour Therapy for Psychiatric Problems: A Practical Guide* (eds K. Hawton, P. Salkovskis, J. Kirk & D. Clark), pp. 52–96. Oxford: Oxford University Press.
—— (1990) Cognitive therapy of depression and anxiety: is it better than drug treatment in the long term? In *Dilemmas and Difficulties in the Management of Psychiatric Patients* (eds K. Hawton & P. Cowen), pp. 55–64. Oxford: Oxford University Press.
—— , SALKOVSKIS, P. M. & CHALKLEY, A. J. (1985) Respiratory control as a treatment of panic attacks. *Journal of Behaviour Therapy and Experimental Psychiatry*, **16**, 23–30.
FENNELL, M. J. (1989) Depression. In *Cognitive Behaviour Therapy for Psychiatric Problems: A Practical Guide* (eds K. Hawton, P. Salkovskis, J. Kirk & D. Clark), pp. 167–234. Oxford: Oxford University Press.
JOHNSTON, D. A. W. (1981) Depression: treatment compliance in general practice. *Acta Psychiatrica Scandinavica*, **63**, (suppl.), 447–453.
LADER, M. (1975) The social implications of psychotropic drugs. *Royal Society of Health Journal*, **95(b)**, 304–305.
LESSER, A. (1985) Problem-based interviewing in general practice. *Medical Education*, **19**, 200–204.
MURPHY, G. E., SIMONS, A. D., WETZEL, R. D., *et al* (1984) Cognitive therapy and pharmacotherapy: singly and together in the treatment of depression. *Archives of General Psychiatry*, **41**, 33–41.
ROSS, S. M. & SCOTT, M. (1985) An evaluation of the effectiveness of individual and group cognitive therapy in the treatment of depressed patients in an inner city health centre. *Journal of the Royal College of General Practitioners*, **35**, 239–242.
SCOTT, A. I. & FREEMAN, C. (1992) Edinburgh primary care depression study: treatment outcome, patient satisfaction, and cost after 16 weeks. *British Medical Journal*, **304**, 883–887.

SCOTT, C., SCOTT, J., TACCHI, M. J., *et al* (1993) Abbreviated cognitive therapy for depression: a pilot study in primary care. *Behavioural and Cognitive Psychotherapy* (in press).

SCOTT, J. (1984) Cognitive behaviour therapy of depressive illness. *Psychiatry in Practice*, **10**, 9–15.

TEASDALE, J., FENNELL, M. J., HIBBERT, G. A. *et al* (1984) Cognitive therapy for major depressive disorder in primary care. *British Journal of Psychiatry*, **144**, 400–406.

TWADDLE, V. & SCOTT, J. (1991) Cognitive theory and therapy of depression. In *Adult Clinical Problems: A Cognitive–Behavioural Approach* (eds W. Dryden & R. Rentoul), pp. 56–85. London: Routledge.

WILLIAMS, J. M. G. & MOOREY, S. (1989) The wider application of cognitive therapy: the end of the beginning. In *Cognitive Therapy in Clinical Practice* (eds J. Scott, J. M. G. Williams & A. T. Beck), pp. 227–250. London: Routledge.

21 The prevention of mental illness in primary care

DENIS PEREIRA GRAY, ALASTAIR WRIGHT, GREG WILKINSON, RACHEL JENKINS and KEITH LLOYD

Reduced infant mortality, increased life expectancy, and the control of many infectious diseases have been major triumphs for preventive medicine. Opportunities for prevention in primary care are great, since general practice is the point of entry to the health care system for most people. This chapter seeks to review the potential contribution of the primary care team and colleagues in secondary care to the prevention of mental illnesses.

Prevention and promotion

The concepts of prevention and health promotion are sometimes confusing. There remains much to be said for Caplan's (1964) established classification of prevention into three levels: primary, secondary, and tertiary. There was logic in this classification when it was first introduced, and it is still of practical use. It has the additional advantage that it is relevant to, and can be shared by, general practitioners, psychiatrists, and other specialities such as public health physicians.

Primary prevention involves measures aimed at reducing the incidence of a disease, and of reducing the likelihood of it starting at all. Enhancing host resistance through immunisation of babies is the classic example. The vast majority of babies are immunised in general practice against diseases like polio, tetanus, diphtheria, measles, and whooping cough. Another example would be eliminating risk factors such as smoking or cholera from the community.

Secondary prevention is preventive action which is taken when a disease condition has just begun, but at a stage where its existence is often or usually unknown to the patient. Originally the term was used to mean the treatment of disease. Increasingly in general practice it is being used to cover the identification and treatment of risk factors or diseases before they cause symptoms. The concept of pre-symptomatic detection of disease is now well established, having originally become best known through the mass X-ray screening service which detected lung disease before it was clinically evident. The millions of cervical smears taken in general practice each year are examples (most practices take smears from over 80% of all the adult women who are eligible and who are registered with them).

Tertiary prevention involves measures to reduce disability resulting from a disorder, and to reduce the chances of complications and relapse. In this sense most rehabilitation is tertiary prevention. For example, prolonged treatment of many mental diseases after the point at which full function is restored is tertiary prevention, most commonly planned to reduce the risk of relapse. Tertiary prevention thus merges with good clinical care. The main thrust of true 'prevention' has to be at the primary and secondary levels, with primary prevention being the most desirable.

More recently, the concept of health promotion has come to prominence (Catford & Nutbeam, 1984). The term is variously defined and is often used synonymously with prevention in general. It includes the idea of enhancing health as a positive concept rather than health being just the absence of disease.

Does prevention work?

Two broad debates have dominated medical thinking about logical approaches to prevention. These are, firstly, the nature/nurture approach, and secondly the population versus the personal approach.

Nature versus nurture

The controversy about how much of health/illness/behaviour is due to inherited characteristics or traits in contrast to how much is associated with patterns of behaviour seen or learnt in life is not specific to medicine but has been long disputed by the scientific community. The debate continues, but there is more clarification as individual genes become identified. It may take decades to clarify precise mechanisms. For example, it has long been known that heavy drinking runs in families. Even with the discovery of a gene associated with this, it may still be true that family culture and attitudes to alcohol may be important factors or even necessary ones for the gene to be expressed.

Thus, in terms of prevention, neither school of thought is likely to have a complete answer in clinical practice. One of the first general conclusions which emerges in the prevention of many diseases is the need for a multi-pronged approach. This principle is particularly important in mental and emotional illness.

The population versus the personal approach

The population or personal approach is another of the great dialogues which have dominated thinking in preventive medicine, especially in the last three decades. In cardiovascular medicine, for example, there has been much work on prevention and many risk factors have been identified. Professor Geoffrey Rose has long championed the population approach (Rose, 1992) and Professor Michael Oliver the opposite, advocating concentration on high-risk groups. On the whole, one fact is self-evident: that the population approach, if possible, reaches the greatest number of people. Successful examples include the compulsory wearing of seat belts in order to reduce damage sustained in traffic accidents and the introduction of legislation regarding the legal limits for alcohol consumption while driving. Some legislation such as banning non-flameproof nightdresses has been notably successful. However, the population approach may not be effective for political, cultural, professional, or financial reasons. It can be difficult to persuade a person to alter a risk behaviour such as smoking because it will benefit the health of the population but may make little difference to that person.

Application of a population approach is acceptable in some areas but is sometimes felt to be less so with mental illnesses. Many practitioners prefer to take an opportunistic approach. Newton (1992) and Lloyd & Jenkins (1994) take the view that the priority on practical grounds should be vulnerable groups. The identification and support of those at high risk for illness is the targeted primary preventive strategy. Early detection and prompt treatment of those who are already ill should be priorities for secondary preventive initiatives. The Oliver high-risk-group approach is preferred because of the difficulty of applying the population approach to the prevention of mental illness in a field where there are still problems of stigma and where the relevant factors are not yet always clearly isolated. Opportunities for legislation are limited (alcohol consumption being a notable exception).

The population-based approach may be more fruitful for mass educational campaigns. Indeed, this is being tested through the Defeat Depression Campaign of the Royal College of Psychiatrists and the Royal College of General Practitioners.

Prevention in general practice

Modern British general practice has found a way of reconciling many, although not all, of the tensions between the personal and the population approach. While they must remain in conflict with some specialist approaches (public health medicine is almost by definition permanently wedded to the population approach, and many leading clinicians permanently wedded to the personal approach), in general practice it is at last now possible to reduce the tension in this dichotomy by doing both at once.

The reasons for this remarkable possibility are fourfold: first, the British tradition of personal doctoring; secondly, the NHS system of the registered list in general practice; thirdly, the guidance of the academic wing of general practice (Watts, 1958; Eimerl, 1960; Royal College of General Practitioners, 1981); and lastly the computer systems (Preece *et al*, 1970). These four factors make integration of personal and population measures possible in preventive medicine in general practice for common diseases and health problems. The tradition of the personal doctor is essentially European, and because of the great strength of the referral system generalists are aware of all illnesses and specialist expertise is concentrated on the conditions they are most likely to be able to help.

The key is that people consult their GPs first for virtually every problem, and so the generalist gains a clear overview of all the problems in the relevant community and can quantify them and classify them by severity. Secondly, the National Health Service (NHS) is based on a registration system in general practice which enables precise numbers of the population at risk for any health problem to be known, and also the invaluable facility of being able to calculate age-specific and sex-specific rates for any condition and to follow these over time. Both these special advantages of the British system are long-standing, going back to 1913.

Until the 1940s, UK general practice was essentially a reactive service. It was based on the idea of patients consulting the doctor when they were sick. It was not until the introduction of immunisations and antenatal care in the 1940s that the same doctors who provided medical care for the sick started to provide personal preventive care. Before this there had been a variety of preventive services available, including health visiting, but always separate from the main medical services. With the introduction of the NHS, another important element was in place: a service free at the point of delivery. In the UK patients do not have to pay the doctor, thus making access to general practice easy for the poorest members of society.

The fusion of medical care for the sick with personal preventive care under the NHS is a historically important feature of British general practice.

An important step towards developing and later implementing a policy on personal preventive care (later called 'anticipatory care') was Tudor Hart's (1975) work on the detection and treatment of high blood pressure in general practice. By covering the whole of his registered population he demonstrated vividly how personal care and 'small-population' epidemiology could be integrated in primary care.

In November 1977, on the occasion of the 25th Jubilee James Mackenzie Lecture of the Royal College of General Practitioners in London, the case was made for a major re-evaluation of the place of personal preventive medicine. Not only was the place of this work presented in a table in which it came at the top, but the idea of personal preventive medicine being not only important but even more important than traditional curative medicine was spelled out explicitly as the doctor's "supreme activity" (Pereira Gray, 1978). Now the policy was conceptualised not as care for one condition or disease, but care across the board. According to this view, all medical activities can be arranged in a hierarchy by the point at which the doctor intervenes in the disease process:

(a) the prevention of disease
(b) the presymptomatic detection of disease
(c) the early diagnosis of disease
(d) the diagnosis of established disease
(e) the management of disease
(f) the management of the complications of disease
(g) rehabilitation after active treatment has been completed
(h) terminal care
(i) counselling the bereaved.

The following year the final stamp of approval was given to the place of preventive care as a part of primary care when the World Health Organization (WHO), in conjunction with the United Nations Children's Fund (UNICEF), published its historically important *Alma Ata Declaration* in 1978. This set out clearly that a major responsibility of primary health care is to provide preventive care to the defined population which it served.

At the same time there has been a transformation of professional attitudes through the academic wing of general practice (the Royal College of General Practitioners and the university general practitioners). Both have advocated the establishment of a research culture in primary care. Subsequently, the advent of desk-top, networked, microcomputer systems in general practice has at last made it possible to gather, recall, and analyse these data academically in reasonable time scales (Wright, 1990).

Building on the special features of general practice in the British NHS, the Royal College of General Practitioners in 1981/82, led by its President Dr John Horder, published a series of important reports on personal preventive medicine. They marked both a professional and a policy turning point. From then on the provision of such care in effect became part of the job of the GP.

Preventive approaches to mental illness

Psychiatry has been slower than some other specialties to adopt a preventive approach. There were, however, important early initiatives such as the mental hygiene movement in the 1920s and 1930s. This involved individual work with children and was not highly successful. It was not until the 1950s and 1960s that preventive care really took off in general practice and in psychiatry.

In 1952 two Leicestershire GPs, Arthur and Beatrice Watts, reported that about one-fifth of patients attending their joint practice had a psychological illness. They went on to publish the first textbook on psychiatry in general practice. Watts continued to lead the literature with his article on the chronic mental patient in general practice in *The Lancet* in 1954. In 1957 Balint's *The Doctor, The Patient and the Illness* was perhaps one of the most important books ever written for general practice. Although not concentrating on preventive action as such, it provided new and then unique insights into the nature of the generalist's role, including the problems of somatisation. In effect, it provided an intellectual platform on which GPs increasingly began to stand with confidence in general practice psychiatry. Balint was the first to suggest that GPs were better placed than specialists to comprehend certain complex patterns in emotional illness. Watts's second book, *Depressive Disorders in the Community*, was published in 1966. The next year also from general practice but from the Balint stable came Ryle's (1967) *Neurosis in the Ordinary Family*.

Paralleling these developments, a new approach was brought to bear on psychiatric epidemiology through the 1950s and 1960s. For a hundred years, asylum-based psychiatrists had been studying the frequency of mental disorders by counting cases entering mental hospitals. In the late 1950s, Michael Shepherd began the epidemiological work in primary-care psychiatry that was to lead to the establishment of the General Practice Research Unit (GPRU) at the Institute of Psychiatry. In 1966, two years after Caplan, a child psychiatrist, formulated the model of primary, secondary, and tertiary prevention, Shepherd recognised the crucial role for the primary health care team in the prevention of mental disorders, observing that:

> "the general practitioner by virtue of his provision of primary care to a population, is well placed to monitor psychiatric disorder in the community as a whole, and to identify those patients serious enough to warrant treatment". (Shepherd *et al*, 1966)

One of the major achievements of the GPRU (now the Section of Epidemiology and General Practice) has been to emphasise that in population terms the most important mental illnesses are depression and anxiety. Across the whole practice list, or the wider population, the large numbers of people with depression and anxiety result in a very significant workload and have considerable public health implications. In the US, Eisenberg (1992) has calculated that minor depression results in 50 million more days lost from work than major depression, with only chronic heart disease producing more disability. As Shepherd's work has shown, the primary health care team are potentially in a position to detect, treat and prevent the whole range of psychiatric disorders.

The general-practice side of the profession did not respond to the challenge of prevention until the Royal College of General Practitioners "Report from General Practice No. 20" entitled *Prevention of Psychiatric Disorders in General Practice*, published in February 1981. This strong Working Party was chaired by Philip Graham, Professor of Child Psychiatry at the University of London, and included Drs Peter Tomson and Andrew Markus from general practice, and Sheila Ball as a health visitor. The other psychiatrist was Dr Murray Parkes, and Professor George Brown was a member as a leading academic sociologist. Unfortunately this report made less of an impact on the practising profession than other such reports, and has been less often cited.

Paykel (1994) has recently edited a book on the scope of prevention in psychiatry covering: prevention and genetic, biological and psychosocial causal factors; the prevention of specific disorders; prevention in special groups; and prevention in certain settings, including general practice.

Service planning and prevention in general practice

As has been stated, GPs come into contact with, and are responsible for treating, the bulk of psychiatric disorder in the population, and only a small proportion of the mentally disordered who consult GPs reach the specialist psychiatric services. Patients consulting GPs with identified psychiatric disorder outnumber consultant out-patient attenders by 10 : 1, and psychiatric admissions by 100 : 1. Demonstrable psychosocial problems are present in one in three of all general practice attenders, and on average, half of these are not detected by the GP (Goldberg & Huxley, 1980). Having emphasised the vast scale of the problem, the particular advantages of the GP's position, and the scope for preventive activity in general practice, how can the busy GP possibly deliver, in the midst of all the other competing obligations? He or she clearly needs help and support, and plenty of it. How can this best be achieved?

Several developments have arisen from this need, and some have been thoroughly evaluated. They have generally built on the practice of attaching secondary care personnel to the primary care team. The World Health Organization has usefully classified services into primary, secondary, and tertiary (Fig. 21.1).

Primary care includes those serving at the front line of the health service in any country, dealing directly with the population and its mass of ills. These doctors and nurses bear the prime responsibility for most of the care of most of the illnesses of most of the people for most of the time. They are usually generalists. Their responsibility is to undertake research on the

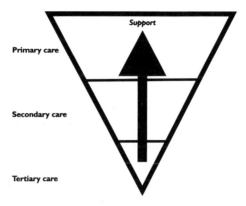

Fig. 21.1. The relative roles of primary, secondary, and tertiary care (from Horder, 1983).

work they do and to advise colleagues in both secondary and tertiary care on priorities. A key feature of the World Health Organization model is that the prime responsibility for personal prevention falls to primary care.

As Shepherd *et al* (1966) had observed, it is only in primary care that large numbers of healthy people are seen regularly, and only there that personal relationships lasting over decades are established which are invaluable in discussing sensitive changes in lifestyle, for example. By 1990, in some British general practices, attendance for some form of personal preventive medicine had become the second commonest reason for coming to the practice.

Secondary care services are essentially specialist. They consist of doctors who concentrate on one group of illnesses and sometimes on single diseases. Their experience is therefore concentrated and they acquire expert knowledge within their field. They have important responsibilities to undertake research in their field and to advise colleagues in both primary and tertiary care.

Tertiary care health staff work in national centres and limit their field even further to specific problems or diseases, or in surgery often to single operations. They become experts on the conditions which they see and have responsibilities to undertake research and to advise colleagues in primary and secondary care.

There are also in all countries a few senior medical and nursing staff in national and regional administrative centres, usually in a planning role. They are usually close to government or part of government, and are either professional advisers or civil servants, although much of their work involves attending meetings and discussions with medical colleagues. They are experts in national statistics and trends and need to be expert in the facts and figures about health care in primary, secondary and tertiary medical care. They are functionally in tertiary care and in practice tend to have close links with other tertiary care workers. Horder (1983) has summarised the relationships between primary, secondary and tertiary care which changed in understanding the roles advocated by the World Health Organization.

Attaching specialists to primary services

Brook & Temperley (1976) were the first to report on the supportive attachment of a psychiatrist to general practice. They also emphasised the educational role of attached mental health professionals. Since those early steps there have been a variety of attachments and arrangements of various health professionals to general practice, including counsellors, social workers, and community psychiatric nurses (CPNs). The attachment of secondary care personnel to the primary care setting cannot solve the problem on a national basis, however, because of the sheer numbers involved. There are approximately 30 000 GPs in the country, each of whom will have 300–600 patients with depression and anxiety in any one year, and there are 2000 consultant psychiatrists. Therefore each psychiatrist would need to have close links with 15 GPs, and could realistically only help each GP with a tiny proportion of all their depressed patients. Strathdee & Williams (1984) have traced the enormous growth in psychiatrists working, in some fashion, within general practice.

Attachments of CPNs are now probably the most common, and the least evaluated. A recent thorough evaluation by Brooking demonstrated the enormous opportunity cost entailed in withdrawing CPNs from the severely mentally ill. Again, there is a numerical problem. There is one CPN between five and ten GPs (the precise ratio varying across the country). If we take the best case of one CPN to every five GPs, we know that, on average, each GP has seven patients with chronic severe mental illness (mostly chronic schizophrenia) who require supervision, support, family interventions, etc., from the CPN (Kendrick *et al*, 1991). He or she thus already should have a caseload of 35. It is easy to see that if each GP also refers three or four depressed patients, the CPN's working week has been overloaded (unless care is withdrawn from those with severe mental illness) and, meanwhile, only a tiny dent has been made on the GP's load of several hundred depressed patients. The severely mentally ill now, more than ever, need concentrated efforts in continuing care during and after they leave hospital. CPNs will often be their case managers or key workers, and there are substantial concerns that this important work is being jeopardised by the shift of CPNs' caseloads from being primarily focused on the severely mentally ill to being primarily focused on those with lesser psychiatric morbidity (White, 1990).

Schemes of attached social workers have proven value in the treatment of people with chronic depression related to chronic social difficulties (Corney & Jenkins, 1992). Schemes of attached psychologists have been evaluated in the treatment of anxiety disorders and in cognitive therapy of depression.

An alternative strategy, instead of shifting secondary care personnel into the primary care setting to see patients for the GP, is rather to use secondary care personnel in a supportive and educational role rather than a direct 'hands on' role in relation to those patients with minor psychiatric morbidity. The GP, meanwhile, needs more 'hands', and these can be obtained by strengthening the primary care team by the employment of practice nurses and counsellors and strategic deployment of health visitors and district nurses.

The growth of counsellors in general practice is now well established, although we still need more careful evaluative studies of the effectiveness of the brief psychotherapies used by counsellors, and the indications for such treatment. The Department of Health sponsored a conference on counselling in primary care (Corney & Jenkins, 1992) which carefully examined many of the issues involved including efficacy, ethics, training issues, deployment within the team and research.

Most practices already employ practice nurses, but these have traditionally only been used for physical and not psychological problems. However, there are now a number of innovative studies of using practice nurses for detection and prevention of psychological problems (Wilkinson, 1992). Health visitors and district nurses are in the front-line for the detection of depression in, respectively, new mothers and the elderly.

For the management of chronic psychotic mental illness there is a need for cooperation between community mental health teams and the primary care team. The care programme approach can be an important focus for this approach.

Primary preventive care

Both universal and selective primary preventive activities already take place in primary care. Many have important implications for promoting mental health. Specifically, health education, immunisation, nutritional advice, dental hygiene, avoidance of alcohol, family planning, and obstetric care can all be used to address psychosocial issues.

Public education campaigns about mental illness are largely unevaluated. For example, there might be scope to evaluate help seeking before and after an educational campaign about the burden on carers in elderly couples or where there is physical illness in the family. Screening can be applied as a primary preventive strategy by focusing on high-risk groups. In practice, however, it is much more difficult to identify high-risk populations than high-risk situations. For example, it would be useful to evaluate the effects of antenatal education on rates of reporting and outcome of postnatal psychological problems.

There is similar scope for continuing medical education initiatives within the remit of primary prevention.

Depression and anxiety

The most interesting possibilities in the *primary* prevention of emotional illness at present lie with depression and anxiety. Two practical approaches involve identifying, first, people at risk, such as women who have lost their mother before the age of 11 years (Brown & Harris, 1978), or those who have recently faced an adverse life event such as a major personal loss (i.e. bereavement, recent separation, or divorce). Targeting or focusing support offers the potential for prevention, and the work of Parkes (1981) on bereavement strongly suggests that adverse medical consequences of inappropriate grieving can be reduced with skilled care.

Computer systems in general practice are now beginning to allow GPs for the first time to identify both at-risk individuals and at-risk situations (Jenkins *et al*, 1992) and to link the two. By the mid-1990s, computerised risk assessment packages are likely to be in use in general practice. Donovan (1988) has introduced the idea of screening adolescents for emotional as well as physical aspects of health in general practice. Sharp (1992) has researched the antecedents for postnatal depression in general practice, and highlighted some risk factors like previous depression or poor marital support. These can be used by health visitors and midwives and doctors alike. Blanchard (1992) has identified screening procedures for the elderly. Finally, and by no means least, the depressive effects of many medications, including many common ones, for example the contraceptive pill, need to be constantly remembered. There is scope for more reviews in general practice, where most drugs are prescribed, since more drugs are being continually prescribed in the UK and with an average of seven prescriptions per person per year in 1991. C. Illingworth (personal communication, 1992) found that as many as 40% of one series of depressives in general practice were also taking at least one drug which was theoretically capable of causing or exacerbating depression. Avoiding iatrogenic depression must be a high priority in general practice prescribing.

Alcohol and substance abuse

The Central Statistical Office (1991) has shown the strong association between the use of alcohol and road accidents, and there is evidence that the numbers consuming alcohol excessively are also related to the numbers drinking in all. The single most effective strategy for the primary prevention of excessive alcohol consumption appears to be raising the price through taxation (Bruun *et al*, 1975). There have been several studies showing that consumption is related to price, and as far as the whole population is concerned it is reasonable to recommend to government that taxes on alcohol should be increased, which is indeed the current policy of responsible professional opinion such as the Royal College of General Practitioners, the

Royal College of Psychiatrists, and the British Medical Association. As far as primary care is concerned the first question is whether or not the public want their GPs to advise them about healthy living and health promotion. Here the evidence from Wallace & Haines (1984) is clear – patients want it and respond significantly.

The primary prevention of drug abuse is a major challenge for society, involving parents and schools as well as the Health Service.

Primary prevention of other mental illnesses

Learning difficulties, schizophrenia, other psychoses and dementia are all associated with considerable stigma. The main primary preventive task at present is public and professional education.

Secondary preventive care

Secondary prevention is discussed below in relation to depression, anxiety, and alcohol consumption, after consideration of some general issues.

Screening

Screening is a key strategy in secondary prevention. Ideally any screening procedure should have a high positive predictive value and a low misclassification rate. Having detected the condition, it should be possible to reverse, alleviate, or modify its effect on a sufferer. There are various types of screening programmes. Selective screening involves the investigation of identified high-risk groups. This can involve those at high risk who develop a single disease (e.g. amniocentesis in older mothers) or multi-phasic, such as antenatal investigations in pregnant women. On the other hand, mass screening programmes such as mammography investigate large populations without specific consideration of individual risk factors. For a detailed discussion of screening, see Lloyd & Jenkins (1994).

Accessibility

If patients are made welcome at their practice, if personal contact from receptionist to doctor and nurse is professional, courteous and indicates interest in the patient as a person, then it is easier for patients to seek help with symptoms which, although often very troubling, are also often embarrassing or frightening. Patients who lack comfortable access tend to present late or to other less appropriate sites, so that encouraging sensitive responses in all members of primary teams is important for secondary prevention of emotional illness in itself. Practice management issues of this kind directly affect clinical care and were raised as early as 1978 by Jones *et al* in their book *Running a Practice*. Another major issue of practice organisation is the use of personal lists (Pereira Gray, 1979), since without them the changes and the arithmetic given in this chapter are considerably diluted.

Time for patients

The question of time is also critical. General practice is faced with rising demand. For example, consultations per person have increased by 20% in the last 20 years (Office of Population Censuses and Surveys (OPCS), 1991). The *General Household Survey 1989* (OPCS, 1991) shows that demand for general practice from children under five years (usually expressed through their mothers) has doubled in the last 20 years.

Time is the GP's most precious asset, and its deployment is a matter of immense organisational importance. The view is sometimes implied that GPs are too busy to look after the depressed well. However, there are powerful reasons why the GP should, while actively building up a multidisciplinary team, play a major role in managing one of the commonest of all conditions in practice.

Among all the members of the primary health care team, GPs have the longest chronological knowledge of patients (they move much less often than health visitors and practice nurses). Doctors do home visits as well as surgery consultations, unlike practice nurses (which can be invaluable both for detecting behavioural change (Pereira Gray, 1978) and some counselling). GPs actually see three times as many patients as practice nurses, since there are three times as many GPs as there are practice nurses. In fact, many of these patients are consulting anyway, in the guise of other health problems and diseases. Good care of depression is more efficient and can actually save the doctor time and frustration, apart from being intellectually and professionally particularly rewarding in general practice.

Finally, contrary to general impressions, GPs have more time in contact with more patients than any other health professional. The two key facts are that first the average consultation now lasts just under nine minutes in general practice, with home visits lasting an average of 12 minutes (Department of Health, 1991), and secondly that the average contact rate is 3.25 consultations per year (Royal College of General Practitioners, OPCS and Department of Health, 1990) for the GP for the whole population.

In addition, there is a rate of 72% contact every year for adult women, a contact rate of 7 per patient per year for those over 75, and ever-increasing expectations and demands, making training in general practice by GPs essential.

The average household unit of four people now sees a GP 13 times a year for an average of 12 years at a time, which is the average duration of registration in the NHS (i.e. $156 \times 8 = 1248$ minutes or 20 hours). This is the arithmetical basis of what Steen (1992) describes as "the climate necessary to gain the patient's trust and confidence". GPs are thus not short of time with their patients, but the challenge is to use the time available efficiently. The Royal College of General Practitioners was ridiculed for its book *The Future General Practitioner* when it was published in 1972, and it remains under criticism, but it became a classic and was notable for introducing much theory in general practice. In particular its emphasis that GPs must make diagnoses in physical, psychological and social terms antedated the types of multi-axial classification systems, now in use in psychiatry.

Depression

In general practice, 5% of attenders have DSM–III–R (American Psychiatric Association, 1987) major depressive disorder, 5% DSM–III–R dysthymia, and 10% significant depressive symptoms which impair functioning. It has been calculated that a GP with a list of 2000 identifies approximately 240 patients with a non-psychotic mental illness per year. Almost as many attenders again have an undiagnosed mental illness. Most commonly that illness is depression or anxiety (Paykel & Priest, 1992).

Value of earlier detection of depression

Depression has a better prognosis if it is detected early and treated effectively. The value of earlier detection of depression in general practice is not as well known as it should be, so some key references are worth listing: Johnstone & Goldberg (1976), Zung *et al* (1983), and Freeling *et al* (1985). Contrary to early expectations, the longer-term outcome of untreated depressive illness in primary care is not as favourable as was originally thought (Mann *et al*, 1981). Effective pharmacological and psychological interventions exist and are excellently summarised by Freemantle *et al* (1993) and Wright (1993).

It is therefore crucial to improve detection and management in order to avoid the consequences of untreated depression, such as suicide and parasuicide, marital breakdown, occupational problems such as sickness absence, labour turn-over, problems with colleagues, poor performance, and accidents. There are also problems for the children of depressed parents; they are more vulnerable to emotional and cognitive impairment, which in turn can predispose to adult mental illness on maturity, as well as having an adverse effect on the children's ultimate intellectual attainment. Chronic non-psychotic illness, such as chronic depression, persistent unresolved grief states, chronic phobias and tranquilliser dependency, leads not only to considerable stress, and a low quality of life, but also may act as a trigger for alcohol and drug abuse, an excessive burden on health services, as well as loss of productive economic activity (Jenkins *et al*, 1992).

The direct and indirect costs of anxiety and depression in England have recently been estimated at about £5.6 billion a year, with the majority of the direct financial burden falling on primary care services. This compares with an estimate of £1.6 billion for schizophrenia (Croft-Jeffreys & Wilkinson, 1989).

Besides persistent morbidity, a small proportion kill themselves. Of those completing suicides: 90% have some form of mental disorder, most frequently depression; 66% have consulted their GP in the previous month; 40% have consulted their GP in the last week; and 33% expressed clear suicidal ideation (Department of Health, 1992).

How to detect depression

It is important to have available a range of methods for detecting depression, so that the GP and other members of the team can choose the one most suited to their needs. Screening instruments are one possibility, the best known being the General Health Questionnaire (GHQ: Goldberg *et al*, 1988). The purpose of the GHQ is to detect a range of psychiatric disorders, and it is *not* a diagnostic instrument. It is well validated and is easy to complete and score. It is a pencil-and-paper self-completion test taking only a few minutes and is widely used as a first-stage screening test. After patients have completed the GHQ, the GP is in a position to review the findings, saving several minutes of consultation time. The Edinburgh Postnatal Depression Scale is a suitable instrument for use with new mothers (Sharp, 1992). The Geriatric Depression Scale (see page 168) is useful as a screening questionnaire in the elderly. The screening role of practice staff other than the GP, such as the practice nurse, requires further evaluation (Wilkinson, 1992).

Educational strategies

The value of continuing medical educational strategies to help improve detection and management are currently being evaluated. The Royal College of General Practitioners, in collaboration with the Department of Health, the Mental Health Foundation and the Gatsby Charitable Foundation has recently appointed Dr André Tylee as Senior GP Fellow in continuing education of GPs in mental health. The overall objective of the Fellowship is to take a national cascade approach to improving the mental health component of continuing medical education, so that GPs will be educated and supported to manage the large numbers of patients who present to them with psychological problems of varying degrees. The aim is to plan a good mental health course in knowledge and skills for each region targeted at GP tutors. All regional advisers in England and Wales have been consulted with a view to appointing regional fellows, who in turn will be responsible for disseminating knowledge and skills to GP tutors and course organisers.

Depression has interesting parallels with conditions like hypertension, asthma and diabetes, where there is a range of abnormality, from mild to severe, where the threshold for medical management is arbitrary, but can be subjected to evaluation studies. For some of these conditions, protocols have been found to be helpful, and Elaine Fullard in Oxford pioneered the use of the GP facilitator in assisting general practices to develop protocols for the screening and management of hypertension. There are now several hundred GP facilitators in England. It was with this in mind that the Department of Health has funded a three-year trial exploring whether a GP facilitator can take on the task of mental illness in a similar way, developing protocols to help the practice team improve management (Armstrong, 1992). Others have explored the use of video feedback techniques in continuing medical education (Gask, 1992).

Somatisation

Many people who are depressed express their distress through physical rather than psychological symptoms. This process is called somatisation. A major field for the reduction of suffering and ill-health is improved detection, recognition and treatment of depression in this group.

Such patients go to the doctor seeking help for symptoms which they believe represent physical illness. Skilled assessment, which often properly includes enough investigation to exclude physical disease to both the GP's and the patient's satisfaction, is necessary, and this needs to be done simultaneously with starting as soon as possible the management of the depressive disorder. This calls for good communication and clinical skills, and is an interesting example of the efficiency of the generalist system in British medicine. By operating simultaneously in both the physical and psychological dimensions of care, the medical generalist is at a great advantage in taking a diagnostic overview and steering treatment onto the most productive lines (Wright, 1990). There is a need for general practice to teach the skills of such diagnosis and such management to psychiatric registrars.

Depression combined with physical illness

A related and equally taxing clinical challenge arises when depression occurs, as it frequently does, in the presence of significant physical, often chronic, disease. Indeed, in a personal series of the first author, as many as half of 114 patients with depression had co-existing physical disease. Secondary prevention in general practice offers the possibility of seeking out the so-called hidden morbidity of depression in both somatisers and those with chronic disease, which makes it possible to make diagnoses before patients even complain. This then becomes true secondary prevention of the depressive disorder.

General practitioners have now started to use psychiatric questionnaires in their clinical practice in tackling the problem of hidden psychiatric illness (Wright & Perini, 1987). One recent use was by Crossley *et al* (1992), who not only showed substantial under-diagnosis in a rural area for the first time, but drew attention to seven patients with ''a high degree of psychological distress that they had not revealed on the general health questionnaire but had disclosed to the doctor''.

Alcohol consumption

Alcohol consumption falls on a spectrum of activity which runs from social drinking, which is certainly acceptable, and may well be desirable, at one end, to gross alcoholism which is a severe, often lethal form of addiction, at the other.

Detection and intervention are possible at any stage in the natural history of alcohol dependence, according to the patients' willingness to own the problem and accept intervention. Whether patients will respond to advice on drinking habits (i.e. can GPs effectively alter lifestyle) was investigated by Wallace *et al* (1988), who found that the advice was effective.

In terms of patterns of behaviour such as heavy drinking, leading on to problems of alcohol consumption in various degrees up to chronic alcoholism, it is now possible for many GPs (e.g some of the authors of this chapter) to know the drinking consumption of over 90% of all registered adults, and to quantify and categorise alcohol consumption by the number of units in each level of consumption. There are also several screening instruments which have been extensively evaluated, such as the MAST and CAGE questionnaires (Chapter 9) which are simple and quick to apply. There are suggestive haematological and biochemical findings which may be detected on routine blood testing.

Thus, a logical plan for preventive activity can be constructed which is relevant for secondary prevention (those patients drinking satisfactory and reasonable amounts can be identified and excluded). Advice can then be tailored and aimed at those drinking over the recommended rates of 15 units for adult women and 21 for adult men (Royal College of General Practitioners, 1986; Royal College of Psychiatrists, 1986; Royal College of Physicians, 1987). These patients are usually symptom-free and often unaware of any health risk (i.e. this is presymptomatic detection and the advice is secondary prevention).

Childhood and adolescent disorders

In children, evidence of disturbance is based more on the observations of behaviour made by parents, teachers and others than on the accounts of children themselves. The treatment of childhood psychiatric disorders differs from that of adult disorders in that it often involves other members of the family and the broader network. Psychological treatments are commonly used. Effective treatment strategies have been developed for conditions such as enuresis and encopresis.

Learning difficulties

Between 2% and 3.5% of the population have an IQ below 70. The average general practice list has 10 patients with severe learning difficulties. Severe learning difficulties are associated with intrauterine and perinatal problems, Down's syndrome, inherited abnormalities, and congenital malformations.

General practitioners and health visitors are already involved in early postnatal biochemical checks such as those available for phenylketonuria (PKU) and hypothyroidism, which can be effectively treated. Regular postnatal and developmental checks are important ongoing screening opportunities. Screening for PKU or congenital hypothyroidisim provides an interesting contrast to most other forms of psychiatric screening. Both conditions are very rare, and, unlike the neuroses, both have specific aetiologies. Both are readily treatable and therefore it is highly cost-effective to screen for them.

Schizophrenia

The lifetime risk of schizophrenia is in the order of 1%. It is generally assumed that the vast majority of first presentations will be detected with relative ease and managed initially by the psychiatric services. The majority of the work in general practice involves the maintenance and monitoring of patients who have already been diagnosed and who are in the poor-prognosis group, with persistent handicaps and in need of rehabilitation and support. Ten per cent of schizophrenic people commit suicide.

Detection of the first episode is generally not difficult. Subsequent monitoring should focus on the re-emergence of symptoms. Here, close links with secondary services are valuable, and community psychiatric nurses have a key role to play. The care programme approach can play a useful part in this process. To date, little emphasis has been placed on the need to monitor for long-term complications of drug treatment, such as dystonia and tardive dyskinesia. With the increasing trend towards GP prescribing for long-term patients, this will become an increasing area of concern.

Tertiary prevention

Depression

The main practical, recent development in the tertiary prevention of depression in primary care is the growing amount of evidence that treatment with therapeutic doses of antidepressant medication for much longer than had previously been thought necessary is beneficial. This appears to hold good both for adults in the middle years (Manning & Frances, 1990) and for the elderly (Blanchard, 1992), while for the tertiary prevention of depression in secondary care, Evans *et al* (1992) have shown that cognitive therapy reduces relapses.

A currently controversial issue is the choice of antidepressant medication in general practice. Traditionally, most GPs have used tricyclic antidepressants such as amitriptyline and, increasingly, dothiepin, on which most of the research on effectiveness had been undertaken in general practice (Hollyman *et al*, 1988). However, Henry (1992*a*, *b*) has calculated a 'fatal toxicity index' which shows that the death rate (about 5% of suicides use antidepressant drugs) by drug used is higher for the older tricyclics than for the newer, and much more expensive, selective serotonin reuptake inhibitors (SSRIs). Other experts suggest that these findings should be treated with caution, as we do not yet have a full picture of long-term safety of the much more costly SSRIs (Song *et al*, 1993; Freemantle *et al*, 1993). Song *et al* conclude that the use of SSRIs as "the first line treatment of depressive illness may greatly increase cost with only questionable benefit".

Alcohol consumption

General practitioners can be more effective in counselling heavy-drinking patients than many have thought. Drummond *et al* (1990) showed that GPs could be almost as effective with problem drinkers as specialists, and are of course much less expensive.

Schizophrenia

Tertiary prevention means not only good initial treatment but good follow-up, especially for psychotic patients. Administrative systems which provide *systematic* primary care, with any injections being given there, are optimal, as are a single nurse and single doctor to provide as much of the follow-up as possible, so that personal relationships are built up and fostered. Systems must be promptly reactive, so that failure to arrive for an appointment triggers a response, and if necessary follow through to the home quite quickly. Again, the care programme approach should be of help here.

Dementia

Only 5% of the elderly and only 14% of those with dementia are in any form of institutional care. It is generally estimated that about 6% of the elderly population (20% of those over 80) suffer from dementia. Community studies show that not all patients with cognitive impairment undergo much further decline. With an increasing elderly population, dementia is going to become more common (Jacoby & Bergman, 1986).

Apart from those patients who are worried about their memories, the vast majority of cases are brought to the attention of the GP by relatives, or come to light when some change in the patient's circumstances means that he/she can no longer function independently. It is particularly difficult to distinguish the effects of mild dementia from the effects of normal ageing or lifelong poor cognitive performance. Williamson *et al* (1964) found that GPs were unaware of 87% of the cases of mild to moderate dementia on their lists. Results from a large identification and intervention study among over-75s in East Anglia suggest that although the quality of life of dementia sufferers can be improved by early detection, admission rates are not reduced (O'Connor *et al*, 1991).

Alzheimer's disease is not reversible. Its social and psychological accompaniments are amenable to treatment. Underlying physical conditions can also be treated as part of secondary and tertiary prevention. Accompanying toxic confusional states (from infections or drugs) are not uncommon, and are important to treat as they greatly exacerbate problems with cognitive function. Routine measurement of blood pressure and checks for evidence of atherosclerotic disease are of value in the detection of risk factors for atherosclerotic dementia.

The resource implications of an ageing population are immense. It is not clear how effective earlier intervention in the dementing process will be. Certainly, early identification may allow early, effective support to be offered to sufferers and carers.

Conclusions

A preventive approach to emotional and mental problems in primary care is an idea whose time has come. The far-sighted book by Caplan (1964) and the Royal College of General Practitioners' report of 1981 were signposts, but were ahead of their time. The major body of work conducted by Shepherd and the General Practice Research Unit has established the epidemiological underpinnings for much current thinking. More than 40 years after Watts & Watts (1952) first identified the scale of the clinical challenge of emotional medicine in general practice, GPs have a better research base (although still all too little from GPs themselves) from which to work. Detecting and treating depression well and reducing suicides are principal targets in 1993, along with reduction of alcohol consumption. Both are partly possible in general practice, now that multidisciplinary teams are forming and with computerisation occurring in more and more practices.

General practice is the first point of contact for the vast majority of patients with a psychiatric disorder. The key to successful primary preventive strategies lies with increasing detection in groups who are at risk of developing psychiatric disorders. One of the aims behind the 1990 contract for GPs was to give prevention of illness and health promotion greater emphasis. Particular emphasis was given to screening procedures, although these are primarily for physical disorders, immunisation procedures, and health checks.

There are no financial incentives in the contract to detect and treat psychological disorders, and it is important not to place too high or impossible expectations on the "front line of the Health Service" (Royal College of General Practitioners, 1987). Yet population disorders are part of the bread and butter of primary care. General practice faces the problems of the society it serves. Much of the misery and suffering seen in the consulting-room stems from bad personal relationships and inappropriate expectations and values. In improving these, and in reducing violence, nothing short of a national campaign integrating families, schools, and health professionals will be enough, but that must be the subject for a different book! In the meantime we have the tools at our disposal to engage in the preventive care of common mental illnesses in general practice.

References

AMERICAN PSYCHIATRIC ASSOCIATION (1987) *Diagnostic and Statistical Manual of Mental Disorders* (3rd edn, revised) (DSM–III–R). Washington, DC: APA.

ARMSTRONG, E. (1992) Facilitators in primary care. *International Review of Psychiatry*, **4**, 339–342.

BALINT, M. (1957) *The Doctor, His Patient and the Illness*. London: Pitman Medical.

BLANCHARD, M. (1992) The elderly. *International Review of Psychiatry*, **4**, 251–256.

BROOK, A. & TEMPERLEY, J. (1976) Contribution of psychotherapists to general practice. *Journal of the Royal College of General Practitioners*, **26**, 86–94.

BROWN, G. W. & HARRIS, T. O. (1978) *The Social Origins of Depression*. London: Tavistock.

BRUUN, K., EDWARDS, G., MALEKA, K., et al (1975) *Alcohol Controlled Policies in Public Health Perspective*. Helsinki: WHO, Finnish Foundation for Alcohol Studies.

CAPLAN, G. (1964) *Principles of Preventive Psychiatry*. New York: Basic Books.

CATFORD, J. & NUTBEAM, D. (1984) Towards a definition of health education and health promotion. *Health Education Journal*, **43**, 2–3.

CENTRAL STATISTICAL OFFICE (1991) *Social Trends*. London: HMSO.

CORNEY, R. & JENKINS, R. (1992) *Counselling in General Practice*. London: Routledge.

CROFT-JEFFREYS, C. & WILKINSON, G. (1989) Costs of neurotic disorder in UK general practice (Editorial). *Psychological Medicine*, **19**, 551–558.

CROSSLEY, D., MYRES, M. P. & WILKINSON, G. (1992) Assessment of psychological care in general practice. *British Medical Journal*, **305**, 1333–1336.

DEPARTMENT OF HEALTH STATISTICAL AND INFORMATION DIVISION (1991) *General Medical Practitioners Workload Survey 1989–90*. London: Department of Health.

DEPARTMENT OF HEALTH (1992) *The Health of the Nation Key Area Handbook. Mental Illness*. London: Department of Health.

DONOVAN, C. F. (1988) Is there a place for adolescent screening in general practice? *Health Trends*, **2**, 64.

DRUMMOND, D. C., THOM, B. & BROWN, C., et al (1990) Specialist versus general practitioner treatment of problem drinkers. *Lancet*, **336**, 915–918.

EIMERL, T. S. (1960) Organised curiosity. *Journal of the Royal College of General Practitioners*, **3**, 346–352.

EISENBERG, L. (1992) Treating depression and anxiety in primary care. Closing the gap between knowledge and practice. *New England Journal of Medicine*, **326**, 1080–1084.

EVANS, M. D., HOLLON, S. D., DeRUBEIS, R. J., *et al* (1992) Differential relapse following cognitive therapy and pharmacotherapy for depression. *Archives of General Psychiatry*, **49**, 802–808.

FREELING, P., RAO, B. M., PAYKEL, E. S., *et al* (1985) Unrecognised depression in general practice. *British Medical Journal*, **290**, 1880–1883.

FREEMANTLE, N., *et al* (1993) The treatment of depression in primary care. *Effective Health Care*, **5**, 2–12.

GASK, L. (1992) Training general practitioners to detect and manage emotional disorders. *International Review of Psychiatry*, **4**, 293–300.

GOLDBERG, D. & HUXLEY, P. (1980) *Mental Illness in the Community: The Pathways to Psychiatric Care*. London: Tavistock.

——— , BRIDGES, K., DUNCAN-JONES, P., *et al* (1988) Detecting anxiety and depression in general practice settings. *British Medical Journal*, **297**, 897–899.

——— & HUXLEY, P. (1992) *Common Mental Disorders: A Biosocial Model*. London: Routledge.

HENRY, J. A. (1992a) The safety of antidepressants. *British Journal of Psychiatry*, **160**, 439–441.

——— (1992b) *Contemporary Topics in Psychiatry*. London: Pfizer Ltd.

HOLLYMAN, J. A., FREELING, P., PAYKEL, E. S., *et al* (1988) Double-blind placebo-controlled trial of amitriptyline among depressed patients in general practice. *Journal of the Royal College of General Practitioners*, **38**, 393–397.

HORDER, J. (1983) Alma-Ata Declaration. *British Medical Journal*, **286**, 191–194.

JACOBY, R. & BERGMAN, I. (1986) The psychiatry of old age. *Essentials of Postgraduate Psychiatry*, (eds R. Murray *et al*). London: Grune & Stratton.

JENKINS, R., NEWTON, J. & YOUNG, R. (eds) (1992) *The Prevention of Depression and Anxiety: The Role of the Primary Care Team*. London: HMSO.

JOHNSTONE, A. & GOLDBERG, D. (1976) Psychiatric screening in general practice. *Lancet*, **i**, 605–608.

JONES, R. V. H., BOLDEN, K. J., PEREIRA GRAY, D. J., *et al* (1978) *Running a Practice*. London: Croom Helm.

KENDRICK, T., SIBBALD, P., BURNS, T., *et al* (1991) Role of general practitioners in care of long-term mentally ill. *British Medical Journal*, **302**, 508–510.

LLOYD, K., & JENKINS, R. (1994) The prevention of psychiatric illness in general practice settings. In *Preventive Approaches in Psychiatry* (ed. E. Paykel). London: Gaskell.

MANN, A. H., *et al* (1981) The twelve-month outcome of patients with neurotic illness in general practice. *Psychological Medicine*, **11**, 535–550.

MANNING, D. & FRANCES, A. (1990) *Combined Pharmacotherapy and Psychotherapy for Depression*. Washington, DC: American Psychiatric Association.

NEWTON, J. (1992) *Preventing Mental Illness in Practice*. London: Routledge.

O'CONNOR, D. W., *et al* (1991) Does early intervention reduce the number of people with dementia admitted to institutions for long term care? *British Medical Journal*, **302**, 871–875.

OFFICE OF POPULATION CENSUSES AND SURVEYS (1991) *General Household Survey 1989*. London: HMSO.

PARKES, C. M. (1981) Evaluation of a bereavement service. *Journal of Preventive Psychiatry*, **1**, 179–188.

PAYKEL, E. (1994) *The Place of Prevention in Psychiatry*. London: Gaskell.

——— & PRIEST, R. G. (1992) Recognition and management of depression and general practice: consensus statement. *British Medical Journal*, **305**, 1198–1202.

PEREIRA GRAY, D. J. (1978) Feeling at home. James Mackenzie Lecture. *Journal of the Royal College of General Practitioners*, **28**, 6–17.

——— (1979) The key to personal care. *Journal of the Royal College of General Practitioners*, **29**, 666–678.

PREECE, J. F., GILLINGS, D. B., LIPPMAN, E. O., *et al* (1970) An on-line record maintenance and retrieval system in general practice. *International Journal of Biomedical Computing*, **1**.

ROSE, G. (1992) *Strategies for Prevention*.

ROYAL COLLEGE OF GENERAL PRACTITIONERS (1972) *The Future General Practitioner – Learning and Teaching*. London: British Medical Journal.

——— (1981) *Prevention of Psychiatric Disorders in General Practice*. Report from General Practice 20. London: RCGP.

—— (1981/82) *Combined Reports on Prevention*. Reports from General Practice 18–21. London: RCGP.

—— (1986) *Alcohol – A Balanced View*. Report from General Practice 24. London: RCGP.

—— (1987) *The Front Line of the Health Service*. Report from General Practice 25. London: RCGP.

——, OFFICE OF POPULATION CENSUSES AND SURVEYS & DEPARTMENT OF HEALTH (1990) *Morbidity Statistics from General Practice 1981–1982. Third National Study: Socio-economic Analyses*. London: HMSO.

ROYAL COLLEGE OF PHYSICIANS (1987) *A Great and Growing Evil*. London: Tavistock.

ROYAL COLLEGE OF PSYCHIATRISTS (1986) *Alcohol – Our Favourite Drug*. London: Tavistock.

RYLE, A. (1967) *Neurosis in the Ordinary Family*. London: Tavistock.

SHARP, D. (1992) Liaison between providers of primary care: early detection of difficulties. B. Predicting postnatal depression. In *The Prevention of Depression and Anxiety, The Role of the Primary Care Team* (eds R. Jenkins, J. Newton & R. Young). London: HMSO.

SHEPHERD, M., COOPER, B., BROWN, A. C., *et al* (1966) *Psychiatric Illness in General Practice*. Oxford: Oxford University Press.

SONG, F., FREEMANTLE, N., SHELDON, T. A., *et al* (1993) Selective serotonin re-uptake inhibitors: meta analysis of efficacy and acceptability. *British Medical Journal*, **306**, 683–687.

STEEN, C. (1992) Mental health promotion in general practice. In *The Prevention of Depression and Anxiety* (eds R. Jenkins, J. Newton & R. Young). London: HMSO.

STRATHDEE, G. & WILLIAMS, P. (1984) A survey of psychiatrists in primary care: the silent growth of a new service. *Journal of the Royal College of General Practitioners*, **34**, 615–618.

TUDOR HART, J. (1975) The management of high blood pressure in general practice. *Journal of the Royal College of General Practitioners*, **25**, 160–192.

WALLACE, P. & HAINES, A. (1984) General practitioners and health promotion: what patients think. *British Medical Journal*, **289**, 534–536.

——, CUTLER, S. & HAINES, A. (1988) Randomised controlled trial of general practitioner intervention in patients with excessive alcohol consumption. *British Medical Journal*, **297**, 398–400.

WATTS, C. A. H. (1954) The chronic mental patient in general practice. *Lancet, ii*, 85.

—— (1958) How to compile an age–sex register. *Between Ourselves*, no. 8, 1–12.

—— (1966) *Depressive Disorders in the Community*. Bristol: Wright.

—— & WATTS, B. (1952) *Psychiatry in General Practice*. London: Churchill.

WHEATLEY, D. (1973) *Psychopharmacology in Family Practice*. London: William Heinemann.

WHITE, E. (1990) *The Third Quinquennial Survey of Community Psychiatric Nurses*. Manchester: Manchester University Press.

WILKINSON, G. (1992) The role of the practice nurse in the management of depression. *International Review of Psychiatry*, **4**, 311–316.

WILLIAMSON, *et al* (1964) Old people at home – unreported needs. *Lancet, i*, 1117–1120.

WORLD HEALTH ORGANIZATION AND UNITED NATIONS CHILDREN'S FUND (1978) *The Alma-Ata Declaration*. Geneva: WHO and UNICEF.

WRIGHT, A. F. (1990) A study of the presentation of somatic symptoms in general practice by patients with psychiatric disturbance. *British Journal of General Practice*, **40**, 459–463.

—— & PERINI, A. F. (1987) Hidden psychiatric illness in general practice: use of the general health questionnaire in general practice. *Journal of the Royal College of General Practitioners*, **37**, 164–167.

ZUNG, L., MAGILL, M. & MOORE, J. (1983) Recognition and treatment of depression in a family medicine practice. *Journal of Clinical Psychiatry*, **4**, 1–9.

Part IV. Training and research

22 Training for general practitioners in psychiatry

LINDA GASK

In this chapter, the training available to GPs in psychiatry, at all stages of their career, from student to experienced doctor, is described. Training opportunities vary from centre to centre, but specific psychiatric training essentially takes place in three main settings: during an attachment in psychiatry as part of a vocational training scheme; during the one-year trainee appointment; and then during continuing medical education, as an experienced GP.

Some training in psychiatry is also provided by departments of general practice at medical school, and although this is not explicitly dealt with in this chapter, there is often considerable overlap between teaching in psychiatry and that provided in general practice. One obvious common area is that both departments may offer training in communication skills, and in some medical schools the training has been coordinated to avoid duplication. Also, those parts of psychiatry that are appropriate to general medical practice, such as how to break bad news, management of normal and abnormal grief, dealing with drug and alcohol abuse in the community (to offer a few examples), may be given more time in the general practice curriculum than the time allocated to psychiatry, which at many medical schools is often heavily devoted to diagnosis and management of major mental illness. Some liaison between departments can ensure that there is no undue duplication. Both departments may then offer their own specialist viewpoint, which may be best done in the form of a series of jointly run seminars or workshops.

Vocational training

This period of training offers two opportunities for training in psychiatry, during a senior house officer post in psychiatry, and during the vocational trainee year, when training in psychiatry may be provided during the day-release course, and also in 'hands-on' training with supervision by the trainer.

The senior house officer post in psychiatry

Not all GP trainees carry out such a post during their training, but a senior house officer post in psychiatry is an option on most GP training schemes and is also frequently included by many trainees who are putting together their own training 'package' which does not form part of a recognised scheme. The Royal Colleges of General Practitioners and Psychiatrists operate a system of approval whereby a scheme cannot be approved for GP training if it is not approved for psychiatric career training. However, the needs of psychiatric and GP trainees are different, and the training received by many GP trainees during their psychiatric attachment does not necessarily prepare them for their future work in primary care.

Ideally GP trainees in psychiatry should have an opportunity to learn as far as possible to identify and manage the same range of morbidity that they will see in primary care. This means that their jobs should not consist entirely of managing in-patient psychotic illness, or even out-patient chronic neurotic illness. It is of course important that the trainee feels able to recognise and manage a new episode of psychotic illness, and knows how to plan a care programme for a chronic patient, but this must *not* be all that he/she learns.

The best attachment is that which offers a varied general experience, with opportunities especially for work in liaison psychiatry in the general hospital, liaison with primary care, and also, if possible, old age psychiatry (perceived as particularly useful by many GP trainees). It is of course difficult to arrange for all experiences in one six-month job, but some experience can be gained by spending for example one day per week with the old-age psychiatry team for three months. An individual programme for each trainee should be planned with his/her participation and active choice of speciality experience.

The trainee should be free to attend the local vocational training scheme (VTS) course during the attachment, which ensures a continuing link with peers. The course attended by trainee psychiatrists is generally inappropriate for GP trainees, with its heavy emphasis on psychopathology and other more specialised aspects of psychiatric training. Each region should attempt to meet the needs specific of its GP trainees in psychiatry by offering them a course in psychiatry for family doctors. Such a course has been successfully run in the North West Region now for several years (Creed, 1987). This can be attended both by GPs currently working in psychiatric posts and by trainees working in general practice who do not have a psychiatric attachment in their training scheme. In order to be accepted on such a course trainees must agree to bring with them video-recordings of their encounters with patients. Those trainees who are attached to primary care are particularly important to such courses, since they give access to actual encounters between doctor and patient in the setting in which all the trainees will ultimately be working themselves.

In planning such a course, formal lectures should be limited in number, and should emphasise problems rather than diagnoses. For example, topics included might be:

anxiety and depression
somatisation
dealing with a new episode of psychotic illness
chronic psychotic illness: the role of the GP
common psychiatric disorders in childhood
problems related to pregnancy and childbirth
confused elderly patients
alcohol problems
drug problems
sexual and marital problems
dealing with suicidal behaviour.

There should be opportunities to present and discuss particularly difficult patients, preferably in a conference where both a senior GP and a psychiatrist who works in the community are present. Trainees also welcome the opportunity to develop a repertoire of useful management skills, such as bereavement counselling, and assessing marital and family problems. Above all, when psychiatrists, psychologists, or other specialist mental health workers teach, it is essential that they do not simply say what the mental health professional could do if the problem were referred, an approach which has been common in much postgraduate teaching but which de-skills and undervalues the GP. Instead, they must provide guidelines for recognition and treatment in primary care by GPs themselves, with straightforward guidance on when and how to use the specialist services (see below).

All trainees attending such a course should also have the opportunity to view their own interviews, recorded in a primary care or psychiatric out-patient setting, in order to provide specific training in psychiatric interviewing skills. It has been shown that GP trainees can be trained to be more accurate in detecting psychiatric illness, that improved detection is linked to objective changes in behaviour, and that such changes improve patient care (Gask *et al*, 1988). Those attending such a course can be encouraged, if they are working in general practice, to bring a videotape of a real patient, or, if this is not possible, role-played interviews can be specially recorded. A range of skills for both detecting and managing patient problems can be taught during group feedback sessions. The skills learned during these sessions can be built upon and further developed during the vocational training course.

In the course which runs in both Manchester and Preston, we have introduced training in specific management skills relating to two commonly encountered problems in primary care, somatisation and depression. The teaching session on the management of somatisation, entitled "Reattribution" (Goldberg *et al*, 1989), employs a specially produced videotape which demonstrates a model for such a consultation and the component skills required to enable patients presenting with somatic complaints who are suffering from psychological illness to re-attribute the aetiology of their symptoms to a psychological rather than a physical cause. In order to treat such patients successfully, doctors must be able to help a patient to *feel understood,* and then to *change the agenda* of the interview to include the psychological symptoms that they have elicited, and *make the link* for the patient between their physical and psychological symptoms (words in italics refer to the components of the teaching model).

A second videotape gives the trainees, who work in pairs taking it in turns to role-play doctor or patient, the opportunity to practise the specific 'microskills' of the model. The tape is stopped, and the trainees practise responding to cues delivered by 'patients' on the videotape, in the presence of a group of teachers, who each work with and listen to the responses of three or four pairs of trainees. After the practice session the tape is restarted and one possible correct response is demonstrated.

A similar approach to teaching the skills required for assessing and managing depression in a one-day workshop has also recently been introduced on this course; it is currently being evaluated, and has proved popular with trainees. The teaching on depression emphasises the tasks and skills necessary for a primary care assessment. This can be completed in ten minutes, unlike a full psychiatric assessment, which takes much longer, primarily because it is necessary to explore aetiological factors in the family and personal history. In primary care, this can usually in the first instance be omitted. It becomes important when a patient fails to respond to simple first-line therapies (and hence requires referral). It is crucial that both teachers and trainees appreciate this, otherwise trainees will attempt a fuller assessment, fail because of shortage of time, and never learn how to use the time efficiently to get useful information.

The tasks that we have found appropriate to teach for assessing depression and negotiating the initial treatment contract with the patient are:

(a) key assessment tasks
   (i) severity
   (ii) duration
   (iii) past history
   (iv) views of self, world, and future
   (v) suicidal ideation
   (vi) exacerbating and ameliorating factors

      (vii) social support

      (viii) range of depressive symptoms present/absent

  (b) key tasks in negotiating treatment

      (i) positively re-frame as 'depression' (common and treatable)

      (ii) link to life events (if appropriate)

      (iii) offer antidepressants (if appropriate); explain delayed action and side-effects

      (iv) draw up problem list with order of priority

      (v) agree date for review and frequency of consultations.

The vocational training scheme

On the day-release course

The day-release course of the vocational training scheme (VTS) plays a central role in the education of the GP trainee. During the course, trainees will again have many opportunities for increasing their knowledge of psychiatry, and it is important that sessions devoted to psychiatry are not simply 'consultant' presentations of what local services can offer, but instead are interactive, relevant, and aimed at improving knowledge of and skills in dealing with commonly presenting problems in primary care. If there is no local course available in psychiatry, such as the one described above, many of the topic areas listed could be dealt with on the day-release course. However, the major advantage of this year for training is that the trainees now have first-hand experience of the presentation of psychiatric problems in primary care. They are faced with *undifferentiated illness* and discover that, unlike in psychiatric out-patient departments, the patient does not necessarily present with emotional distress if he/she has a psychiatric problem. They are also understandably now concerned about how to help patients in the limited time available to them.

Most VTS courses now incorporate an element of communication skills training using videotape feedback, and the model described by Pendleton *et al* (1983), which seeks to clarify the *ideas*, *concerns* and *expectations* of the patient, has been particularly influential. Pendleton's rules for giving feedback are well known, but deserve repetition.

  (a) After the consultation has been observed, the doctor concerned should be allowed to make the first comments about the consultation and his/her strengths and weaknesses.

  (b) The teacher should first comment on the strengths of the consultation, the tasks that have been achieved, and the skills and strategies that were effective in doing so.

  (c) Negative comments about tasks which have been less well achieved should always be coupled with constructive comment about skills and strategies that may be more helpful or effective.

Many trainees are hesitant about video feedback, and although teaching in communication skills is now more widespread within medical schools it is often not carried out sensitively. A useful way to begin is for the course organiser to agree to show one of his/her tapes initially, perhaps with a visiting psychiatrist or psychologist facilitating the group teaching. Trainees respond much more willingly when they realise that teachers rarely carry out perfect interviews.

The problem-based approach to teaching communication skills with video or audiotape (Lesser, 1981, 1985) provides a practical model for then learning new skills and strategies. It has also been used to teach more specifically psychiatric interviewing skills to GP trainees. During the group teaching sessions, which can be facilitated by a psychiatrist, a GP, or both working together, tapes of real consultations are used specifically for the rehearsal of new skills, and not to assess performance of the doctor, rate the consultation in any way, or as a focus for interpreting the patient's behaviour. The tape is stopped throughout to learn how to recognise key verbal and non-verbal cues of emotional distress, to discuss how particular cues given by the patient might have been responded to differently, and to label particular skills and strategies and practise alternatives.

Ideally, such a group should run on a number of occasions during the VTS course year, so that everyone has an opportunity to show at least two interviews. It is helpful if trainees get an opportunity to go away and practise new skills and then show another tape later, when they will be able to discuss difficulties they have experienced. This rarely happens on many courses after new skills such as counselling have been taught, and the increased time that trainees usually take over consultations after their first training experience can result in them rejecting rather than absorbing new skills if a follow-up 'trouble-shooting' session is not organised.

The course organiser can ask members of the group to try to select material before the session, and to bring material of patients with whom they are experiencing some difficulty assessing or managing. However, if members of the group *always* select patients to be discussed during the session, they are highly unlikely to choose patients with hidden psychiatric morbidity, since they cannot be expected to select such patients if they are unaware of their disorders. A way around this is to ask a member of the group to make videotapes of an entire clinic. Each patient seen completes a psychiatric screening questionnaire such as the General Health Questionnaire, and the teacher is presented with a list showing the names of the patients in the order in which they appear, the questionnaires, and the videotape. The trainer/ facilitator views the tape before the teaching session, looking only at the interviews between the trainees and patients who score highly on the screening questionnaire. Teaching can then focus on these consultations, where emotional disorder is likely to have been missed by the practitioner, and can focus both on missed 'cues' and on the doctor's behaviour which may have discouraged the patient from discussing his/her problems. This approach, combined with a brief presentation on the basic research demonstrating which patients are missed in primary care and why, can form a particularly useful workshop on 'improving detection of psychiatric illness'.

It is an essential part of the process that members of the group are responsible for their own learning. If the teacher constantly stops the tape and points out everything to the group, then they will never improve their own powers of observation or skills. Teachers should practise how to use a hierarchy of prompts: for example, "Why do you think I stopped the tape? Did you notice anything happening at that point? What did you notice about the patient's voice? Did you notice how her voice changed when she started talking about her husband? How did it change?" If necessary the tape can be rewound in order to listen to or watch the relevant section a second time. New ways of phrasing statements, or different strategies, can be handled in a similar way.

Group teaching should initially focus on three important sources of information, which have been described in detail by Lesser (1985). These are:

(a) *what the patient says* to the doctor – the events, symptoms and feelings that the patient talks about
(b) *what the doctor 'sees'* – in other words the appearance and non-verbal behaviour of the patient
(c) *how the doctor feels* – feelings are in themselves a useful source of information and may tell something about how other key people in the patient's life might react to him/her.

A number of basic 'problem-detection' and 'problem-management' skills can be taught during the group teaching sessions (Gask *et al*, 1991*a*):

(a) Key problem-detection skills
    (i) picking up verbal cues (e.g. "I feel down about things . . .")
    (ii) responding to verbal cues
        (1) with open questions (e.g. "Tell me about that . . .")
        (2) with clarification (e.g. "Tell me what you mean by 'down'")
        (3) by asking for examples (e.g. "Tell me about the last time you felt down . . .")
    (iii) picking up non-verbal cues
    (iv) responding to non-verbal cues (e.g. "You look quite tense . . .")
    (v) making empathic comments (e.g. "I can see it's been tough for you recently")
    (vi) asking about health beliefs (e.g. "Is there anything in particular you've been worried about?")
(b) Key problem-management skills
    (i) ventilation of feelings
    (ii) negotiation

   (iii) making links (e.g. between physical symptoms and psychosocial
        problems)
   (iv) motivational interviewing (helping patients to change their
        behaviour, e.g. reduce alcohol)
    (v) problem solving
   (vi) special types of interviewing (e.g. seeing couples and families).

Specific therapeutic skills can also be taught in these sessions, building
on what may already have been learned during the attachment in psychiatry.
It is crucially important that trainees get some grasp of management
strategies for patients with emotional and psychiatric problems during the
trainee year. It is not simply enough to learn how to clarify the 'ideas,
concerns and expectations' of the patient if you do not know what to do
next. Teaching about psychiatric illness should incorporate four components:

   (a) *The diagnostic criteria and the skills involved in detection.*
   (b) *Factual information about treatment strategies* (e.g. the respective roles of
       drug treatment and psychological treatment in depression, what to
       prescribe, when to refer, etc.). This can often be provided by a
       psychiatrist who has an interest in psychiatric illness in primary care.
   (c) *The skills involved in carrying out the treatment* (e.g. how to negotiate about
       treatment, simple problem-solving skills, ensuring compliance with
       medication). These skills are best taught using video feedback, as
       described above, with recordings of real or role-played consultations.
       If professional actors (such as the group ''Spanner'', who are based
       in the north-west and specialise in this approach to teaching) are used,
       they can often provide useful and sensitive personal feedback about
       what it was like to be interviewed by the doctor (Whitehouse *et al*, 1984).
   (d) *The local resources available for consultation and referral.* This can be provided
       by both psychologists and psychiatrists, but should include not only
       facilities for out-patient consultations but also what other resources are
       available locally, for example, self-help groups, social service agencies
       and welfare rights agencies, and patient self-help reading lists and
       literature available, for example, from health promotion departments.

Teaching should thus build on or complement that provided during a six-
month attachment in psychiatry, at a time when the content seems more
clinically relevant to the trainee.

The counselling model, rooted in the client-centred approach of Carl
Rodgers, has been particularly influential in training on vocational training
courses for GP trainees. Bensing & Sluijs (1985), in The Netherlands, found
that their training was undoubtedly effective in providing the doctors with
new skills. However, patients presenting with somatic complaints were no
more likely to talk about their emotional problems when given more space

and time than before the doctors received training, and instead the patient used the extra time to talk even more about their physical symptoms! This finding suggests that the counselling model may not be appropriate for the early stages of consultation in primary care, when the problem is 'undifferentiated', and at this stage a more active approach in which cues are picked up and clarified seems to work more effectively.

Counselling comes into its own when a 'marital' or 'bereavement' problem is clarified, but it may not then be possible or appropriate for GPs to offer this themselves unless they are prepared to undergo full training and receive supervision (see Chapter 17). For this reason, it is probably better that trainees learn and master basic consultation skills rather than, for example, have brief exposure to formal counselling during the trainee year, which may in fact be counterproductive. Counselling cannot be taught in a couple of sessions and to suggest this may be both harmful to patients, misleading to trainees who may try out some of the skills learned and then get into deep emotional water which they need to be rescued from (an experience which may further put them off exploring psychological issues again), and undervalues the skills of the professional counsellor.

With the GP trainer

The crucial part played by the general practice trainer in shaping the attitudes and skills of the trainee cannot be underestimated. During the trainee year, a number of teaching sessions will be devoted to psychiatric topics, and at this stage it is important that teaching is broadly based and emphasises the role that psychological factors can play in many common situations in primary care.

Real problems brought by the trainee should be capitalised upon to discuss feelings and attitudes as well as knowledge. For example, having to arrange for the compulsory admission to hospital of a patient that he/she has spent time building up a relationship with can be a harrowing experience for the trainee. Such an episode could provide a wealth of related psychiatric topics to teach on such as how to use the Mental Health Act, the presentation and treatment of the illness concerned, the impact of psychiatric illness on the patient and the family. However, perhaps most important will be the attitudes of the trainee to compulsory treatment and his/her feelings about the effect of the admission on the ongoing relationship with the patient.

Continuing medical education

This section looks at the training available for the GP trainer, particularly in teaching consultation skills, and psychiatric education for experienced practitioners.

Training for the GP trainer

General practitioner trainers are now being encouraged to play an active role in teaching communication skills using video, and the approach to teaching interviewing skills described above can also be carried out one-to-one between trainer and trainee. Such sessions have the advantage of being 'safer' for the trainee and more personal, but the absence of the group to make a range of suggestions means that both trainer and trainee have to work hard at providing suggestions. Many trainers do not feel comfortable using the technology of video, and may feel unsure how the medium can most effectively be used. A method for training GP trainers how to teach communication skills using video has been developed, and it has been shown that the teaching skills of trainers can be significantly improved by an experiential learning intervention, in which they present their own consultations to a group, facilitated in the way described above (Gask *et al*, 1991*b*). Further specific teaching on 'how to teach' had no further significant effect on their skills. In other words, if you want to learn how to do something you have to experience it yourself, and there is a great deal to be said therefore for not submitting our trainees to video feedback until we have undergone this ourselves!

In some regions seminars for trainers are underway to enable them to improve their use of video in the teaching of communication skills. Clearly, an important first step in disseminating these skills is for trainers to bring their own recordings of consultations to trainer groups in order to clarify both what they want to teach using video or audio feedback, and what skills are required to teach the skills.

Both 'live' and 'video' methods can be used to improve teaching skills (Gask *et al*, 1992). In the 'live' feedback group, one trainer elects to show his/her videotape and play the 'trainee' and another agrees to play the role of the 'trainer'. One other member of the group assumes a leadership role. The teaching session proceeds while other members of the group silently observe and are asked not to intervene. At suitable intervals, usually every 15 minutes or so, the group leader calls "time out", and asks for feedback. He/she first asks the 'trainee' to give feedback to the 'trainer' on how it felt to be taught using the taped consultation, and then the 'trainer' is asked for comments on how he/she felt as the teaching progressed. Both 'trainee' and 'trainer' are asked to comment on the strengths as well as the weaknesses of the tutorial exercise. After both have spoken, the rest of the group are similarly asked to comment, and are particularly asked for observations on both the teaching skills employed by the 'trainer' and also on possible missed opportunities for teaching consultation skills which, as observers, they are in the best position to notice. Group members can focus on what they would have done or said themselves at a particular point in the teaching exercise, so that new teaching skills can be rehearsed by group members.

Videotapes of a trainer teaching a trainee consultation skills using video or audio can also be watched by the group, and treated in exactly the same way as a consultation (see above). This approach has an advantage over 'live' feedback in that the person taking the role of the trainer is actually able to see him/herself on video, which can be a powerful factor in bringing about changes in teaching style.

Psychiatric training for the experienced practitioner

A wide range of training opportunities are available for the experienced GP through the continuing medical education programme organised with postgraduate education allowance funding at local postgraduate centres, departments of general practice, and elsewhere. Psychiatric topics have to compete with a wide range of other interests, but topical issues such as depression, anxiety, and somatisation, as well as more controversial topics such as 'ME', are often popular subjects for courses. The Health Education Board for Scotland (1990) is attempting to disseminate training in the management of alcohol problems by organising training in the DRAMS scheme in each district. It is not generally clear how effective such courses actually are in imparting knowledge or changing practice, although recent research has shown that brief training interventions can improve the ability of GPs both to detect and to diagnose psychiatric disorder. It has also been demonstrated that group teaching of the type described above, where participants bring recordings of their own consultations, can appeal to and improve the psychiatric interviewing skills even of experienced GPs (Gask *et al*, 1987; Whewell *et al*, 1988), and the skills learned persist over time (Bowman *et al*, 1992).

It is not easy however to find convincing evidence elsewhere that existing models of education change behaviour (Horder *et al*, 1986). Experience suggests that courses are probably most effective if they have clear objectives and employ effective teaching strategies: carrying out pre-course work, brief and clear didactic presentations using good quality visual aids, focused group discussion relating if possible to real clinical examples provided by the participants, demonstration, using videotape and video or audio feedback teaching. Most postgraduate teaching however continues to be carried out in the well-tried one-hour 'expert' lecture over lunchtime, and the effectiveness of this is questionable. Periodic reinforcement is almost certainly required to ensure that objective gains in knowledge and skills are maintained (Evered & Williams, 1980).

For practitioners who want to take time to develop particular psycho-therapeutic skills, a number of options are available. The best-known approach is that of the Balint group, and these operate in a number of centres throughout Britain. Other courses teach basic counselling skills, or the more specialised skills of sexual, family, or marital counselling. Most training available is of a multidisciplinary nature, and these courses are clearly of interest to only a minority of GPs.

Related to the Balint group's approach are specific groups to help doctors manage 'heart-sink' patients. Such groups meet for a limited number of sessions, and seek to provide participants with a helpful framework and management strategies. Corney *et al* (1988) have described such a workshop, and recent experiences of similar groups in the Department of General Practice in Sheffield suggest increased feelings of competency in participants after attending.

Conclusions

Opportunities exist for training in psychiatry during an attachment in psychiatry, on the VTS course, and during continuing medical education. Training can address attitudes, knowledge, or skills, and there is now convincing evidence that training interventions can bring about changes. Effective training, however, requires commitment, enthusiasm and interest, and small-group work needs skilled facilitation. Training of the sort described above can be provided most effectively by GPs and psychiatrists working together. The Royal College of General Practitioners has shown considerable commitment to improving the training available nationally, with the welcome recent appointment of a Senior Educational Fellow in Mental Health.

References

BENSING, J. M. & SLUIJS, E. M. (1985) Evaluation of an interview training course for general practitioners. *Social Science and Medicine*, **20**, 737–744.

BOWMAN, F., MILLAR, T., GOLDBERG, D., *et al* (1992) Improving the psychiatric skills of general practitioners: is the effect of training maintained? *Medical Education*, **26**, 63–68.

CORNEY, R. H., STRATHDEE, G. P., HIGG, R., *et al* (1988) Managing the difficult patient: practical suggestions from a study day. *Journal of the Royal College of General Practitioners*, **38**, 349–352.

CREED, F. (1987) Course in psychiatry for family doctors. *Bulletin of the Royal College of Psychiatrists*, **11**, 193–194.

EVERED, D. C. & WILLIAMS, H. D. (1980) Postgraduate education and the doctor. *British Medical Journal*, **280**, 626–628.

GASK, L., McGRATH, G., GOLDBERG, D., *et al* (1987) Improving the psychiatric skills of established general practitioners. *Medical Education*, **21**, 362–368.

——, GOLDBERG, D., LESSER, A. L. *et al* (1988) Improving the psychiatric skills of the general practice trainee: an evaluation of a group training course. *Medical Education*, **22**, 132–138.

——, BOARDMAN, J. & STANDART, S. (1991*a*) Teaching communication skills: a problem-based approach. *Postgraduate Education for General Practice*, **2**, 7–15.

——, GOLDBERG, D., BOARDMAN, J., *et al* (1991*b*) Training general practitioners to teach psychiatric interviewing skills: an evaluation of group training. *Medical Education*, **25**, 444–451.

——, USHERWOOD, T. & STANDART, S., (1992) Training teachers how to teach communication skills: a problem-based approach. *Postgraduate Education for General Practice*, **3**, 89–166.

GOLDBERG, D., GASK, L. & O'DOWD, T. (1989) The treatment of somatisation: teaching the techniques of reattribution. *Journal of Psychosomatic Research*, **33**, 689–695.
HEALTH EDUCATION BOARD FOR SCOTLAND (1990) *DRAMS Skills for Helping Problem Drinkers*. Instructional videotapes and patient booklets. Edinburgh: HEBS.
HORDER, J., BOSANQUET, N. & STOCKING, B. (1986) Ways of influencing the behaviour of general practitioners. *Journal of the Royal College of General Practitioners*, **36**, 517–521.
LESSER, A. L. (1981) The psychiatrist and family medicine: a different training approach. *Medical Education*, **15**, 398–406.
——— (1985) Problem-based interviewing in general practice: a model. *Medical Education*, **19**, 299–304.
PENDLETON, D., SCHOFIELD, T., TATE, P., *et al* (1983) *The Consultation: An Approach to Learning and Teaching*. Oxford: Oxford University Press.
WHEWELL, P., GORE, V. & LEACH, C. (1988) Training general practitioners to improve their recognition of emotional disturbance in the consultation. *Journal of the Royal College of General Practitioners*, **38**, 259–262.
WHITEHOUSE, C., MORRIS, P. & MARKS, B. (1984) The role of actors in teaching communication. *Medical Education*, **8**, 262–268.

Further reading

BALINT, M. (1964) *The Doctor, his Patient and the Illness* (2nd edn). London: Pitman.
GASK, L. & McGRATH, G. (1989) Psychotherapy and general practice. *British Journal of Psychiatry*, **154**, 445–453.

23 Training for psychiatrists in general practice

TOM BURNS

It is becoming increasingly difficult for young doctors to sample different specialties before they make a decision about their careers. Within the hospital system the best training posts have been incorporated into carefully organised and structured rotational training schemes. The educational content and the balance of the jobs in these schemes are often carefully monitored. It has become just as important for hospital consultants as for trainees to be incorporated into them, and they have become highly competitive.

More recently the same development has been taking place in general practice. Training posts are becoming incorporated into vocational training schemes, which incorporate day-release courses and are tailored to the needs of career trainees in general practice. Like the hospital rotations, they are highly organised and highly competitive. They cannot easily accommodate doctors who wish to 'dip in'. Having a number of disparate jobs on a curriculum vitae has sometimes been judged as lack of commitment by a trainee, and may prove a liability in some interviews. These developments within hospital and general practice training have combined to oblige newly qualified doctors to decide on their careers increasingly early, and often directly after house jobs.

The General Medical Council's Education Committee (1987), however, in *Recommendations on the Training of Specialists*, stresses the need to maintain breadth and flexibility in training. The Committee states: "it is often desirable for a component of experience in general practice to be included" (para. 68). Similarly, the Royal College of Psychiatrists allows up to one year of general practice experience as approved training for its membership examinations (MRCPsych). A group of senior clinicians in South West Thames advanced suggestions for the incorporation of general practice training into specialist training in 1984 (Crisp *et al*).

Despite agreement on the value of breadth of basic specialist training, consultants will increasingly be appointed without experience outside their discipline. Failure to have experience outside hospital practice is particularly regrettable in psychiatry. Both the profession's and the government's avowed policy is to shift activity into the community (Griffiths, 1988). While the benefits of GPs receiving additional training in psychiatric skills have been reported (Goldberg *et al*, 1980; Gask *et al*, 1988), little attention has been paid to a need for psychiatrists to acquire general practice skills.

This chapter reports the experience gained in a pilot study of such training for psychiatrists.

Establishing the study

After negotiation with the Medical Manpower and Education Division of the Department of Health, the Departments of Psychiatry and General Practice at St George's Hospital Medical School were awarded a grant to pilot GP placement for psychiatric trainees. This was to be supervised by the heads of the two departments but to be managed and conducted by the clinical tutor (TB) and the regional adviser in general practice (Dr Trevor Silver). The study was originally for 12 trainees to fill two places in general practice consecutively for over three years. Additional money became available and the study expanded to 18 trainees in three practices. The purpose was to evaluate the feasibility and acceptability of the experience to trainees, trainers, and managers. An evaluation of any changes in consultation style and educational benefit is the subject of an ongoing study.

Selection of training practices and trainees

Three locally practising senior trainers were selected by the regional adviser in general practice, and briefed on the aims and objectives of the study. One trainer was part-time, but there were two trainers and another trainee in the same practice, permitting cross-supervision. Each of the three psychiatric training rotations at St George's Hospital was allocated a practice, thereby ensuring close contact between clinical tutor and the practice, and thus accurate and detailed feedback.

To exclude trainees uncertain about their long-term plans (we aimed to explore the impact on career psychiatrists) we required a minimum of one year in psychiatry and preferably Part I of the two-part MRCPsych. Those with previous general practice experience were also excluded.

We were surprised to find considerable resistance to the GP placement from trainees. There were two principal concerns: firstly, that six months out of the rotation would damage their academic training; and secondly, that it would reduce their opportunities to obtain highly sought after subspecialty posts. To overcome this resistance the first two cohorts were offered an extra post on the rotation. Subsequent trainees were informed of the GP placements at appointment.

As a result there was greater variation in trainee seniority than intended. While all had completed a minimum of two six-month posts, three had completed all their basic specialist training. Thirteen had MRCPsych Part I, and two passed during the placement.

Conditions of appointment

Trainees were appointed on the same terms as normal GP trainees (Department of Health, 1989; SFA paras 38.1–38.43). Thus the six months in GP training could be recognised for vocational training should a trainee change course. To avoid disruption to superannuation and ensure continuity of employment, the trainees remained employees of Wandsworth Health Authority. Payment was made annually in arrears from the Department of Health to the district treasurer's department. Expenditure was monitored by the finance section of Wandsworth Health Authority. Specific financial codes were allocated to cover transactions, thereby ensuring that the costs could be identified as an 'agency payment' on behalf of the department. Expenditure was subsequently recorded under a distinct heading on the official annual accounts. This included:

(a) a training grant (SFA, part 1/schedule 1) for the trainer
(b) salaries and employer's national insurance contributions
(c) car allowance
(d) telephone installation if needed
(e) London weighting.

A trainee model agreement from the British Medical Association was provided. Leave entitlement was as for GP trainees – five weeks per year *pro rata*, and a half-day study leave per week for the vocational training course and a half-day leave. Additional study leave was negotiated individually. Trainees were encouraged to attend:

(a) the local vocational training (VT) course at St George's Hospital
(b) the local trainer/trainee group
(c) one or two tutorials per week.

Formal assessment in the practice is encouraged, and the trainees completed the local trainee questionnaire. They were provided with an emergency bag, an auriscope, and an ophthalmoscope.

Experience of the placements

The trainees met monthly for 90 minutes with the clinical tutor (TB) and the regional adviser in general practice. These meetings were to supervise progress and resolve any difficulties. They rarely dealt with clinical matters. Attendance was good, with invariably two and usually all three trainees present. It rapidly became clear that absence for more than two consecutive meetings indicated serious difficulties for the trainee. This occurred twice.

The main areas of discussion concerned adaption to those professional relationships in general practice which were unfamiliar to the trainees and which compounded the anxiety from their new clinical demands. They found general practice warmer and more informal than the hospital, but less open to questioning. They encountered powerful, often unspoken, rules of conduct in primary care, unlike the more obvious hospital hierarchy with which they were more familiar. They had to learn about these without necessarily acknowledging them. The roles of the practice manager and receptionists caused some problems, as they had no obvious equivalent in the hospital.

The quality and extent of supervision from trainers was warmly praised by trainees. The form of supervision varied between and within practices according to the confidence and ability of the trainee. All reported a couple of weeks of sitting in with their trainer before beginning reduced, parallel clinics. Problems did arise with the part-time trainer. Despite cross-supervision of the two trainees by both trainers in that practice, the psychiatric trainee felt second best, 'an outsider'. Discussing their experiences together highlighted the differences between practices as much as their similarities. These differences stimulated greater understanding of the issues and generated a more rounded discussion.

Attendance at the MRCPsych course soon became a major issue. Initially we had planned for the trainees not to attend the MRCPsych course (to emphasise the 'difference' of the experience). They were unable to accept this, however, and it required negotiation with the trainers, some of whom felt that they expected too much time away from clinical contact. Postgraduate training could account for two to three sessions per week (one for the MRCPsych course, one for the local VT course, and one for psychotherapy patients and research projects). Afternoons off had to be used initially, but with time the issues became less contentious.

The content of our local VT course caused some problems. Psychiatric trainees felt that course modules concentrating heavily on consultation techniques, and psychological aspects of the doctor–patient relationship, were unnecessary given the detailed attention to such issues in psychiatric training. Those modules which focused on practice management (the financial or 'business' side of the practice) were also unappreciated. They were less used to the more interactive-style VT course teaching, which generated mixed feelings among them. Their GP colleagues were clearly more comfortable with peer-group feedback and video exercises.

Three trainees lived too far away from their practice to be on call from home. Accommodation was difficult to fund, and the solutions (borrowing an on-call room in a local hospital and boarding with a practice receptionist) were unsatisfactory. The three trainees involved considered this problem a very serious one. Night calls are an essential component of GP training. Where practices used deputising services, trainees also used them, but were expected to obtain some out-of-hours experience. In the one inner-city practice, female trainees were not prepared to make night calls unaccompanied.

Two placements were not completed. One trainee tragically drowned just over a month before the end of his placement. A second obtained his senior registrar post and left early. He reported being questioned at length at his interview about his general practice experience, which was viewed very positively. He negotiated extended notice to avoid inconveniencing the practice. Leaving early proved less disruptive than expected, and confirmed that GP trainees really are 'paid learners' and not just a pair of hands.

Local arrangements for recovering MRCPsych course fees are already complex, because of the rotational arrangements. It was decided to write these off for the pilot study. The issues of study-leave payments and differing entitlements in hospital and general practice were not resolved.

Reports from trainers and trainees

At the conclusion of the study, letters were sent to the trainers and the trainees to collect their impressions of the project. Because one trainer had left, only two trainers could be questioned. Their differing replies are quoted extensively:

> "After three years of this interesting attachment I have no doubt about its value. I feel it could be justifiably applied to other specialties and can only be helpful on both sides.
>
> "I was surprised by the enthusiasm for practice shown by all trainees. They may have had reservations initially but that disappeared over the 6 months. They were uniformly anxious about paediatrics and out-of-hours work but their confidence visibly grew during the attachment. The main weakness was dermatology which also improved. They were obviously different from our normal trainees. The structure and financing of practice are of no interest to them. In general they needed about the same supervision as normal trainees. They were uniformly good in consultation – the basis of general practice. Their experience of interviewing psychiatric patients, albeit over a longer period of time, was obviously very helpful. They enjoyed home visiting. They were pleased by their patient's appreciation which I gather is not usual in psychiatry.

"The release courses presented a problem every time. It is important that they keep attending their own release courses and only attend practice courses where the clinical content is strong. They all attended the Family Planning course which they enjoyed and felt was relevant and helpful.

"There is no doubt that this attachment has not been a one way process. We have all learned more about psychiatry and the use of drugs for psychiatric patients."

"It was notable that three out of the six trainees had not had SHO experience in any discipline other than psychiatry. The value to them of a six month period in general practice was closely related to this, the learning process retarded in those with least SHO experience. The ability to solve problems and learning judgement between options were the two areas of maximum weakness.

"Each trainee was preparing for his/her Part I MRCPsych. Exam and until this was over their commitment to general practice training was less than wholehearted. There were other commitments to continuing psychiatric training, psychotherapy training, personal analysis and the MRCPsych course, which also intruded to varying degrees.

"Regular contact between GP trainers and the psychiatric tutors would be valuable. Relationships between psychiatric trainees and myself have been considerably more stressful than with normal trainees, this has particularly centred on their attitudes to service commitment."

It is clear that both trainers found problems with the ongoing commitments which their trainees brought. They were experienced as 'different' in their working and relating styles, 'pushier' and less conforming than GP trainees. Some of this assertiveness may have reflected the trainees' awareness that this was a pilot study, allowing more questioning.

Eleven of the 15 trainees who had finished their placements and could be traced were written to between 3 and 24 months later. As with the trainers, the letters encouraged a broad response, and eight replied. They were asked to report on those aspects they found most valuable, most difficult, and most unexpected. Two of the three who did not reply were known to have experienced considerable difficulties.

Most valuable aspects

The very high level of supervision by the trainer, who was *constantly* available for advice, taking the 'anxiety' out of the post.

Brief, problem-solving psychotherapy.

Meeting healthy people (pregnancy, filling in passport forms, administration, etc.).

The coordinating role of the GP with community health services.

The value of the 'common-sense' approach of patient-centred care.

'Worm's eye view' of the interface between primary and secondary care.

Positive feedback from patients.

Being the 'first port of call' and having to 'filter' and decide on appropriate courses of action.

Experience of psychiatric symptoms and minor psychiatric illnesses (and especially somatisation) which do not usually find their way to psychiatry.

Meeting different members of the same family.

Medical skills and knowledge improved ('good for me back in psychiatry').

Learning what sort of information is useful for GPs.

Ease of access, home visits, and learning about the family.

Most difficult aspects

Obstetrics, gynaecology and paediatrics.

The time factor.

Knowing the appropriate time to refer on . . . especially in paediatrics.

Missing the institution.

Adjusting back to psychiatry.

Disruption of my specialty training.

Most unexpected aspects

The effectiveness of liaison.

The extent of somatisation.

The power of desk staff in determining who sees a doctor/nurse.

Ease of access to old learning . . . usefulness of my psychiatry training.

Vast difference between primary and secondary care.

How unhelpful hospitals can be.

How nice GPs want to be to their patients.

How patients can determine their treatment.

Many of these observations have been quoted verbatim to give a flavour of the trainees' experience. *Every one of these trainees rated the experience as positive.* They were glad they did the placement, despite missing some psychiatric training.

Conclusions

This mechanism for employing the psychiatric trainees during their GP post functioned without problems. Overall income level was about the same for our trainees (higher than that for a post in a mental hospital, and slightly lower than that for a post in a district general hospital unit, with a one-in-four rota). A fall in gross income might be a problem for trainees in specialities with heavier on-call rotas.

Administrative matters such as extra payment for accommodation and installation of a telephone worked well, but not automatically. These required rapid and effective intervention from the regional adviser in general practice. This was easily obtained in an intensively supervised pilot project, but might not be so if the scheme were routine. Some of these problems arose from the pilot study's requirements (e.g. linking specific practices to rotations) which would be unnecessary when careful monitoring was not needed.

Allocating trainees to practices too distant to be on call from home should not be accepted in any subsequent arrangements. A balance must be struck between trainee convenience and the value of practices which are used to specialist trainees. Psychiatric trainees were experienced by trainers as 'different'. Other hospital specialties (e.g. surgeons) might also be experienced as 'different', and practices familiar with their style would provide better training. Familiarity with the practice generated increasingly positive attitudes towards the placement among trainees, and the posts became easier to fill over time.

Clinical supervision worked exceptionally well and was warmly appreciated by the trainees. Trainers, however, need to be alerted to the paradoxically greater level of early supervision required by these 'senior' trainees. With specialist trainees, seniority means less familiarity with general medicine, needing greater preparation.

The problems encountered with the regional course may be a purely local phenomenon. Course content varies, and the local emphasis on the doctor–patient relationship (not welcomed by the psychiatric trainees) might be particularly welcome to trainees from disciplines without a tradition of focusing on these areas. Local circumstances and individual trainees' backgrounds need to be carefully assessed.

Trainees welcomed didactic clinical instruction, and were pleasantly surprised by the ease with which old knowledge was revived and updated. Psychiatric trainees would still benefit from preparation in gynaecology, paediatrics, and dermatology. A suggested plan is attendance at antenatal or contraception clinics to practise gynaecological examinations and the use of a speculum, some paediatric experience of asthma and diabetes, and re-exposure to common skin disorders. Such an induction (most easily arranged while still working in the hospital) could be spread over the month before the GP placement. A one-day course in family planning proved essential. Some forward planning is required, as these courses are infrequent and often heavily subscribed.

The trainees' anxieties about general practice were considerably greater than we had expected. This was expressed mainly in terms of missing the local MRCPsych course, de-skilling, losing their ability to exert pressure in local training matters, etc. Many of these worries reflect realistic concerns in an increasingly competitive specialty.

Virtually all of our trainees valued the GP post and were glad they did it. Many would not, however, have elected for it, despite positive feedback from colleagues. Establishing the post as one option in a training scheme might generate poor take-up. It probably needs to be a structural requirement of the training programme (as in this project), or to be offered as an 'extra' which does not reduce the trainees' access to other posts.

Trainees' fear of isolation from their peer group (most marked in newer trainees) proved an unexpectedly severe cause of resistance. The more senior ones experienced less disruption in their professional training, felt more secure in their professional identity, and more prepared to experiment.

Greater discussion with the trainers about the practicalities of the placement is needed. The trainees' ongoing professional obligations need to be agreed in advance and spelled out more clearly than we did. They did not cause great disruption, but avoidable irritation was caused by not addressing them in advance.

The model of joint supervision used here appeared to be successful. Whether meeting jointly with trainees from different specialties would work remains to be seen. Joint supervision by the GP adviser alternating with contact with their specialty tutor is a possibility.

This pilot study has established the feasibility and acceptability of such an experience for psychiatric trainees. Identifying more specific educational goals and objectives involved is clearly the next priority. These are varied and should include understanding of the specialist/general practice interface, the early presentation of psychiatric disorders, and the interplay of physical and psychological processes in health and disease. Techniques for assessing achievement of these goals will require further elaboration if the educational task is to be efficiently discharged. This task is complex and time-consuming, but is of the utmost importance to postgraduate medical education in an exciting period of development and change.

As a result of this study, a number of recommendations have been made in a report to the Department of Health. These include recommending provision for GP experience of at least four months' duration in the basic training of all hospital specialists, and that regulatory bodies for specialty training should be encouraged to recognise that experience. Further consideration is needed about the optimal organisation of this experience. Arranging a 'knock-for-knock' replication of the programme described here is one possibility. This has the advantage of incurring only minimal extra costs. The possibilities of imaginative part-time solutions (in which general practice trainees and hospital specialty trainees job-share for a fixed period) may prove to be more feasible in the long term. Whichever of these models, or other alternatives, eventually shows greatest promise, it is important that this opportunity of increasing interprofessional awareness and improving the quality of training of hospital specialists should not be missed.

References

CRISP, A. H., HEMSI, L. K., PAYKEL, E. S., *et al* (1984) A future pattern of psychiatric services and its educational implications: some suggestions. *Medical Education*, **18**, 110–116.

DEPARTMENT OF HEALTH (1989) *Statement of Fees and Allowances (SFA) Payable to General Medical Practitioners in England and Wales*. London: Department of Health.

GASK, L., GOLDBERG, D. P., LESSER, A. L., *et al* (1988) Improving the psychiatric skills of the general practice trainee: an evaluation of a group training course. *Medical Education*, **19**, 299–304.

GENERAL MEDICAL COUNCIL EDUCATION COMMITTEE (1987) *Recommendations on the Training of Specialists, October 1987*. London: GMC.

GOLDBERG, D. P., STEELE, J. J. & SMITH, C. (1980) Teaching psychiatric interview techniques to family doctors. *Acta Psychiatrica Scandinavica*, **62**, 41–47.

GRIFFITHS, R. (1988) *Community Care: Agenda for Action*. Report to the Secretary of State for Social Services. London: HMSO.

24 Research potential in general practice

GREG WILKINSON and
ALASTAIR WRIGHT

Impetus to the empirical study of mental health and disorder in general practice arose from the work of Shepherd and his colleagues in London. Their seminal work, *Psychiatric Illness in General Practice* (Shepherd *et al*, 1966), led to a significant conclusion:

> "that the cardinal requirement for improvement of the mental health services in this country is not a large expansion and proliferation of psychiatric agencies, but rather a strengthening of the family doctor in his therapeutic role."

In the US a similar verdict has been reached (National Institute of Mental Health, 1980), and the World Health Organization (1973) endorsed the principle in 1973:

> "The crucial question is not how the general practitioner can fit into the mental health services but rather how the psychiatrist can collaborate most effectively with primary care medical services and reinforce the effectiveness of the primary physician as a member of the mental health team."

These considerations have had a far-reaching effect on health service planners, and on the subsequent rapid, and still growing, development of clinical and research activity in this field.

Much of this is detailed in two annotated bibliographies: *Mental Disorder and Primary Medical Care: An Analytical Review of the Literature* (National Institute of Mental Health, 1979), which deals with English-language articles and books published between 1959 and 1975; and *Mental Health Practices in Primary Care Settings* (Wilkinson, 1985), which details some 500 publications published between 1977 and 1985.

As Shepherd (1982) and Burns *et al* (1986) contend, the case for intensive investigation along a broad front has now been established, and a large-scale research effort is necessary in this important but so far poorly developed field of inquiry. Attention has become focused on the roles, attitudes, knowledge and skills of GPs, but, in addition, studies are required on the role of non-medical health professionals in the management of mental disorders in general practice.

There are abundant opportunities for collaboration among individual clinicians and between the Royal College of Psychiatrists and the Royal College of General Practitioners; such research could well begin to develop on a large canvas in relation to the current joint "Defeat Depression" campaign (Priest, 1991) and the Joint Working Party on Shared Care (RCP & RCGP, 1983).

With appropriate education and training, to what extent could the primary care team be able to detect, assess, and treat the majority of people with depression, anxiety, and psychotic disorders? Which skills do members of the primary care team need in the use of supportive counselling, antidepressants for depression, behaviour therapy for anxiety disorders, and education about the recognition of early psychotic symptoms and the continuing case management of people with chronic psychoses? How much psychosocial intervention can be delegated by the GP to adequately trained nurse therapists, health visitors, district nurses, community psychiatric nurses (CPNs), and counsellors?

Mental health and medical consultation in general practice

It has long been recognised that the way in which illness expresses itself is shaped to a great extent by sociocultural and psychological factors. This perspective has been incorporated in the concept of 'illness behaviour'. The act of consulting a doctor is part of illness behaviour, and is itself also influenced not only by the presence of symptoms but also by a range of non-medical factors.

One of today's main issues in health services research is whether primary care services are used in an appropriate manner and according to the needs of patients. This is largely because 25–40% of all patients in general practice have no major medical disorder, and that 30–60% of all visits to GPs are for symptoms for which no serious underlying medical cause is found.

While this illness behaviour may not necessarily be inappropriate, it accounts for a large proportion of expenditure on medical care, and can result in the development of iatrogenic morbidity. Thus, factors which influence the use of medical services in the absence of serious organic disease should be investigated.

Moreover, research should: identify more precisely factors which affect the use, misuse and non-use of health resources by people with mental disorders; and develop health and educational strategies aimed at improving the process by which people with mental disorders presenting in general practice become more easily identified, better treated, and experience more beneficial health outcomes.

Patient (and doctor) personality factors are important influences in all doctor–patient contacts. We all recognise this, but there seems to be little consensus on the measurement of such factors.

Epidemiology of mental disorders in general practice

Leighton (1979) has conveniently summarised research directions in psychiatric epidemiology:

> "A sufficient number of studies of geographically defined populations have now been done so as to make it clear that when all the various kinds of mental illnesses are lumped together, the total prevalence rates commonly amount to 20% or more. These findings imply major challenges to theory, policy, administration, and practice in the health field, and point to a need for vastly more information and understanding."

This point of view is apposite to the field of mental health in general practice.

Clearly, standardised research instruments used in epidemiological inquiries in general practice require continuous evaluation and development, but the fundamental obstacles to further progress are the current imprecision in clinical and research terminology, and the dubious reliability and validity of present systems of classification. Studies on the classification of psychiatric disorders in general practice should be a main focus of future research effort within this area.

The concept of neurotic disorders should be re-examined in general practice, concentrating on clinical, behavioural, and social components. Allied to this, studies should be designed to investigate the identification and measurement of social problems in general practice and the effect of sex differences in psychiatric morbidity.

In view of the prevalence of anxiety and depression, more information is required on their causal factors. In relation to this, it is evident that multi-axial systems of classification have particular relevance in general practice.

The most neglected areas requiring epidemiological attention in general practice are: (a) chronic mental disorders, and drug- and alcohol-related morbidity in adults; and, (b) the entire range of mental disorders occurring in children, adolescents, and the elderly – especially affective disorders.

Practice perspectives

(a) Most research takes place in university settings or practices with a special interest; there is a shortage of information on what happens in non-academic primary care.

(b) More research is needed on the natural history and course of illnesses seen and managed in general practice and which are never referred.

(c) Many people who need help do not seek it – at least from professionals; what is effective in countering stigma and breaking down barriers?

(d) Classification is an obstacle: sometimes GPs believe there is a psychiatric illness present yet patients do not meet diagnostic criteria set by psychiatrists.

(e) Some psychiatric terms have proved harmful; for example the endogenous/reactive dichotomy still deprives some depressed patients of treatment because the cause of their depression is understandable to the doctor and leads to the assumption that treatment is not needed.

(f) Many GPs use (but rarely record) an idiosyncratic multi-axial diagnosis.

(g) Much GP diagnostic labelling is directly related to management possibilities.

Diagnostic practices

Priority should be given to establishing the place of information and computer technology in aiding GPs' diagnostic practices and their skills in detecting, recognising, and assessing mental disorders.

Empirical attention should be directed to the elucidation of the complex question of the validity, nature, and purpose of psychiatric diagnosis in general practice. There are differences between the diagnostic practices of GPs and psychiatrists and, consequently, there is a need for research which leads not merely to the increased reliability of diagnoses, but also to increased diagnostic validity in general practice.

The GP is particularly well placed to assume the role of clinical epidemiologist in the investigation of psychiatric disorders: the relationship of adversity and distress to affective disorder; the relationship of personality traits and states to personality disorders; and of symptom patterns like eating behaviour to eating disorders, and of drinking patterns to alcohol-related morbidity.

Small-scale studies have shown that GPs can be trained to improve their detection, recogntion, assessment, and treatment of mental disorders, but further research is indicated to establish the general feasibility, efficacy, and effectiveness of training large groups of GPs, and other primary care workers, in these skills. In particular, GPs could be trained in better ways of detecting patients with chronic mental disorders, how to organise and provide early and continuing treatment for them, and to recognise when specialist psychiatric consultation and referral is likely to be helpful in their care.

Screening for mental disorder should be directed only at 'high-risk' groups in general practice, who have been identified for particular study purposes, and for whom economic analysis provides justification.

Practice perspectives

- (a) Computerised assessments such as that by Lewis *et al* (1988) may have more than research value.
- (b) Use of simple, cheap psychiatric questionnaires can sensitise GPs to psychiatric thinking and make them more aware of psychiatric problems during the consultation.
- (c) Which psychiatric instruments are most effective for use by primary care teams?
- (d) Are psychiatric educational programmes beneficial in terms of changed attitudes of GPs as well as knowledge?
- (e) Most studies involving psychiatric screening questionnaires are short term (sometimes involving only a single contact), but general practice involves long-term relationships, continuing care and multiple contacts over time.
- (f) What are we screening for in depression in primary care? Has a 'case' of depression presenting first to a GP been defined satisfactorily?
- (g) Should GPs look at whole populations or defined subsets? Case finding may be more effective than screening.
- (h) Depression associated with true physical illness can be difficult to diagnose in primary care.

Therapeutic practices

The top priority for research on mental health in general practice is research on the clinical and economic effectiveness and efficiency of treatment. Double-blind, randomised, controlled clinical trials are required of psychological, social, and pharmacological treatments, both alone and in combination. Small-scale, local, exploratory evaluation of therapy remains lacking.

Studies could include investigation of: new patterns of working relationships between primary care staff and mental health service staff, which have been neglected; reasons for the initial prescription and use of psychotropic drugs; the definition of clinical criteria for appropriate use of psychotropic drugs in general practice and the variation in use of psychotropic drugs; the effect of factors such as personality and therapeutic setting on the effectiveness of psychotropic drugs in general practice; and the epidemiological investigation of the extent and determinants of long-term psychotropic drug use in general practice.

There is relatively little compelling evidence that supports the use of dynamic or behavioural psychotherapy by GPs. Since forms of these activities (such as counselling and relaxation) are widespread in general practice, their efficacy should be examined in relation to other treatment methods delivered by members of primary care and psychiatric teams.

The prospects for therapeutic evaluation may be improved by large studies involving the collaboration of networks of GPs, such as the General Practice Research Framework of the Medical Research Council (MRC). Such an approach could also make it feasible to examine the role of the GP in the prevention of mental disorder.

In addition, there is a lack of investigations which shed light on the relationship between GPs' diagnostic practices and their therapeutic strategies. Factors which influence GPs' management plans for patients with mental disorders are largely unknown, as are the factors which determine the long-term use of psychotropic drugs by practitioners and patients. Additional, detailed information should be gathered about adherence to treatment by patients with mental disorders in general practice.

Finally, Balint's (1971) challenge remains: in what dose should the doctor be prescribed, in what form, how frequently, what is the curative and the maintenance dose, and what are the side-effects?

Practice perspectives

(a) In considering non-directive counselling versus GP traditional support, how can cases be selected for the more expensive option? Less formal GP counselling often continues over years and, as is said: "listening does wonders for the doctor–patient relationship."

(b) To what extent does counselling work in depression? There is pressure from patient groups who do not like drugs, yet we know anti-depressants do work.

(c) How effective can practice nurses and CPNs be in general practice, and how well do different members of the team actually coordinate their contribution?

(d) MRC-type research is effective but heavily 'top-down' in emphasis. GP participation should occur in design and planning of research, as well as in data collection.

Long-term mental disorders

Patients with chronic, long-lasting, and incurable disorders make up about 25% of the patients consulting in general practice, and they require much time, support, and resources, over many years. The most frequent of such conditions are high blood pressure, followed by rheumatic and mental disorders.

However, in contrast to acute psychiatric disorder, little attention has been paid to long-term mental disorder in general practice. This is also the more surprising in view of the movement towards providing health and social care in the community for people with mental disorders. More information is required on the balance between specialist and primary care in meeting the needs of people with long-term mental disorders in the future – especially as general practice is central to the provision of comprehensive health and mental health services.

Extent of long-term mental disorders

Shepherd *et al* (1966) found that of the 14% of patients who consulted their GP at least once in a 12-month period for a condition diagnosed as largely or entirely psychiatric in nature, just over half had chronic conditions, defined as those continuously present for at least one year or recurring with sufficient frequency to cause continuous disability or to require continuous prophylactic treatment.

Within this heterogeneous group of disorders, anxiety and depression have the highest overall rates of occurrence, but psychotic and personality disorders contribute the greatest proportion of severe disability. Such chronic mental disorder is also positively associated with other forms of chronic ill health and a range of social disabilities.

The burden of care

Much of the burden of medical care for patients with long-term disorders falls, inevitably, on the GP. The magnitude is not easy to measure. Parkes *et al* (1962) studied patients with schizophrenia discharged from London mental hospitals and concluded that:

> "While mental hospitals and outpatient clinics were responsible for initiating most of the treatment required for maintaining the patients' health, it was the general practitioners who played the major part in dealing with the crises and relapses that occurred in over half the cases."

The converse is that many people with chronic mental disorders either do not come to the attention of GPs or psychiatrists, or subsequently lose contact with primary and mental health care services.

Shared care

Mental health care for patients with long-term mental disorder provided by members of the mental health and primary care teams can result in fragmentation and confusion. The roles and responsibilities of patients' carers and professionals may be ill defined. Treatment may be started, stopped, and changed by the patient, psychiatrist, or GP without one letting the others know, and problems in communication often arise following discharge from follow-up in the practice or clinic. This has led to the widespread use of shared-care cards in antenatal care and for people with diabetes mellitus;

the application of this concept to patients with mental disorders is discussed in Chapter 22.

Many GPs remain unclear about their role in caring for the expanding numbers of patients with long-term psychiatric disorders previously resident in hospital and now living in community settings. This lack of clarity is only now beginning to be tackled, and much further work is required. The questions of how to determine what balance of physical, social and psychological care is appropriate for specific patients, and who should give appropriate care, are still largely unanswered. Care, in this context, also means including attention to patients' employment, education, and housing. Initially, studies should be directed at the identification, treatment, care, and rehabilitation of patients with these disorders, and towards secondary and tertiary preventive interventions.

Practice perspectives

(a) What is the value of personal lists in effective follow-up in schizophrenia and, especially, in dealing with marital and family conflicts?

(b) How great is the burden on carers and how can GPs help them more effectively?

(c) Can long-term, 'heart-sink' patients be helped by intensive management from the community psychiatric team, then handed back to GP care?

(d) What is the definition of a 'case' of chronic fatigue syndrome and what is the place of antidepressants in its treatment?

Referral and consultation

Surprisingly little research has been done on the processes of referral and consultation between GPs and psychiatrists and other mental health professionals. Although it is evident that consultation rates to GPs for mental health problems are consistently high, there appears to be great variation in the extent of referral and consultation between GPs and psychiatrists and other mental health professionals. The determinants of this variability (e.g. patient's age, sex, marital status, and diagnosis; and doctor's personal and practice characteristics, including number of years in practice and interest in psychiatry) have been virtually unexplored. In consequence, the effect on treatment and outcome is largely unknown.

Further research is necessary. Firstly, there is a need to identify the medical, psychosocial, and demographic factors influencing the formal and informal help-seeking behaviour and self-referral practices of patients with mental disorders in general practice. Secondly, the behaviour of GPs during their professional consultations requires study since the relationship between their assessment, management, and referral procedures is so poorly understood. Thirdly, a number of different models of referral and consultation between GPs and psychiatrists are in operation (e.g. psychiatric clinics in general practice, community mental health care based on the primary care team, psychiatry/family practice liaison programmes, and linkage between primary care projects and community mental health centres). Research is lacking on the comparative clinical and economic effectiveness of these different models in a variety of general practice settings. Finally, evaluative studies are required of the effectiveness and efficiency of patient self-referral and GP referral and consultation with non-psychiatrist mental health professionals, voluntary bodies, and patient self-help groups. In essence, what are the long-term outcomes of GP care only of depressives, specialist liaison care, and traditional referral to a specialist?

Outcome of mental disorder in general practice

Results from the few studies done so far indicate a need for further research into the short- and long-term course and outcome of specific mental disorders in general practice, and, in particular, a need for the adoption of multi-axial systems of classification of health and mental health disorders, with assessments of social stress and support and personality factors, as well as measures of psychiatric symptoms and physical health status.

The main priority in this area is for investigations on the course and outcome of anxiety and depression in general practice. However, there is a continuing requirement for the study of other chronic mental disorders, and drug- and alcohol-related morbidity. In addition, from the vantage of general practice, the course and outcome of mental disorders in childhood, adolescence, and old age is virtually unknown.

The focus here should be on the impact of therapeutic and rehabilitative interventions on the outcome of mental disorders. In practice, what is the best mix between GP and specialist care for common disorders such as depression and schizophrenia? How long should treatment (e.g. with antidepressants) be continued in general practice? If placebo-controlled trials are not feasible, what other methods might be useful?

Conclusions

Research priorities for the next decade should be viewed in the light of the probable effects of government health strategy and changes in Health Service administration. The shift in the balance of care from hospital to the community continues unabated, making it less important where the patient is treated. The White Paper *Health of the Nation* outlines a ''health strategy for England'', with companion papers for Scotland, Northern Ireland and Wales, and previews major changes which will affect general practice. Mental illness is listed among key areas for action; much of the data necessary to monitor progress in the key areas will come from general practice. The government aims to reduce suicide rates. There will be interest in exploring educational support for GPs to enhance expertise in identifying and assessing patients with mental illness. Progress is to be expected in developing local clinical guidelines and in methods for the audit of the quality of care provided for patients.

General practitioners are encouraged by the White Paper to organise health promotion, tailored to the needs of their patients. The concept of 'anticipatory care' may be more appropriate for general practice than the term 'prevention'. The former encompasses preventive and therapeutic care, recognising that the two are complementary and that care is enhanced by better management of existing disease.

So that rational health care decisions may be made, more research is essential on all aspects of mental health in general practice: epidemiologically based study of defined disorders; investigation of determinants and inter-relationships of diagnostic and management decisions; assessment of therapeutic efficacy; evaluation of preventive, screening, and educational interventions; and efficient organisation of service delivery, including the role of non-medical members of the primary care team.

Simple, practical questions remain largely unanswered. What are the effects of illness labelling in general practice? To what extent does counselling affect the course of mood disorders? What is the optimal management for patients with a somatic presentation of affective illness?

There are demonstrable differences, which are largely unaccounted for, in the abilities of GPs to recognise, treat, and refer patients with mental disorders appropriately. Although there are indications that training can improve attitudes, knowledge, and skills, the effects of these differences among GPs on patient care and outcome are virtually unknown. It is not even clearly established that the increased recognition of mental disorders by GPs is associated with improvements in their clinical management of such disorders and in the clinical outcome for patients.

Techniques are available for evaluating GPs' clinical practices with respect to patients with mental disorders, but there are insufficient studies comparing the clinical and economic effectiveness of GPs and specialists with such patients in general practice. It is difficult to identify specific mental disorders for which GPs' current clinical practices are apparently most effective. Problems in the classification of mental disorders in general practice make it difficult to identify mental disorders reliably and validly, and GPs' clinical practices are diverse.

There is some welcome evidence that clinicians and research workers are beginning, belatedly, to focus on longitudinal studies relevant to the causes, courses, and outcomes of psychiatric disorders presenting in general practice. The main focus of future research should be on efforts to improve GPs' treatment practices for patients with mental disorders, rather than on increasing referral of patients to mental health specialists. A wider use of medical audit to monitor process and outcome of care by primary care teams (and an acceptance that psychiatric disorder can be subjected to systematic audit in general practice in the same way as asthma and hypertension) is likely to improve patient care directly, and help take the results of research in psychiatry from the journals to the bedside.

Crossley *et al* (1992) have published a method of audit of psychological care in general practice using a prospective design, a simple practical instrument (the General Health Questionnaire) and predetermined and case-specific indices of outcome established at the initial consultation. The most pertinent conclusion was that quantifiable methods of evaluating psychological care can be achieved in general practice.

References

BALINT, M. (1971) *The Doctor, His Patient and The Illness*. London: Pitman.
BURNS, G. J., TAUBE, C. A. & REGIER, D. A. (1986) Building primary care/mental health research in the United States. In *Mental Illness in Primary Care Settings* (eds M. Shepherd, G. Wilkinson & P. Williams). London: Tavistock.
CROSSLEY, D., MYRES, M. P. & WILKINSON, G. (1992) Assessment of psychological care in general practice. *British Medical Journal*, **305**, 1333–1336.
HANKIN, J. & OKTAY, J. S. (1979) *Mental Disorder and Primary Medical Care: An Analytical Review of the Literature*. Series D, No. 5, DHEW Publication No. (ADM) 78-661. Washington, DC: US Government Printing Office.
LEIGHTON, A. H. (1979) Research directions in psychiatric epidemiology. *Psychological Medicine*, **9**, 235–247.
LEWIS, G., PELOSI, A. J., GLOVER, E., *et al* (1988) The development of a computerised assessment for minor psychiatric disorder. *Psychological Medicine*, **18**, 737–745.
PARKES, C. M., BROWN, G. W. & MONCK, E. M. (1962) The general practitioner and the schizophrenic patient. *British Medical Journal*, **ii**, 972–976.
PARRON, D. L. & SOLOMON, F. (eds) (1980) *Mental Health Services in Primary Care Settings: Report of a Conference*. Series DN, Health/Mental Health Research, DHHS Publication No. (ADM) 80-995. Washington, DC: US Government Printing Office.
PRIEST, R. G. (1991) A new initiative on depression. *British Journal of General Practice*, **41**, 487.
ROYAL COLLEGE OF PSYCHIATRISTS & ROYAL COLLEGE OF GENERAL PRACTITIONERS (1983) *Shared Care of Patients with Mental Health Problems*. London: Royal College of General Practitioners.
SHEPHERD, M. (1982) Psychiatric research and primary care in Britain – past, present and future. *Psychological Medicine*, **12**, 493–499.
—— , COOPER, B., BROWN, A. C., *et al* (1966) *Psychiatric Illness in General Practice*. Oxford: Oxford University Press.
WILKINSON, G. (1985) *Mental Health Practices in Primary Care Settings*. London: Tavistock.
WORLD HEALTH ORGANIZATION (1973) *Psychiatry and Primary Care*. Copenhagen: WHO.

Index

Compiled by JOHN GIBSON

A Fortunate Man (Berger, J. & Mohr, J. 1969) 17
Abbreviated Mental Test Scale (AMTS) 168
Acts of Parliament
Abortion Act 1968 83
Access to Health Records Act 1990 262
Community Care Act 275
Enduring Powers of Attorney Act 1985 55
Mental Health Act 1983 46, 57–8
compulsory treatment in community 49–50
emergency admission 47
guardianship 50
mental disorder definition 46–7
treatment in hospital 48–9
Mental Health (Scotland) Act 1984 46, 58–9
National Health Service and Community Care Act 1990 xiii, 167
Road Traffic Act 1972 54
acute confusional state 158–60
adolescence 97
depression in 96–7
adrenal insufficiency 115
ageing, psychology of 153–6

agoraphobia 115, 123 (table)
drug treatment 124–5
alcohol abuse 115, 135–51
abstinence or controlled drinking? 145
alcohol content of drinks 137 (table)
'at risk' patient identification 140–2
hidden diagnosis 140
screening programmes 140–1
benzodiazepine – associated alcohol increase 236
blood alcohol concentration 144
consumption pattern, benzodiazepines associated 236
dependent drinkers 139
detoxification 146
DRAMS kit 145
drinking and driving 148
effects in workplace 146–7
follow-up 145
gamma-glutamyl transpeptidase screening 136, 143
general practitioners' views 135–6
hazards of alcohol abuse (RC Physicians, 1987) 149–51
high-risk patients 141–2
history taking 142
identifying 'at-risk' patients 140–4

alcohol abuse *(contd)*
  laboratory investigations 143
  low-risk patients 141
  moderate drinkers 139, 141
  older people 164
  outcome 144–5
    spouse's role 145
  patient secrecy 136
  people with a problem 136–9
  physical signs 143
  primary prevention 321–2
  problem drinkers 139
    driving 148
  public health problem 135
  referral 145–6
    self- 142–4
    third party 142–4
  relapse 145
  screening programme 140–1
  self-help materials 151
  sex differences 138–9
  social drinkers 139
  tertiary prevention 329
  what constitutes abuse? 139–40
  women drinkers 138–9
alcometer 144
Alzheimer's disease *see* dementia
amitriptyline 105, 120, 329
amniocentesis 322
amphetamines 115
amputees 65
animal phobia, specific 123
anti-male sex hormone implantation 48
anticholinergics 205
anticipatory care 314
antidepressants 104, 329
  fatal toxicity index 329
  for:
    antisocial personality disorders 186–7
    anxiety disorders 190
  long term 106
  subtherapeutic doses 190

  tricyclic 104–5, 120, 329
antipsychotic drugs, for antisocial personality disorders 186–7
anxiety 112–33
  classification 114
  differential diagnosis 114–15
  evolutionary terms factor 113
  function 113
    conditioned response 113
    negative reinforcer 113
    secondary drive state 113
  old patients 163
  physical conditions mimicking 115
  primary prevention 321
  symptoms 113
  trait 112
anxiety states 112, 114
  management 116–20
    avoiding avoidance 117
    cognitive treatments 119
    controlled breathing 119
    drugs 120
    lifestyle management 116–17
    prediction testing 117–18
    relaxation training 119
    voluntary hyperventilation 118–19
  prognosis 121
assessment services 26–7
asthma 15

Balint, M.
  analysis of doctor–patient relationship 77
  The Doctor, His Patient and the Illness (1957) 5–6, 17
Belbin instruments 85
benzodiazepines 120, 189, 235–45
  contraindication 187
  dependence 215–16, 240
  effects on performance 240–1
  elderly patients 237–8
  indications 238–40
  patterns of use 235–6

alcohol pattern compared 236
pharmacology 236–7
  absorption 236–7
  fate 237
  interactions with other drugs
      238 (table)
  metabolism in elderly people
      237–8
  prescribing 241–2
  repeat 242
  prevention of long–term use
      242–5
  small groups 244
  reduction guidelines 244
  WITHDRAW Project 244–5
  withdrawal 115, 240
bereavement 63, 98–9
  benzodiazepines contraindicated
      240
bereavement *see also* loss
Bereger, J., Mohr, J. *A Fortunate Man* (1969) 17
Berne, E. *Games People Play* (1964) 6
β-adrenoceptors agonists 120
Better Services for the Mentally Ill (1975)
    xiii
blood phobia 123 (table)
British Association for Counselling
    291
British Social Attitudes, 7th report
    (Jowell *et al*, 1990) 11
burn-out 69
buspirone 120

caffeine excess 115
Camberwell GPs, community-
    oriented service planning 26, 27
cannabis 115
carbamazepine 186
carcinoid syndrome 115
care coordination clinic 29
care manager xiv
case/care management xiv

Castelnuovo-Tedesco P. *The Twenty Minute Hour* (1965) 6
Centre for the Advancement of
    Interprofessional Education 276
child
  bereaved 74
  depression 96–7
  psychiatric disorders 327–8
  psychosocial factors in consulta-
      tions 177
  registration with mother's doctor
      78
  school refusal 96
  stealing by 86
  surveillance 78, 85–6
chlordiazepoxide 237
chlormethiazole (Heminevrin) 189
chlorpromazine (Largactil) 120, 205
Chron's disease 108
class 84
classifications 39–44
  DSM-IV 40
  ICD-10 40–2
  ICD-10(PHC) 42–4
  ICPC 40
clinical psychologist 237
clobazam 238–9
clomipramine 128
clonazepam 238–9
clozapine (Clozaril) 205
cognitive behaviour therapy 294–308
  adaption to primary care 307–8
    adjunctive techniques 308
    bibliotherapy 307–8
    interview style 307
  adjunct to pharmacotherapy 296
  behavioural techniques 301–2
    graded task assignment 302
    mastery/pleasure ratings 301
    task assigment 302
    weekly activity scheduling 301
  characteristics 298
  cognitive techniques 302–6
  core therapy techniques 300–6

cognitive behaviour therapy *(contd)*
  for depression 306
  eliciting automatic thoughts 302–3
    dysfunctional thought record 303, 304 (table)
    guided discovery 303
    imagery 303
    increasing awareness 302
    role plays 302
  engagement in therapy 299–300
  event-thought–feeling links 299
  goals 298–9
  identifying schemas 305–6
  problem reduction exercise 299
  session structure 300
  testing automatic thoughts 303–5
    decatastrophising 305
    examining evidence 303–5
    generating alternatives 305
    reattribution 305
  types of patients who seem to do well 300
  why use? 295–6
cognitive theory of emotional disorders 296–8
collaboration models, psychiatry-primary care 27–31
  Falloon model 30
  Greenwich sector model 29–30
  Norwegian integrated model 30–1
  primary care clinics 28
  Tyrer "hive" model 29
colour 82–3
combined–list systems 80
Committee on Child Health Services (1976) 85
communication, general practitioner-psychiatrist 251–63
  face-to-face contact 254–6
  formal 252
  hospital admissions, discharges, deaths 262
  letters 257–63
    education in writting 263

follow-up 261–2
  psychiatric reply 259–61
  referral 259
  notes fit for patient to read 262–3
  telephone contact 252–4
  verbal 251, 252
community care
  countdown to xiv
  potential short comings xv
community care xiii–xvi
Community Care – Agenda for Action (Griffith Report, 1988) xiii
community drug agencies 218–19
community mental health services development 24–5
community psychiatric nurse 24, 196, 273–4, 319
community psychiatry, neuroses 27
compulsory admission to hospital 10, 46–8, 174, 175 (fig.)
  discharge of detained patients 50
  treatment in hospital 48–9
compulsory treatment 48–50
  in community 49–50
  in hospital 48–9
  supervised discharge 50
computer record 83–4
consent to treatment 48–9
consulting privacy 4–5
contraceptive pill 321
coronary artery bypass surgery 108
counselling 12, 64, 82, 280–93, 320
  best theory 291
  confidentiality 292
  couples 89–90
  for depression 107
  formal 283–4
  in general practice 287–90
    supervision 290
    training 290
  medical 285
  patients benefiting from 287
  in primary care 290–1
  record keeping 292

responsibility for patient 291–2
skills in primary care 283
specialist 285
stages 284–5
counselling information folder 291
counsellors 10, 271
  qualifications 291
  training 291
Court of Protection 55, 166
creed 83
criminal behaviour 86
crisis *see also* emergencies 26–7
CRUISE 25, 64
cry for help 86
culture 83
customs 84

Defeat Depression Campaign 361
deinstitutionalisation 25–6
dementia 160–2, 329–30
  tertiary prevention 329–30
Depixol (flupenthixol) 205
depression
  adolescent 96–7
  assessment 340–1
  auditing management 109
  bereavement 98–9
  bipolar (mania–depression) 98
  care systems, organisation 100–1
  childhood 96–7
  clinical features 94, 95–6
  cognitive model of development
    297 (fig.)
  computer-administered interview
    101
  definition 93–6
  diagnostic register 14
  doctor factors 100
  dysthymia 98
  early detection 324–5
  educational strategies 325–6
  how to detect 325
  iatrogenic 321

initial treatment/training 340–1
management in community
    102–8
  antidepressants 104–5
  cognitive therapy 107
  counselling 107
  long-term 106
  psychosocial 106–7
  relapse prevention 105–6
  selective serotonin inhibitors
    (5-HT antagonists) 105
  suicide risk assessment 102–3
missed 13
  reasons for 99–100
neurotic 114
number of GP's patients 324
older people 97–8, 162
patient factors 100
physical illness associated 108,
    326–7
postnatal 269
prevalence 99
primary prevention 321
questionnaires 101
recognition improvement 101
referral to secondary care 107–8
sleep disturbance 231–2
somatisation 326
specimen card for major episode
    [ICD-10(PHC)] 42, 43 (fig.)
subtypes 96
suicide 325
tertiary prevention 328–9
desmethyldiazepam 237
diabetes mellitus 108
  poorly controlled 115
Diazemuls 188
diazepam 236–7
  antisocial personality disorder 188
  elderly people taking 237
  reduction 244
  severe muscle spasm 239
  status epilepticus 238
discharge from hospital planning xiv

district mental health services 24
district nurse 268, 270
disulfiram 146
doxepin 120
DRAMS kit 145
drinking and driving 148
droperidol 188
drug abuse 115, 209–20
    benzodiazepines 211 (table), 214–20
    classification 210
    clinical ambivalence 211–12
    health education 213
    identification 210–11
    management strategies for dependent users 214–20
        community drug agencies 218–19
        drug treatment (detoxification/ withdrawal from drugs) 217–18
        generic services 218
        minimisation of harm 215, 219–20
        prescribing guidelines 215–16
        psychiatric services 219
        residential establishments 219
        terms of agreement 216–17
    medical complications 212
    opiates 211 (table), 214–20
    physical examination/investigation 212–13
    preliminary assessment of users 212–13
    primary prevention 322
    safer sex need 213
    self-parenting role of doctor 214
    solvents 211 (table), 213–14
    stimulants 211 (table), 213–14
    withdrawal symptoms 218
Drug Problems. Where to Get Help (SCODA) 219
drug(s)
    charges 9
    given for more than 3 months during compulsory detention 48–9
    prescription 9
        per person per year 321
dysthymia 98

early morning waking 231–2
Edinburgh Postnatal Depression Scale 325
Eimerl, T. S., diagnostic register (1960) 8
electroconvulsive therapy (ECT)
    consent 48–9
eltoprazine 186
emergencies 170–9
    classification 171–2
    compulsory admission 174, 175 (fig.)
    crisis intervention technique 176
    drug administration 176
    management 172–8
        immediate crisis 172–6
        long-term 177–8
encopresis 328
enuresis 328
epidemiology in general practice 36–44
    mental disorder and reason for consultation 38 (table)
    morbidity in primary care 38
    research 362–3
    practice perspectives 362–3
epilepsy, benzodiazepines for 238–9
ethical problems in practice 51–4
ethics of mental health legislation 45–6
Eysenck Personality Questionnaire 184

Falloon model 30
family, dysfunctional 70

Family Medicine – A Medical Life History of Families (Hygen, F. J. A., 1978) 17
family planning care 77–8
family structure 82
family/household charts 82
family/marital relationships 77–91
  general practice features relevant 77–9
fat-file patients 100
filters 36, 37 (table)
FIRO-B 85
fluoxetine 129
flupenthixol (depixol) 205
fluphenazine (Modecate) 205
flurazepam 240
fluvoxamine 129
future care policies 31–2

General Health Questionnaire (Goldberg *et al*, 1988) 325
General Household Survey 1989 (Office of Population, Censuses and Surveys, 1991) 9, 10, 323
general practice organisation 16–18
  biographical approach 17
  microcomputers 16–17
  personal factors 16
  personal lists 17–18
  records 16
  service planning/prevention in 317–20
  summaries 16
General Practice Research Unit 316–17
general practice/practitioners in British National Health Service 8–19
  antenatal care 78
  availability 8–9
  care of people with severe/long-term mental desorder 25–6
  children/adolescents contact rate 10

contact rate with patients 78
continuity of care 9
counselling parallels 82
countering stigma 11
debt to psychiatry 5
development as scientific discipline 5–6
drug prescription 9
education for GPs 15
encouragement 79
failure to be systemic 91
family care over generations 10
fund-holding xv–xvi
generalist approach 79–84
group practices 80
home visiting 9
home/household understanding 81
lack of information/audit 14
length of consultations 12, 81
life-long care 78
local environment knowledge 9
long-term view 81
medical consultation in 361–2
mental health in 361–2
missed diagnoses 13
multiprofessional team 10
mutual training 10–11
organisation *see* general practice organisation
patient satisfaction 11–12
people as people 79–80
personal care 9
personal lists 80
practice perspectives 367
prevention of disease 313–15
publications dearth 14
records 81
registration
  children 78
  couples 9
  duration 78
  family groups 9
research *see* research in general practice

general practice/practitioners in British National Health Service (*contd*)
  system 8–11
  systematic approach need 15–16
  training *see* training for GPs
  undressing by patient 13
  whole population care 11
  working with members of secondary care services 271–3
generalised anxiety *see* anxiety states
Geriatric Depression Scale 168, 325
Goldberg, D. *et al.*
  framework for understanding mentally ill pathway 36
  operational definition of psychiatric illness 37
  screening for psychiatric illness 16
Greenwich sector model 29–30
grief 64
  chronic 66
  conflicted 67
  outcome/prognosis 75–6
  pathological, treatment of 73–5
grief work 65
group homes, patients in 26
guardianship 50

haloperidol 188
Hansen, V., Norwegian integrated model (1987) 30–1
health promotion 311–12
health visitor 177, 268, 269
heartsink patients 98
Heminevrin (chlormethiazole) 189
hepatic cirrhosis 146
hidden psychiatric disorders 37
home visiting 9
Hospital Plan–1962 xiii
hostel, patients in 26
5-HT antagonists (selective serotonin reuptake inhibitors) 105
5-hydroxytryptophan reuptake inhibitors 105, 129

hypnotics 229–31
  dependence 230
  safe prescribing 230–1
  tolerance 230
  withdrawal 230, 231
hypochondriasis 114, 129–30, 163, 164
  cognitive–behavioural models 130, 131 (fig.)
  diagnostic criteria 129–30
  management 131–2
  prognosis 132
hypomania 98
hypothyroidism, congenital 328

ill-defined conditions 3
immunisation of babies 311
imipramine 124, 125
influenza 108
injury phobia 123
institutional neurosis 164
International Classification of Disease, 10th revision 40–4
  assessment 42–4
  mental disorders 41–4
  specimen card for major depressive episode 42, 43 (fig.)
irreversible treatments 48
isocarboxazid 189

Kemadrin (procyclidine) 205
Kendrick, A. (1990, 1991), practice policies for long-term disorders 31–2

Largactil (chlorpromazine) 120, 205
law xiii–xvi, 45–60
  driving 54
  making a will 55
  managing properties/affairs 54–5
  see also Acts of Parliament
learned fear 69
learned helplessness 69
learning difficulties 328

Learning Styles Questionnaire 85
life-long care in general practice 78
lithium 186
Living with Fear (Marks, I. M.,
     1978) 124, 128
long-term mentally ill patients
     365–7
   care 366–7
   extent 366
   practice policies 31–2
   registers 31–2
lorazepam 237, 244
loss 63–73
   assessment of risk 67–70
      personal vulnerability 69–70
      situational factors 67–68
   bereaved attachment to counsellor
      73
   bereaved children at risk 74
   family suport 63–4
   management by primary care
      team 70–3
      preparation for loss 70–2
      support in course of loss 72
   outcome/prognosis 75–6
   reaction to 64–7
      chronic grief 66
      classification 65–6
      compulsive care giving 66–7, 74
      delayed/inhibited 66
      identification with lost person 66
      non-specific stress reactions 66
      psychosomatic disorder 66
   see also bereavement; grief

mammography 322
mania 98, 174
marital/man–woman problems
     87–91
   outcome 90
   patient–doctor synthesis 88
   patient's perception of cause 88
   planning 89–90
      counselling couples 89–90

seeing partner 89
   style 90
   telling partner 89
   presenting patient's experience
      87–8
Markus, A. G. *et al Psychological
   Problems in General Practice* (1989)
      64
Maudsley Personality Inventory 184
medical audit 10
mental disorder, definition (Mental
   Health Act) 46
*Mental Disorder and Primary Medical
   Care: An Analytical Review of the
   Literature* (National Institute of
   Mental Health, US) 360
mental functions tests 167
Mental Health Act Commission 51
Mental Health Foundation 31, 252
Mental Health (Northern Ireland)
   Order 1986 46, 47, 59–60
Mental Health Practices in Primary
   Care Settings (G. Wilkinson,
   1985) 360
Mental Health Review Tribunal 51
mentally disordered offenders 56–7
migraine 115
missed diagnoses 13
Modecate (fluphenazine) 205
monoamine oxidase inhibitors 120
multi-infarct dementia (arteriosclerotic dementia) 161
mutual training, general practice-
   psychiatry 10–11
myocardial infarct 108

National Health Service, British
   emotional illness ideals 6–8
   registration system 314
National Institute of Mental Health
   (US) 360
needs assessment by local authority
   xiv
neuroleptics 205–6

neuroses, community psychiatric care 27
Neurosis in the Ordinary Family (A. Ryle, 1967) 316
neurotic depression 114
nicotine excess 115
nitrazepam 237, 238–9, 240
Norwegian integrated model (Hansen) 30–1
notes fit for patient to read 262–3
nurse therapists 31, 270

obsessive–compulsive disorders 114, 121, 125–9, 164
  differential diagnosis 126
  management 126–9
    drugs 128–9
    prolonged gradual exposure plus self-imposed response prevention 126–7
  prognosis 129
older people 153–68
  affective disorders 162–3
  alcoholism 164
  anxiety 163
  behavioural disorders 163–4
  community care 166–7
  depression 97–8, 162
  history taking 157
  hypochondriasis 163, 164
  institutional neurosis 164
  investigations 158
  legal protection 166
  mental state examination 157–8
  metabolism 237–8
  obsessive neurosis 164
  personality problems 164
  physical examination 157
  prevention care 164–5
  psychoneurosis 163–4
oxazepam 237, 240

panic attack 39
paranoid personality disorder 188

paraphrenia 163
parasuicide 173–4
parent–child relationship 9, 85–6
parental influences 5
parental insecurity 69
paroxysmal atrial tachycardia 115
people as people 79–80
personality 84–5
  tests 84–5
Personality Assessment Schedule 185
Personality Disorder Examination 185
personality disorders 180–91
  anankastic 182 (table), 183
  antisocial (dyssocial) 182 (table), 183, 184 (table)
    drug treatment 185–8
    management 187–8
    psychological treatment 187
  anxious 182 (table), 183
    drug treatment 189–90
    psychological treatment 190–1
  assessment 184–5
  avoidant 182 (table)
  borderline 182 (table)
    treatment 191
  dependent 182, 184 (table)
  diagnosis 181–5
  histrionic 182 (table)
  impulsive 182 (table)
  inhibited 184 (table)
  initial assessment 180–1
  narcissistic 182 (table)
  obsessive–compulsive perfectionism/inflexibility 182 (table)
  paranoid 182 (table)
  passive–aggressive–persuasive 182 (table)
  schizoid 182 (table)
  schizotypal 182 (table)
  withdrawn 183, 184 (table)
    treatment 188–9
phantom limb 65

phenelzine 125, 190
phenothiazines 120
phenylketonuria 328
pheochromocytoma 115
phobic disorder 114, 121–5
  post-traumatic 125
  prognosis 25
  treatment 122–3
    drugs 124–5
    prolonged graduated exposure 122–3
    self-help organisations 124–5
  types 123 (table)
population needs 3–5
post-traumatic stress disorder (phobia) 114, 125
post-viral syndrome 108
power of attorney 54–5
practice counsellor 271
practice nurse 270, 320
pre-symptomatic detection of disease 311–12
prescription charges 9
prevalence of mental illness 99
prevention of disease 311–13
  nature v. nurture 312
  population v. personal approach 313
prevention of mental illness 315–31
Prevention of Psychiatric Disorders in General Practice (Royal College of GPs, 1981) 317
primary care 265–7, 317–18
  preventive 320–2
    alcohol abuse 321–2
    anxiety 321
    depression 321
    mental illness 311–12
    substance abuse 322
  specialist attachment 319–20
primary care clinics 28
primary care team 26, 27, 267–8
  five-level model 268
procyclidine (Kemadrin) 205

propranolol 120
Psychiatric Illness in General Practice (M. Shepherd *et al.* 1966) 6, 360
psychiatric morbidity 22
psychiatric questionnaires 327
psychiatrist, working with members of secondary care services 271–3
psychoanalysis 82
Psychological Problems in General Practice (A. G. Markus *et al.*, 1989) 64
psychological treatments, GPs to undertake 27
psychosocial transition 65
psychosurgery 48
psychotherapy 280–93
  brief-intervention 285–6
  clinical 286
public education campaigns 320

questionnaires 327

rapid tranquillisation 187–8
Recommendations on the Training of Specialists (General Mediacal Council, Education Committee 1987) 350
Relate 25
relationship, primary-secondary services 23–7
  changes to service provision 23–4
  traditional 23
relaxation 119
research diagnoses v. clinical diagnoses 39
research in general practice 10, 14, 360–70
  diagnostic practices 363–70
  epidemiology of mental disorders 365–7
  outcome of mental disorders in general practice 368
  referral/consultation 367–8
  therapeutic practices 364–5

risperidone (Risperdal) 205
Royal College of General
    Practitioners
  James Mackenzie lectures 80
  national morbidity study,
    1981/82 3
  The Future GP (1972) 83

scapegoating 87
schizophrenia 194–207, 328
  acute 194, 197
  acute paranoid 197
  audit 206
  call/recall systems 199
  chronic 194
  community care 23, 25
  continuity of care 199–200
  disease register 198–9
  GP's role 195–6
  home visit 200
  lifetime risk 328
  periodic review 200–4
    mental state 200–3
    physical health 203–4
    social needs 204
  practice management 197–206
    proactive approach 197–8
  record cards 200
  special sessions 200
  suicide risk 328
  tertiary prevention 329
  violent patient 174
screening programmes 322
secondary care 318
secondary preventive care 311,
    322–8
  screening 322
  time for patients 324
secondary team 266–7
selective serotonin reuptake
    inhibitors (5–HT antagonists)
    105, 329
senile dementia *see* dementia

senior house officer post in
    psychiatry 338–41
senior medical/nursing staff 318
sertraline 129
sex differences 5
sheltered accommodation 30
shifted out-patient model 28
shortage of texts 80
sibling relationship 87
sleep 221–34
  diary 226–8
  disorders 231–2
  education about 228
  factors affecting 222–4
  information for patients 232–4
  management plan 228–9
  normal 221–2
  "poor" 225–6
  purpose of 222
*So You Want to Cut Down on Your
    Drinking?* (Health Education
    Authority, London) 141
social phobia 115, 123 (table)
social workers 274–5
somatisation 4, 37, 326
  management 340
Standardised Assessment of
    Personality 185
status epilepticus 238
Stelazine (trifluoperazine) 120, 205
stigma of psychiatric illness 4
  countering 11
stroke 108
Structural Clinical Interview for
    Personality Disorders 185
Structured Interview for DSM-III-R
    Personality Disorders 185
suicide 13–14, 325, 328
  attempts 14
  risk assessment 102–3
supervised discharge for detained
    patients 50

talking therapies 281–2, 286–7

Tansella, M. (1989), community service planning 27-8
tarvide dyskinesia 186, 187
teamwork in community 265-77
temazepam 237
temporal lobe epilepsy 115
tertiary prevention 312, 328-30
  alcohol abuse 329
  dementia 329-30
  depression 328-9
  health staff work 318
  schizophrenia 329
testamentary capacity 55
The Future General Practicioner (RCGP, 1972) 83
The Longest Art (K. Lane, 1969) 17
The Twenty Minute Hour (P. Castelnuovo-Tedesco, 1965) 6
thyrotoxicosis 115
To Heal or To Harm (Grol, R., 1981) 4
training for general practicioners 337-48
  medical education continuing 345-8
  psychiatric training for experienced GPs 347-8
  training for GP trainer 346-7
  senior house officer post in psychiatry 338-41
  vocational 337-45
  day-release course 341-5
  with GP trainer 345
training for psychiatrists 350-8
  conditions of appointment 352
  experience of placements 353-4
  reports from trainees/trainers 354-6

  selection of training practices/trainees 351-2
Transcultural Medicine (B. Ouershi, 1989) 83
triazolam 241
trifluoperazine (Stelazine) 120, 205
trimipramine 105
Tudor Hart, J. (1975), blood pressure talking 8
Tuke, D., classification as a fiction 39
Tyrer's "hive" model 29

United Nations Children's Fund (UNICEF) 315

violence 174

Walls, C. A. H. *Depressive Illness in the Community* (1966) 316
Watts, Arthur, Beatrice 316
Welldorm 189
widows 65
will making 55
witnessing a document 55-6
women 5, 9
"won't do" syndromes 78, 86
World Health Organization 360
  Alma Ata Declaration (1978) 315
  primary care 24, 266
"worried well" 24, 28

Zimorane (zopiclone) 189
Zollinger-Ellison syndrome 115
zopiclone (Zimorane) 189

WM100PUL X